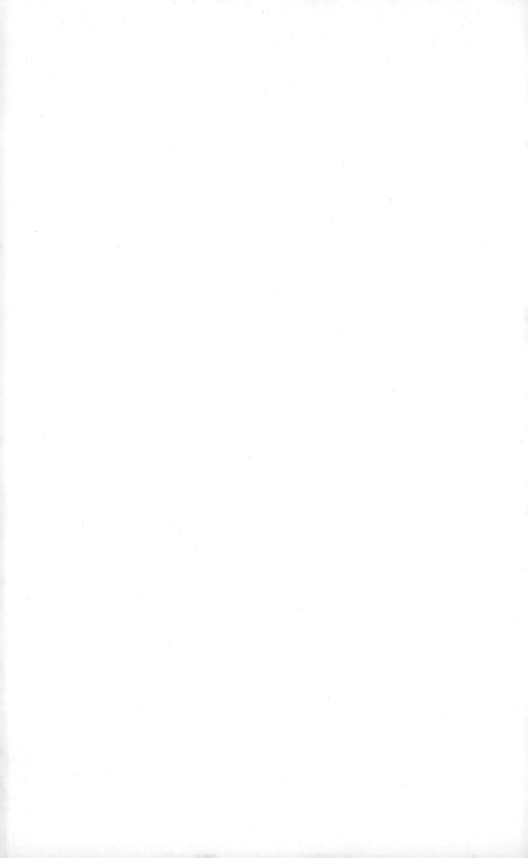

# HUMAN FACTORS IN
# JET AND SPACE TRAVEL

*A Medical-Psychological Analysis*

EDITED BY

## S. B. SELLS, PH.D.

PROFESSOR OF PSYCHOLOGY
TEXAS CHRISTIAN UNIVERSITY

and

## CHARLES A. BERRY, M.D.

LIEUTENANT COLONEL, USAF, MC
CHIEF, FLIGHT MEDICINE BRANCH
AEROSPACE MEDICINE DIVISION
OFFICE OF THE SURGEON GENERAL, USAF

FOREWORD BY

## OLIVER K. NIESS, M.D.

MAJOR GENERAL, USAF, MC
SURGEON GENERAL, USAF

THE RONALD PRESS COMPANY · NEW YORK

*To Helen and Del*
*With love*

# List of Contributors

Charles A. Berry, M.D., M.P.H., Lieutenant Colonel, USAF, MC, Chief, Flight Medicine Branch, Aerospace Medicine Division, Office of the Surgeon General, USAF, Washington, D.C.

Hans G. Clamann, M.D., Professor of Biophysics, School of Aviation Medicine, USAF, Brooks Air Force Base, Texas

Ashton Graybiel, M.D., Captain, MC, USN, Director of Research, U.S. Naval School of Aviation Medicine, U.S. Naval Aviation Medical Center, Pensacola, Florida

Henry B. Hale, Ph.D., Associate Professor of Physiology, School of Aviation Medicine, USAF, Brooks Air Force Base, Texas

Thrift G. Hanks, M.D., Director of Health and Safety, Boeing Airplane Company, Seattle, Washington

Gerrit L. Hekhuis, M.D., Colonel, USAF, MC, Chief, Department of Radiobiology, School of Aviation Medicine, USAF, Brooks Air Force Base, Texas

W. Guy Matheny, Ph.D., Chief, Human Factors Division, Bell Helicopter Corporation, Fort Worth, Texas

Alfred M. Mayo, Assistant Director for Bioengineering, Office of Life Science Programs, National Aeronautics and Space Administration, Washington, D.C. *Formerly*, Chief, Equipment and Safety Research Section, Engineering Department, El Segundo Division, Douglas Aircraft Company, Inc., El Segundo, California

Harry G. Moseley, M.D., Colonel, USAF, MC, (Late) Chief, Aeromedical Safety Division, Directorate of Flight Safety Research, Office of The Inspector General, USAF, Norton Air Force Base, California

John A. Norton, M.D., Colonel, USAF, MC, Director of Medical Operations, Aerospace Medical Center, Brooks Air Force Base, Texas

S. B. Sells, Ph.D., Professor of Psychology, Texas Christian University, Fort Worth, Texas. *Formerly*, Chief, Department of Medical Psychology, School of Aviation Medicine, USAF, Randolph Air Force Base, Texas

Hamilton B. Webb, M.D., Colonel, USAF, MC, Director of Base Medical Services, Otis Air Force Base, Massachusetts

William A. Wilbanks, Ph.D., Associate Professor of Psychology, University of Mississippi, University, Mississippi. *Formerly*, Human Factors Engineer, Bell Helicopter Corporation, Fort Worth, Texas

v

# *Foreword*

Although our time is commonly called the "Space Age," it might more accurately be termed the "Aerospace Age." It is well to remember that there is no sharp dividing line between the problems of atmospheric flight and those of space flight. The areas and the problems are a continuum. The United States Air Force has some fifty years' experience in this area, having progressed from the biwing Wright Brothers' aircraft through high-performance jet aircraft and now to spacecraft. During this entire period the maintenance of the good health of those who fly has been the job of the flight surgeon. The realm of flight has expanded to the point that almost every person has some awareness of the vehicles and their problems. The expanded use of jet airliners brings to the civilian population many of the problems previously faced only by military organizations, whose solutions to some of these should be of great value to the airlines.

This expansion of the horizon of flight has vividly demonstrated the necessity of team effort in meeting the challenge of these new vehicles and of the environment they are capable of reaching. The flight surgeon, psychologist, engineer, physiologist, and others must join in concentrated effort if man is to conquer safely the problems of this hostile environment.

This book makes its timely appearance as jet airliners are going into general service and space probes and satellites assume increasing importance in the ever-advancing progress of powered flight. It should be of interest to all those engaged in furthering these endeavors.

In these programs, human-factors problems loom as hurdles to overcome, and their solutions depend on the cooperative effort of the many disciplines mentioned above. The editors have rendered a service to the profession and to the general public in presenting a broad view of aviation medicine through this skillfully organized collection of papers. The book has points of concern to airline

medical directors, practicing physicians, aircraft builders and operators, and others in the aerospace field. The authors give their
opinions, supported by evidence, on controversial issues. Various
contributors do not always agree, but provocative opinions on complex issues are always worthy of note.

OLIVER K. NIESS
Major General, USAF, MC
Surgeon General, USAF

# Preface

Despite the popularity of flying as the preferred mode of travel, there is astonishingly little up-to-date information available in systematic form on the human problems of high-performance flight. This book has been prepared to meet that need. It is intended to present a comprehensive view of the human factors, to give physicians, physiologists, engineers, flight crews, and other interested persons a better perspective of what is involved in putting man in a foreign environment and then insuring his well-being there.

A second purpose of *Human Factors in Jet and Space Travel* is to provide physicians with a reference book on aviation medicine and related human-factors problems. As more jet airliners go into commercial service, physicians will increasingly be treating patients whose physical and psychological complaints may be critical in relation to flying or attributable to experiences in flight. The most important problems are discussed in scientific and clinical contexts, and references are cited for more detailed study.

Third, the treatment of most topics should be of interest to students who desire information concerning scientific careers in specialties related to aviation and the approaching era of space travel. The dramatic accomplishments in missiles, satellites, and space vehicles to date have often been treated in the press as though the problems of space travel were different from those of aviation. Actually, this is not so. It is true that in the rarefied air at high altitudes, over 80,000 ft., jet engines cannot function, but rocket engines, which carry their own oxygen as a component of their fuel, are efficient in the void of space. It is true also that problems have arisen at higher altitudes and speeds that were not particularly bothersome at lower-performance levels. Thus, while the most important aeromedical problems of the piston-propeller era were in the areas of respiratory physiology and acceleration, high-speed, high-altitude jet flight has called attention to additional problems of neurocirculatory functions and spatial orientation. In space travel, weightlessness, isolation, and alertness may be of outstanding interest. These differences are variations along a continuum determined by distance from the zone of optimal adaptation, however, and are not qualitatively different problems. Emphasis may shift, but the coordinated efforts of the human-factors team will be required to provide solutions to the problems encountered.

Developments in space travel reflect a heroic struggle of man not only to overcome gravitational forces but also to survive and perform efficiently in situations in which natural adaptation is impaired or impossible. His success reflects the contributions of aviation medicine and human-factors sciences to the understanding of human requirements for various conditions of flight and to the development of means to compensate for them.

The human-factors support of aviation has thus required the solution of problems of human adaptation to the environment of flight and of equipment. Human-factors problems derive from discrepancies between human limitations, on the one hand, and the conditions of human exposure in flight on the other. These discrepancies may be reduced by selection of flight personnel with superior tolerances for the particular stresses encountered and aptitudes for the tasks to be performed. This is the rationale for physical and psychological standards in aviation. This approach is only a partial solution, particularly with reference to survival at altitudes at which present-day jets operate routinely.

The residual discrepancy, after selection of the most suitable personnel, must be resolved by equipment design. With reference to environmental protection, it implies the development of conditioning and protective provisions in the aircraft to enable the occupants to live and function effectively. On flights of long duration in a scaled cabin, these requirements virtually prescribe a self-contained, recycling system, analogous to that of the mother spacecraft, earth. Considerations of comfort, habitability, and adaptation of task configurations to operator limitations have been extensively investigated. Although the importance of these problems has never been contested, and solutions superior to those commonly used have been developed, progress in securing their adoption has lagged until recently. However, the greater demands of jet aircraft and the prospect of sustained flight with air-borne refueling have convinced many operators that comfort, habitability, and task simplification are necessities rather than luxuries. As one looks ahead to even greater demands in space travel, these problems loom much larger.

Human-factors research and development in aviation have been a joint effort of many disciplines. Medicine, physiology, psychology, engineering, physical anthropology, physics, chemistry, and astronomy have developed specialties in the field of aviation problems. Until recently aviation was regarded as a pioneering field. Today, however, it is a universal mode of transportation. At the same time aviation may be only on the threshold of its accomplishments. Rocket ships are just beginning to be tested. It is not too fantastic to predict that the performance capabilities attained in the next ten years will be as far ahead of today's jet airliners as these are ahead of the Wright Brothers' plane of Kitty Hawk.

The opinions expressed in the chapters written by members of the Armed Forces are solely those of the authors and do not necessarily reflect the views or endorsement of the Armed Forces.

S. B. SELLS
CHARLES A. BERRY

# *Acknowledgments*

Grateful appreciation is expressed to the following persons and organizations for permission to include copyrighted material: Dr. Donald O. Hebb and W. B. Saunders Company, Philadelphia, for Table 4–1, from Hebb's *A Textbook of Psychology;* Holt, Rinehart and Winston, Inc., for the quotation in Chapter 6, from *Up Front* by Bill Mauldin; Commander A. P. Webster and *Aerospace Medicine* for Table 2–3; the American Society of Heating, Refrigerating and Air Conditioning Engineers, Inc., for Fig. 5–8; Wright Air Development Center, USAF, for the photographic illustrations in Chapter 5; and the Douglas Aircraft Company, Inc., for the illustrations in Chapter 13.

Chapters 8 and 12 were published originally in slightly different form in the *Air University Quarterly Review* and are included with the permission of Lt. Col. Kenneth F. Gantz, USAF, Editor. Chapter 6 appeared in the *United States Armed Forces Medical Journal* and is included with the permission of Col. Robert J. Benford, USAF, Editor.

The preparation of the manuscript was materially aided by a grant by the Faculty Research Committee of Texas Christian University. Mrs. Pat Adrion and Elizabeth Koenig, Mary Littlejohn, and Linda Varner assisted competently in typing various portions of the final manuscript. The editors owe a great debt to Mrs. Helen F. Sells for editorial advice and for preparation of the index.

S. B. S.
C. A. B.

# Contents

CONTENTS

# HUMAN FACTORS
## IN
## JET AND SPACE TRAVEL

# 1

# Medical Aspects of Jet and Space Travel

ASHTON GRAYBIEL, M.D.[*]

Artificial flight has enabled man to extend his activities into the atmosphere and beyond. These activities cover a wide range from peaceful utility to hostile intent. Political and economic interests have fostered the creation of large civil, military, and space flight programs. Such programs include research and development, fabrication of equipment and vehicle, the establishment of far-flung facilities, and flight operations. All these vast preparations and undertakings have a common focus in the actual flight itself. Success or failure in a particular flight reflects back on the preparation, and the measure of success in individual flights, taken together, determines the over-all success in such major endeavors as the transport of man and goods, the military posture, and the exploration of space.

The human element touches nearly all aspects of these flight activities, and, in turn, these activities have important reciprocal influences on the well-being of mankind. The broadest concept of flight medicine takes into consideration all these influences (14). When these aspects and influences affect mankind, the medical profession may be concerned; and when they affect the individual, the flight surgeon or physician may have important responsibilities.

In the early days of aviation, the primary emphasis was on the physical fitness of the flyer, and it was natural to turn to the physician for help and advice in this regard (16). The physician, devoting himself to these new responsibilities and new problems, soon received the special designation of flight surgeon. The flight surgeon

[*] Captain, MC, USN, Director of Research, U.S. Naval School of Aviation Medicine, U.S. Naval Aviation Medical Center, Pensacola, Florida.

sought the help of physiologists and allied scientists as environmental flight stress increased and the help of psychologists as the complexity of the flyer's task increased. The clinically oriented flight surgeons had the opportunity to apply the knowledge gained from specialists in many allied disciplines and to discover new problems requiring solution. Some flight surgeons after experience in aviation physiology, aviation psychology, and, indeed, in the aeronautical sciences as well, evolved as cross-trained generalists. As a result the competent generalist became qualified to act as a representative of the several disciplines in coordinating human factors in programs and activities.

The medical profession has recognized that certain problems are properly within its area of interest and still other problems await such recognition. Matters properly a concern of the profession include every by-product of flight that causes or may cause harm to mankind. Old problems reappear in new forms, such as health hazards due to communicable disease when travel time is short. New problems range from flight safety in commercial operations to the propriety of the physicians' aiding in the selection and care of men in a man-plane-weapon system. The medical profession has recognized that the problems in this field constitute a medical specialty, and those in this specialty recognize the problem of keeping pace with the dramatic advances in the design and exploitation of new vehicles. Although here we are not dealing with the broad concept of flight medicine, it is worth emphasizing that some appreciation of this broad concept is necessary to a proper understanding of the narrower concept, "success in flight."

The flight surgeon's primary responsibility is for man in actual flight. In the case of jet and space travel, he is directly charged with the physical and mental fitness of the participants. More specifically, he is expected to maintain and also to predict reliability of human performance insofar as it is dependent on *general fitness*. This prediction is made after evaluating the flyer in the light of his task aloft. In certain instances an evaluation may be carried out prior to a specific flight, but ordinarily it has longer-range implications.

This general fitness of the individual is very closely related to his professional qualifications; together these comprise the *total fitness* for his task aloft. The development of over-all fitness of the flyer begins with the initial selection for flight training and includes the nature and extent of the subsequent training and experience. The effort and cost of ensuring this over-all fitness is so great that it can be justified only on a career-long basis, and the flight surgeon in his role of medical examiner is responsible for selecting men most likely to remain fit over their professional lifetime. Subsequently, the flight surgeon, from the clinical standpoint, has two responsibilities which are in some respects antithetical. One is concerned with preventive medicine, medical care, and such other measures that ensure the best performance of the flyer over the longest possible period. The other is concerned with "quality control," the detection of disease, defect, functional disorder, and other factors that disqualify the flyer. The flight surgeon's dual role as physician and monitor has great disadvantages, and a separation of these roles is always desirable.

## The Flight

Before entering into a more detailed discussion of medical problems, it is advantageous, if not essential, to discuss very briefly the major elements concerned in manned flight, their principal interactions, and important implications for man. That this will be concerned with well-known facts and statements adds rather than detracts from its importance inasmuch as it is precisely these things which may be overlooked because of their familiarity.

**The Distinction Between the Purpose and Act of Flight.** The purpose and act of flight are distinguishable though inseparable. The purpose may be transportation or the execution of some mission from a vantage point aloft. The act of flight is an instrument essential to these purposes. The distinction between purpose and act is best made clear by example. Assume that the purpose is transportation from point A to B, but that the flight is redirected to C. The original purpose was not accomplished even though the act of flying may have been carried out properly. This failure of purpose is also subject to a quantitative evaluation. The difficulty of getting from C to B, i.e., fulfilling the original purpose, may be greater than that involved in going from A to B or so small as to be almost negligible. Further, let us assume that the flight landed at B with destruction of landing gear but no damage to the cargo. The original purpose was accomplished, but the act of flight was not a complete success. Still another example is needed. Assume that the purpose is to drop a bomb at point A. If, after a successful bombing, the vehicle is lost, the mission will have been fulfilled but at a cost of vehicle and crew. Alternatively, the bombing may not have been on target, although the vehicle may have returned. This distinction has important implications for everyone concerned with the human element as a limiting factor in flight. Flight safety may be compromised in many ways by the demands of the mission (6, 11, 39). Success of the mission may be compromised by overensuring success in actual flight. In large operations calculated risks are taken in accordance with the purpose of the operation as a whole. The opinion of the flight surgeon regarding these risks and the evaluation of pilot-error in case of mishap should be based on a firm appreciation of the distinction between act and purpose of the flight.

**The Act of Flight.** Inasmuch as the act of flying may serve different purposes, it is the more general factor and the one on which our attention will mainly center. In its simplest form the act of flight represents a state of dynamic equilibrium resulting from interactions between the vehicle, the meteorological environment, and the force of gravity. The compliance in this interaction is almost entirely on the part of the vehicle; nothing can be done to alter gravitational force and little to alter the meteorological environment.

GRAVITATIONAL FORCE. Gravitational force is the only element consisting of a single factor. The laws governing the mutual attraction of bodies in the universe are known and make it possible to calculate gravitational field gradients in advance of travel. For low-level flights it may be regarded as a constant, although the flattening at the poles and whatever altitude is reached introduce small variations.

The decrease in the earth's gravitational field as one ascends into space is readily determined, and the influence of other planets has been calculated with sufficient accuracy for most space flights (37). The inertial forces required to overcome or balance gravitational force are governed by the laws of motion, and the two forces are equitable. The interaction between these forces and the vehicle has important implications not only for compliance in flight but also with regard to the effects on man. Compliance on the one hand represents a continuous requirement * and on the other a danger

---

* Under orbital conditions or when the flight path of a vehicle describes a Keplerian trajectory, the gravitational attraction of the earth is counterbalanced by the centrifugal force of the vehicle, and a state of zero force results. If the orbiting

lest the structural limitations of the vehicle be exceeded under high accelerations or equipment fail to function under zero g or sub-gravity states. The effects of these forces on man are only known in part and will be discussed in detail later on.

THE METEOROLOGICAL ENVIRONMENT. The medium in which flight occurs represents the unique component in the act of flight. The meteorological environment consists of many factors, some of which vary in any given location and some with change in altitude or geographical location. A number of these changes can be predicted with great accuracy, while others are predictable either with difficulty or not at all. The changing conditions in this outer environment present a continual problem in terms of compliance and guidance of the vehicle.

The decrease in density of the atmosphere with increasing altitude has a profound influence. A good example is given in the next section in discussing the rocket plane. There are practical limitations to the speed of flight in the dense turbulent air near sea level, but as one rises above the earth's atmosphere, speed is no longer limited by friction and, theoretically, near-relativity speeds are possible. The composition of the atmosphere near sea level is favorable for man, and the density provides a protective shield from ionizing radiation and meteorites. As one ascends, the hostility of the outer environment increases, and man becomes more dependent on the functional integrity of the vehicle and the life-support systems.

THE VEHICLE. The essential features of the vehicle are the physical structure, the propulsion system, the means for guidance, and the accommodation for man. While none of these characteristics are unique, they all differ greatly from their counterparts in other types of vehicles.

Human ingenuity has led to the construction of a wide variety of vehicles of great structural integrity, responsive to controls, and containing accommodations for man. The engines for propulsion have high reliability in performance; the limiting factor today is fuel supply. The control equipment includes complex devices to aid in guidance and to provide environmental control.

---

vehicle is above the atmosphere, it no longer requires power for propulsion because friction is absent. This "steady state" represents the exception to the rule that a vehicle aloft has no "resting place."

Provision for man creates great demands in terms of his need for cabin space and proper environment. These aspects are discussed in detail in later chapters. It is sufficient here to emphasize the concept of *limiting factors* in preserving the constancy of his internal environment and in the preservation of his efficiency for the tasks assigned to him.

Man in Flight. Man in flight represents a system within a system. He may be an essential link in the control system of the vehicle, but in addition he always represents an independent system. The constancy of his internal environment is dependent on the fitness of the outer environment. It is here that one may distinguish between man as an instrument in the act of flight and man as an individual (17). His ability to carry out specific tasks aloft constitutes his professional qualifications, and his availability to do this is dependent on the integrity of the underlying physiological and psychological mechanisms. The distinction between his professional and non-professional qualifications is of more than academic interest, partly because their overlap represents a sort of no man's land where lines of responsibility are unclear. Some of the elements of specific fitness for the task are not separable from his general fitness for which the physician is directly responsible.

**Interactions in Flight.** These fall into two categories which, though distinguishable, are inseparable, namely, compliance and destination guidance. Compliance refers to the behavior of those factors that ensure a state of dynamic equilibrium aloft. This involves guidance but not necessarily directional guidance toward a specific destination. Compliance and guidance are always dependent on man or man-made devices. Compliance depends on the functional integrity of every significant component of the system and on their proper interaction or coordination. Guidance toward some specific destination or in some particular maneuver is something superimposed on compliance.

**Implications for the Human Operator.** A consideration of the essential phenomena of flight discloses important implications for man. Although briefly mentioned now, these topics will form a large part of the subject matter that follows as well as that of later chapters.

Environment for Man in Flight. Provision must be made for an adequate environment. There is a close relationship between the fitness of the outer environment and the preservation of the constancy of man's internal environment, and in turn his ability to perform efficiently (21).

PROFESSIONAL QUALIFICATIONS OF THE HUMAN OPERATOR. Man is poorly fitted by his inheritance and ordinary experiences for the tasks incidental to compliance, guidance, and carrying out a mission aloft. The requirements place demands on human skill, intelligence, and temperament. In certain instances the requirements are so great as to require years of training and experience. Obviously, such preparations are justifiable only on the basis that these skills are utilized over a period of years.

CONTINUAL NATURE OF DEMANDS ON THE HUMAN OPERATOR. Man has limits for continuous operation and, within these limits, limitations. A human operator can work continuously only for relatively short periods, and within these limits he is prone to error and may become unfit for certain of his tasks. The tendency is for the capacity of the flyer to fall during flight. A certain decrement may still allow him to perform his tasks efficiently, but a point may be reached at which he becomes inefficient. This loss in efficiency may result from the spontaneous development of disease or disorder, the precipitation of disease or disorder by some factor aloft, or from the lowering of efficiency caused by fatigue or unfavorable conditions aloft in the absence of defect or disease. Take-off and landing are critical periods in the operational control of the vehicle and place heavy demands on the human operator. It is essential to ensure the reliability of human performance at the end of a flight when efficiency may be lower than at any other time.

Worthwhile attempts are being made in the direction of defining man's capabilities as part of a man-machine system in engineering terms (29, 38). This is useful only up to a certain point, inasmuch as man may fail in carrying out very simple tasks. It would seem that the best solution would take into account man's unique abilities and inherent weaknesses.

Inasmuch as the reliability of a single person for constant performance is not perfect, adding a copilot, for example, represents an attempt to increase reliability. Two persons constitute a social system, and, as additional crew members are added, not only the complexity of this system increases, but also new problems arise involving such different factors as cabin design, providing adequate environmental conditions and operational facilities, task engineering, personnel training and placement, and mission planning, among others (35).

DURATION OF FLIGHT. There is a time limitation on every flight. The duration is arbitrarily set within the safety period of factors that limit the duration of flight. The "set time" can be exceeded only up to the point at which one of these factors becomes critical. The human operator is one of these limiting factors. Of all the limiting factors that can be anticipated in advance, the safety period of the human operator is least susceptible to precise measurement.

SPEED IN FLIGHT. Some important implications for man center around the problems imposed by time as a function of speed in carrying out tasks aloft. Man has a remarkable facility for adjusting to different rates at which he receives, decodes, and acts on new information. However, as natural limits are exceeded, compensatory accommodations are required (38). Unless these are adequate, efficiency falls and error increases. High speed has a tendency toward causing "time stress" which has important implications for man aloft. Moreover, it adds to the number and complexity of the instrumental aids which have a tendency toward creating "load stress" and problems incidental to equipment failure. Escape from aircraft becomes more difficult and more dangerous with increasing speeds (20).

ORIENTATION IN FLIGHT. The journey aloft introduces the third dimension in travel and necessitates control over the altitude of the vehicle as well as the vertical profile and the geographical flight path (27, 40). The flyer must be correctly oriented to the vehicle, to the earth, and to the three dimensions of space. The problem is complicated by the linear and angular accelerations generated by the vehicle. The sensory receptors stimulated by the force of gravity and which normally result in orientation to the direction of gravity can be equally effective in reorientation to the direction of a force representing the vector addition of gravitational and inertial force. Moreover, the unusual patterns of angular accelerations aloft may lead to disorientation directly or indirectly through stimulation of the semicircular canals. Disorientation for these and other reasons is a common cause of human error, resulting from misinterpretation or lack of orientational cues (5, 25).

DANGER IN FLIGHT. The interactions of forces during flight represent a state of dynamic equilibrium with a natural tendency for the vehicle to come to rest. The preservation of this state presents a continuous requirement in terms of a source of energy, structural and functional integrity of the vehicle, compliance, and guidance. It is precisely because of these requirements that flight moves in an element of danger. Failure of power or equipment, loss of structural integrity of the vehicle, and human error may lead to disaster. The awareness of danger has an effect on human efficiency. The effect depends on the degree of stress on the one hand and individual differences in reacting to this stress on the other. The implications for selection, training, and monitoring of performance of flyers in this regard are self-evident. Moreover, stress creates demands for safety and escape procedures. Theoretically, every provision may be met regarding safety, but in reality accidents occur.

## Medical Aspects of High-Performance Jet Flight

Here we are primarily concerned with the general fitness of the flyer for his assignment, although his specific fitness or professional qualifications also must be kept in mind. In the preceding section a brief analysis of the flyer's task emphasized the fact that compliance of the vehicle in flight is ordered by human intelligence and that this represents a continuous requirement. Moreover, flight moves in a hostile environment in the three dimensions of space, and safety depends on the functional integrity and proper functioning of all essential components. To all this must now be added the stresses incident to high-performance flight, which center around environmental factors, increase in complexity of the task, and danger. Fitness of the environment within cabin or cockpit is subject to compromise in the interest of high speed, high altitude, maneuverability, and pay load.

Only minimal requirements are met regarding periods of respite from work, nutrition, elimination of bodily wastes, ability to move around in the environment, and freedom from fear and anxiety. The pilot wearing a pressure suit and encumbered with survival equipment is seriously handicapped. Efforts to ensure a wider margin of safety under a given set of conditions are almost immediately offset by increased demands. The difficulty of the task is increased because of the necessary introduction of artificial aids and what has been termed "load stress" and "speed stress," i.e., the need to do many things quickly. Moreover, the flight may be carried out under unfavorable meteorological conditions and, in the military, as a simulated combat sortie. The danger is declared by the high death rate due to accidental injury (8, 15). Even in peacetime, military pilots are engaged in what might be termed "paracombat." In this contest man is carrying out a difficult mission, often under very unfavorable environmental conditions.

Man is inadequately fitted by his inheritance or by his experience for the task just described. Indeed, few men have the potential abilities to become successful pilots of high-powered aircraft. This poses problems in selection and training and in providing experience over a long period of time, an undertaking justifiable only on a career-long basis. Some of the medical aspects of this program are sharply defined and some are not. The former are of a clinical nature and involve physical standards, preventive medicine, hazards to health, and treatment of disease or injury. Less sharply defined are responsibilities involving the professional qualifications of the flyer, his safety, and the effects of stress due to environmental factors and the task aloft.

The objective of medical control is to ensure the reliability of performance of the flyer insofar as it depends on his general fitness. It is absolutely essential that the integrity of his performance be guaranteed beyond reasonable doubt during a particular flight and that it be maintained over as long a period as possible. Although a flyer has a short career as a high-performance jet pilot, this is long in terms of the useful life of equipment that might replace him. Assuming this period to be from age twenty-five to age thirty-five, it would seem at first glance to represent a long period of time. However, it is worth considering for a moment just how much of this period he might actually be expected to spend aloft. At periodic intervals he has need of a vacation or rest from his duty; at irregular intervals he is likely to lose time because of acute illness or injury. In any given day he requires periods set aside for sleep or rest and recreation. At no time can he work very long without fluid, nourishment, and taking care of various bodily needs. Moreover, even during those hours when he is devoting himself exclusively to his task, there are interruptions due to the limitation of his attention span.

**Selection and Quality Control.** Prospective flight students must hold promise of remaining effective over their professional careers. However, the biological cycle is inexorable, and at some point for everyone a time comes when he is no longer fit for assignment to high-performance aircraft. At times he may even be unfit for physical or psychological reasons. Monitoring the general fitness of the flyer, insofar as it is feasible, should be carried out by a trained flight surgeon, not by a physician responsible for medical care. The reason is that the monitor, poised to reject the unfit, may not enjoy the full confidence of the flyer.

The medical examination has the purpose of discovering disease, functional disorder, or defect that renders the subject unfit to fly. The initial evaluation is for the purpose of selecting only those candidates who are fit and likely to retain their general fitness over their professional lifetime. Subsequent examinations are for the purpose of determining whether any changes have occurred which would render the flyer unfit for his task; the term "quality control" (3, 13) best expresses this function.

The several items in the medical evaluation vary greatly in terms of their reliability. The medical history may be unreliable because of the bias of the person examined, and, consequently, greater reliance must be placed on objective methods. Many of these methods are unreliable or inadequate. This is particularly evident in the detection of functional disorders and in the detection of incipient disease (1, 2).

Minimal physical standards should be established as a guide in selection and in monitoring quality control. This is one if the most important and difficult assignments for flight medical specialists. Difficulties include deficiencies in reliability of the methods used, irregularities in carrying out the evaluation, and lack of adequate validation of the findings in terms of actual experience. There exists a great need for more reliable medical procedures and for long-range validation of the medical findings. It has been demonstrated that the cost of research and implementation in this area is more than met by savings in manpower.

**Preventive Medicine.** The dual objective here is the maintenance of a high level of general fitness and prevention of defect, disease, or injury that may disqualify the flyer. This involves the identification of worthwhile measures and their implementation. This program should be based on factual information insofar as it is known, and research should be encouraged in cases in which it is not. Implementation has many aspects, not least of which is the enthusiastic cooperation of the flyer. This cooperation, especially by professional flyers, may be gained through a continual display of factual propaganda. A positive program is needed to increase fitness and efficiency and to prevent, insofar as possible, both acute illness and the effects of aging. The main point that needs to be emphasized here is that the general fitness required for success in high-performance flight need not be present in persons ordinarily regarded as being in good health. These factors stand over and above this concept of health, even though dependent upon it.

**Medical Care.** The care of the flyer should be based on the broadest concept of industrial medicine, in itself a specialized field. It includes the problem of fatigue and the treatment of illness and injury. One important consideration deserves a comment, namely, that even minor illness or functional disturbance, ordinarily regarded as unimportant, may render the flyer unfit for his assignments.

**Protection of the Flyer from Environmental Stress.** The flight surgeon has an important share of the responsibility for protecting the flyer from environmental stresses aloft. This includes the determination of the flyer's tolerances to such stresses, the development of protective equipment, indoctrination and instruction in the use of this equipment, and the attempt to determine any deleterious effects, either from acute or chronic exposure. Survival equipment and procedures are usually considered hand in hand with protective equipment, although it is important to keep the two separate, conceptually. Although protective and survival equipment are essential, they constitute a stress in themselves and decrease the efficiency of the flyer for his task. It is important to be sure that they constitute a gain and not a loss in terms of the efficiency with which the pilot carries out his task.

**Task Stress.** The flight surgeon has some responsibility with respect to the stress imposed on the flyer as a direct result of the task he must carry out aloft. The high-performance jet pilot must carry out a complex mental task, often under hazardous conditions and often to the point of great acute fatigue. Although the flight surgeon is not directly involved in making the flying assignments, his counsel may be an important factor and should be based on thorough knowledge of the effect of this aspect of flying stress. The flight surgeon, probably more than anyone else, should be able to form a balanced opinion as to the effect of all the flying stresses acting in concert and whether or not these may reduce a flyer's efficiency below the safety level by the time the flight has ended. This is a borderline area in which responsibility is divided among the flyer, the flight surgeon, and those in charge of flight operations.

The need for research in the clinical aspects of flight medicine has been emphasized, and it remains to emphasize the need for cooperative research; the broadened problems indicate the value of an interdisciplinary approach.

MEDICAL ASPECTS OF ROCKET-PLANE FLIGHT. The major considerations represent a logical extension or modification of what has been discussed under high-performance jet flight. Thus far only a few vehicles have been developed and tested, and the program has not progressed beyond the research and development stage.

The flight profile will resemble a ballistic trajectory with boost, free flight, and re-entry. As exemplified in the rocket plane X-15, it will have two sets of controls, one for aerodynamic control within the atmosphere and another energized by small rocket motors when above the region of effective aerodynamic control (37). Some of the implications for man are clear-cut and deserve brief comment.

The use of rocket planes for destinations on earth will involve relatively short travel time in view of the high speed, although missions requiring orbiting around the earth will be that much more prolonged. The compliance and directional guidance of X-15 is pilot-controlled and places a heavy demand on the human operator. The problem of orientation is as difficult as it is important. Transition from one set of controls to the other, the speed and load stress, and the danger incidental to the experimental flights all bear heavily on the pilot. Even under "ideal" flight conditions, the environmental stress is great, but certain limits may not be exceeded without impairing dangerously the efficiency of the flyer. This type of flight demands not only good physical and mental fitness but also requires great professional skill and courage (7).

## Medical Aspects of Space Flight

Man's exploration of outer space falls into three major phases, namely, the exploration of solar systems beyond our own, the exploration of our solar system, and the establishment of manned space stations. In all these undertakings, it is a contest between man's ingenuity on the one hand and the hostility of the environment on the other. When man leaves the earth for outer space, despite his ingenuity he will suffer from two basic inadequacies: his inability to control time and gravitational force. Additionally, he will have to take with him an environment of his own making and will have to withstand not only the hazards and stresses of his immediate surroundings but meteorological hazards as well (32).

EXPLORATION BEYOND OUR SOLAR SYSTEM. Such explorations must await new discoveries of a dramatic nature. Propulsion systems for reaching speeds in the relativistic speed range would be required, and even plasma rockets could not fulfill this requirement.

TABLE 1–1

Acceleration Loss Due to Relativistic Mass Increase

| Speed of Vehicle | | Mass in Multiples of Mass at Rest | Acceleration Expressed as Fraction of Classic Value |
|---|---|---|---|
| Per Cent of Speed of Light | Miles/Second | | |
| 1 | 1,860 | 1.00005 | 0.99995 |
| 10 | 18,600 | 1.005 | 0.995 |
| 20 | 37,200 | 1.02 | 0.98 |
| 40 | 74,400 | 1.09 | 0.918 |
| 75 | 139,500 | 1.51 | 0.662 |
| 90 | 167,400 | 2.29 | 0.436 |
| 95 | 176,700 | 3.16 | 0.314 |
| 100 | 186,000 | $\infty$ | 0.0 |

Some new source of energy, such as controlled fusion power, will be necessary not only as a source of energy for propulsion but also to provide an economy adequate to underwrite the cost of the undertaking.

Even if one assumes that full exploitation of atomic fusion provides sufficient energy, the fact still remains that speeds approximating that of light will never be possible because of relativistic acceleration loss (Table 1–1). Travel at velocities considerably below that of light introduces a radiation hazard of serious, if not prohibitive, proportions. Van Allen estimates that, even in positions remote from a star, traveling at velocities three-tenths that of light, the vehicle will be bombarded on its frontal area by protons and electrons creating, in the absence of shielding, an exposure level of the order of 20 million roentgens an hour (42). Shielding is possible, but with minimal shielding the deterioration would soon render it ineffective.

Assuming an effective means of reducing radiation hazard to acceptable limits and sufficient energy to propel a vehicle at three-fourths the speed of light, it would require nearly five months to reach this speed at acceptable (2 g) limits of acceleration. To reach the nearest star and return would require about twelve years. We are not ready to accept this challenge but must pass it on to those who follow.

EXPLORATION OF OUR SOLAR SYSTEM. With regard to the exploration of our solar system, even a limited effort, such as exploration and landing on an inner planet, represents an undertaking which is barely conceivable in terms of present-day technology and bioastronautical skills. The requirements of such an effort as this are indeed formidable. It would demand ion-rocket-powered spaceships with great range and full maneuverability. Not only the structural integrity of such a ship must be assured, but also every element in its power plant and navigational and guidance systems must be continuously operational over periods of many months or even years. The same integrity and reliability would be demanded with respect to every item in the complex representing the biotechnical systems whereby man's needs in a sealed environmental cabin would be met for like periods of time. The world's resources would need to be mobilized to establish the necessary launching platforms in space and to provide a fleet of spaceships.

MANNED SPACE STATIONS. The establishment of manned space stations, despite the magnitude of the undertaking, will soon be a reality (32). They will be useful to man on earth and an essential step in man's exploration of space. Placed outside the earth's atmosphere, they will have unique qualifications as observation posts for the study of the universe. As a staging area for space vehicles, the advantages of a frictionless medium and reduced gravitational drag are apparent.

The medical problems center around purposeful living in a closed ecological environment with man exposed to stresses and hazards from within and without (9, 10, 26). It is impossible here to convey a full and proper appreciation of the number and complexity of the problems involved in providing for man, partly because they have not been satisfactorily identified and partly because a major experiment, including regenerative processing, has not been carried out. A few implications for man may be pointed out.

The long duration of stay aloft brings into consideration processes of adaptation on the one hand and deterioration on the other, if stress multiplied by time has cumulative effects. The great danger in travel to and from the station, as well as while aloft, will have important psychological effects. The environmental stresses include exposure to high acceleration, zero g (or constant rotation), and compromises in terms of an ideal atmospheric environment and the amenities of ordinary living conditions on earth. Prior to the actual experience, less will be known concerning the prolonged effects of zero g than any other stress (22, 43). Although readily tolerated for periods measured in seconds, unpleasant effects may be cumulative, which would require the generation of an artificial field force through rotation of the vehicle. Generation of this force would not be difficult but would have disadvantages and introduce new problems, mainly arising from stimulation of the semicircular canals (24). Adaptation readily occurs, fortunately, if rotational velocities are slow, as would be the case for satellites of large diameter (19, 28). Additional problems will be involved such as work-rest cycles (4), the monotony of prolonged confinement (36), and "space asthenia." The hazards from without include Nature's abhorrence of a vacuum, meteorites, and ionizing radiation. Proper placement with regard to the Van Allen radiation belts, below 1,000 km or above 4–5 earth radii (33), would obviate this hazard, and shielding from auroral radiation is readily accomplished (42). Man will be exposed to the heavy primary cosmic rays which may present deterrents or limitations in length of exposure (34). The only fortunate aspect of the radiation hazard lies in the fact that the energy spectrum may be determined in advance of manned flight.

The establishment of a station on the moon has attractive possibilities, but these may be offset by environmental hazards. Exploitation of solar energy, obtaining water and oxygen from the minerals, use of underground spaces for shielding from cosmic rays and meteorites, and the absence of the forces of erosion have great advantages. Moreover, man might adapt very well to the gravitational field of 0.165 g relative to the earth. This would be sufficient to avoid disorientation having its origin in the otolith apparatus and might have advantages with regard to the cardiovascular system.

Indeed, a lunar laboratory would provide an opportunity to study the possible therapeutic effects of low g and its influence on aging. However, the advantages of a lunar base might come to naught if the terrain is radioactive or otherwise hostile.

**Preliminary Flights.** As a step toward the establishment of space stations, man will be sent aloft in missiles on a ballistic trajectory for a short period of orbiting around the earth and return (37). This program now under way has two main aspects running concurrently, namely, animal experimentation under actual flight conditions and preparations for sending men to follow.

Carrying out a biological experiment aloft represents a prodigious effort in terms of the meager data to be obtained (12, 18, 23). It requires the cooperation of many persons and coordination of their efforts as a single team. Major requirements include the care and training of the animals, the specifications for the construction of the biocapsule and its instrumentation, the provisions for a closed-life support system, the technical requirements for obtaining physiological and performance data, and the training of launch and pickup teams.

Undoubtedly, the biotechnical features present the greatest problems. Here, a degree of reliability is required beyond anything which might be anticipated under ordinary laboratory conditions. Moreover, this reliability must be guaranteed under conditions of high accelerations, zero gravity, and vibration. The difficulties and complications are so numerous and varied that a brief statement cannot convey a proper appreciation of the problem. Nevertheless, these severe conditions provide precisely the experience required prior to sending man aloft. The development of "professionals" in carrying out successful animal experiments in space vehicles covers all aspects of sending man aloft except for modifications in the protection equipment, escape and survival, and selection and training. These experiments present requirements so different from the biotechnical aspect that they can best be met by providing not only special facilities but also specialized workers in this field.

The implications for man resemble in some respects, but are different in others, those incidental to high-performance jet flight or rocket-glide flights as represented by the X-15. They have in common the element of danger, short duration, and some similarities in environmental stress. They differ greatly in terms of the task.

Compliance and directional guidance will not depend on the astronaut, although provisions for escape and some provision for guidance may be under his control. As corollaries he will not be subjected to the speed stress, load stress, and orientational difficulties imposed on the rocket-glide flyer. However, he will be subjected to greater stresses in terms of linear accelerations and the important transitions to and from the zero g state and to the psychological stress of long periods of waiting in case of delay at lift-off. In orbital flights over fairly long periods, the astronaut will undoubtedly be expected to carry out tasks involving maintaining instruments, sending and receiving signals, and making and recording observations of different kinds. Thus, the task is different from that in high-performance jet or rocket flight, but the environmental stress is far greater.

**Examination, Selection, Care, and Indoctrination of Astronauts.** This is a long-range project which would benefit by the establishment of control headquarters for the astronauts with a permanent staff to follow the lines of direction proved to be successful in the case of aviators.

EXAMINATION AND QUALITY CONTROL. The medical and professional qualifications (general and specific fitness) are more closely interrelated than in the case of the high-performance jet flyer and will be considered together. In early flights at least, the emphasis will be on the general fitness. Hence, the chief medical aspects of the examination would be special tests designed to disclose cryptic physical defects, functional disorders, and disease processes not yet overtly manifested.

The successful astronaut must not only be physically fit but must also be able to withstand environmental stress, and here the use of flight simulators and other stress tests are imperative. He must be able to perform under hazardous conditions, and here his personality and development become objects of prime importance.

SELECTION OF THE ASTRONAUT. By limiting the volunteer candidates to those with recent experience in flying high-performance operational aircraft, advantage is taken by ensuring the selection of men not only with experience in flying but also men who can perform under hazardous conditions. With regard to the latter and related characteristics, the use of peer-rating techniques is to be recommended.

A second important factor determining initial selection centers around whether the applicant is or is capable of becoming a student of his profession. Much could be done by means of interview and questionnaire techniques to determine the ability and desire to learn.

CARE OF THE ASTRONAUT. Physicians responsible for day-to-day care, including advice and counsel, should be entirely outside this program. All communications between physicians and astronauts should be regarded as privileged, and any findings arising in connection with this care should be turned over to others only with the consent of the individuals concerned. Insofar as possible, rapport should be established between each astronaut and a particular physician. This would do much to gain his full cooperation.

THE INDOCTRINATION OF THE ASTRONAUT. If the original selection is made from among a group of experienced jet pilots, deficiencies will fall into two main areas or categories: (1) background knowledge of aviation and space medicine and (2) familiarity with the specific task he will be called upon to perform under simulated flight conditions.

*Background Knowledge of Aviation and Space Medicine.* It is hardly necessary to justify a course of instruction that would ensure thorough familiarity with all the equipment incidental to providing an adequate microenvironment in the vehicle. The ability to detect any important changes or the development of a hazardous condition and to interpret correctly subjective symptoms are essential to instituting corrective procedures at the earliest moment. Pertinent knowledge of the human organism and of its physiological and psychological tolerances is essential to survival and a necessity for efficient performance (41, 44). This important training and experience cannot be obtained quickly. Direct application of this information to the task ahead is essential.

*Familiarity with Specific Task.* The advantages of specific indoctrination procedures are obvious. The chief decisions will center around the selection of the tests in the light of the task to be carried out, the magnitude of the stresses to be employed, and attempts to simulate as nearly as possible actual conditions aloft.

*Quality Control.* Frequent complete re-evaluations covering both the general fitness and the professional qualifications are essential. In maintaining quality control, the size of the group is unimportant with regard to general fitness. A large group has advantages with regard to the professional qualifications.

Acknowledgment is made to Dr. Hermann Schaefer for the preparation of Table 1–1 and for helpful suggestions based on a critical reading of the manuscript.

# References

1. ADVISORY GROUP FOR AERONAUTICAL RESEARCH AND DEVELOPMENT. 1953. *Methods and Criteria for the Selection of Flying Personnel.* (AGARDograph No. 2.) Butterworth & Co., Ltd., London.
2. AVIATION MEDICINE RESIDENCY TRAINING PROGRAM. 1957. *Symposium: Physical Standards and Selection.* Air University, School of Aviation Medicine, Randolph Air Force Base, Texas.
3. BERKSHIRE, J. R., and LYON, V. W. 1959. Human quality control in naval air training. *Am. Psychologist 13:* 153–155.
4. BROWN, F. A. 1957. The rhythmic nature of life. *Recent Advances in Invertebrate Physiology.* University of Oregon Publications, Eugene. Pp. 287–304.
5. CLARK, B., and GRAYBIEL, A. 1955. II. Disorientamento: Una della cause di errore del pilota. *Riv. med. aeronaut. 18:* 219–250 and 583–641.
6. CLARK, B., NICHOLSON, M. A., and GRAYBIEL, A. 1953. Fascination: A cause of pilot error. *J. Aviation Med. 24:* 429–440.
7. CROSSFIELD, A. S. 1957. A test pilot's viewpoint. *J. Aviation Med. 28:* 492–495.
8. CUTLER, S. J., and RAFFERTY, J. A. 1949. *Comparison of Life Expectancy, Period of Active Duty and Medical History of Flying and Non-Flying Officers, 1920–1947.* (Project No. 21–02–014, Report No. 1.) USAF, Air University, School of Aviation Medicine, Randolph Air Force Base, Texas.
9. EHRICKE, K. 1959. Atlas: Concept for a manned space station. *Spaceflight 2:* 66–68.
10. FENNO, R. M. 1954. Man's milieu in space: A summary of the physiological requirements of man in a sealed cabin. *J. Aviation Med. 25:* 612–622.
11. FITTS, P. M., and JONES, R. E. 1947. *Analysis of Factors Contributing to 460 "Pilot-Error" Experiences in Operating Aircraft Controls.* (Report TSEA-694–12.) Air Materiel Command, Wright Patterson Air Force Base, Ohio.
12. GALKIN, A. M., GORLOV, O. G., KOTOVA, A. R., KOSOV, I. I., PETROV, A. V., SEROV, A. D., CHERNOV, V. N., and YAKOVLAV, B. I. 1958. *Investigations of the Vital Activity of Animals During Flights in Hermetically-Sealed Cabins to an Altitude of 212 Kilometers.* (U.S. Joint Publications Research Service, JPRS/DC-288.) Pp. 5–28.
13. GRANT, E. L. 1952. *Statistical Quality Control.* McGraw-Hill Book Company, Inc., New York.
14. GRAYBIEL, A. 1954. The concept of aviation medicine. *J. Aviation Med. 25:* 504–514, 522.
15. GRAYBIEL, A. 1955. Flying stress and heart disease in naval aviators. *J. Aviation Med. 26:* 329–336.
16. GRAYBIEL, A. 1956. Problems involving the pilot and his task: The changing emphasis in aviation medicine. *J. Aviation Med. 27:* 397–406.
17. GRAYBIEL, A. 1957. Future trends in military aviation medicine. *Military Med. 120:* 347–352.
18. GRAYBIEL, A., AND OTHERS. 1959. An account of three experiments in which two monkeys were recovered unharmed after ballistic space flight. *J. Aerospace Med. 30:* 871–931.
19. GRAYBIEL, A., CLARK, B., and ZARRIELLO, J. J. 1959. *Clinical Observations on Human Subjects Living in a "Slow Rotation Room" for Periods of Two Days: Canal Sickness.* (Project MR005. 13–6001 [formerly NM 17 01 11],

Subtask 1, Report No. 49.) U.S. Naval School of Aviation Medicine, Pensacola, Florida.

20. HABER, F. 1952. Bailout at very high altitudes. *J. Aviation Med.* 23: 322–329.
21. HABER, H. 1954. *The Physical Environment of the Flyer.* USAF School of Aviation Medicine, Randolph Air Force Base, Texas.
22. HABER, H., and GERATHEWOHL, S. J. 1951. Physics and psychophysics of weightlessness. *J. Aviation Med.* 22: 180–189.
23. HENRY, J. P., BALLINGER, E. R., MAHER, P. J., and SIMONS, D. G. 1952. Animal studies of the subgravity state during rocket flight. *J. Aviation Med.* 23: 421–432.
24. JOHNSON, W. H. 1956. Head movement measurements in relation to spatial disorientation and vestibular stimulation. *J. Aviation Med.* 27: 148–152.
25. JONES, G. M. 1958. *Disorientation in Flight.* (FPRC/Memo 96.) Royal Air Force Institute of Aviation Medicine, Farnborough, England.
26. KONECCI, E. B. 1959. *Manned Space Cabin Systems.* (Engineering Paper No. 376.) Douglas Aircraft Company, Inc., Santa Monica, Calif.
27. KRIJGER, M. W. W. 1954. *De Betekenis Van Het Evenwichtsorgaan Voor De Vlieger.* Drukkerij Fa. Schotanus & Jens., Utrecht.
28. LANSBERG, M. P. 1957. The function of the vestibular sense organ and construction of a satellite. *Aeromedical Acta* (Special Edition) 69.
29. MAYO, A. M. 1956. Improvements for pilot can increase aircraft efficiency. *J. Aviation Med.* 27: 23–26.
30. MOWBRAY, G. H. 1956. Man as a link in complex machine systems. *Sci. Monthly* 83: 269–276.
31. NADEL, A. B. 1958. *Human Factors Requirements of a Manned Space Vehicle.* (RM 58 TMP–10.) General Electric Company, Technical Military Planning Operation, Santa Barbara, Calif.
32. ORR, W. A., and TUCKER, J. W. 1958. Getting man into space. *Aviation Age* 28: 30–31, 102–105.
33. SCHAEFER, H. J. 1959. Radiation and man in space. In ORDWAY, F. I., III (ed.). *Advances in Space Science.* Academic Press, Inc., New York. Vol. 1.
34. SCHAEFER, H. J. 1958. New knowledge of the extra-atmospheric radiation field. *J. Aviation Med.* 29: 492–500.
35. SELLS, S. B. 1959. Human behavior in groups. *U.S. Armed Forces Med. J.* 10: 926–944.
36. SOLOMON, P., LEIDERMAN, H., MENDELSON, J., and WEXLER, D. 1957. Sensory deprivation: A review. *Am. J. Psychiat.* 114: 357–363.
37. STAFF REPORT OF THE SELECT COMMITTEE ON ASTRONAUTICS AND SPACE EXPLORATION. 1959. *A Space Handbook. Astronautics and Its Applications.* U.S. Government Printing Office, Washington, D.C.
38. STRUGHOLD, H. 1949. The human time factor in flight; the latent period of optical perception and its significance in high speed flying. *J. Aviation Med.* 20: 300–307.
39. SYMONDS, C. P. 1949. *Psychological Disorders in Flying Personnel of the Royal Air Force Investigated During the War 1939–1945.* Air Ministry A.P., 3139.
40. TSCHERMAK, A., and SCHUBERT, A. 1931. Über Vertikalorientierung im Rotatorium und im Flugzeuge. *Pflüger's Arch. ges. Physiol.* 228: 234–257.
41. VAETH, J. G. 1954. Training for space. *Astronautics* 1: 1–6, 30–32.
42. VAN ALLEN, J. A. 1959. *On the Radiation Hazards of Space Flight.* (SUI–59–7.) Department of Physics, State University of Iowa, Iowa City.
43. VON BECKH, H. J. 1958. *Flight Experiments About Human Reactions to Accelerations Which Are Followed Or Preceded by the Weightless State.* (AFMDC–TN–58–15.) Space Biology Branch, Aeromedical Field Laboratory, Holloman Air Force Base, New Mex.
44. VON DIRINGSHOFEN, H. 1956. The preventive psychosomatic concept of the flight surgeon in active air defense. *J. Aviation Med.* 27: 153–155.

# 2

# The Natural Environment and the Environment of Flight

HENRY B. HALE, PH.D. *

This topic is basic to much material included in subsequent chapters. It is important, therefore, not only to mention the particular features of the environment that have physiological significance but also to attempt to show in broad perspective the true relationships that exist between the major environmental factors and certain physiological aspects.

Biologists recognize that, as a general rule, there is a degree of *fitness* between a living organism and its environment, and it is believed that the distribution of animal forms over the earth can be explained in part on this basis. Man as a species has a vertical distribution which is usually wide. Human communities range from sea level (or slightly below) to levels as high as 15,000 ft. or thereabouts. Furthermore, many individuals routinely perform their daily labors at levels that are still lower and higher than these limits. Mining, diving, submarine, and aviation operations all represent extensions of the vertical distribution of man.

In the opinion of the physiologist, the ideal environment in the entire vertical range is that found at sea level. It is here that the "physiologic cost of living" is lowest. The particular combinations of physical factors that go to make up weather can be ignored for the present purpose.

The natural environment is a complex of dynamic factors, of which gravity, moisture, pressure, temperature, and electromagnetic radiations are important components. Air, by virtue of its pressure,

* Associate Professor of Physiology, School of Aviation Medicine, USAF, Brooks Air Force Base, Texas.

temperature, water-vapor content, chemical constituents, and other properties, constitutes a major part of the environment. The environment should never be regarded as passive in any respect, although, when environmental conditions are optimal for the human being, it may seem that no physical forces are in play. The environment is rich in energy, and the human being is dependent upon it for energy supplies.

The balance between internal (physiological) and external (environmental) energy utilized in the delivery of oxygen to the tissues is an outstanding example of the dependence of the organism on the environment. The average, relatively inactive adult normally requires approximately 300 ml of oxygen per minute, and this is theoretically the same at sea level and at altitude. At sea level the external pressure is sufficient to provide the major share of the energy required, and the energy balance for oxygen is optimal. The pressure is that exerted by oxygen molecules in the external air, which reflects the kinetic energy of these molecules and is mechanically important for transportation of oxygen to the tissues.

As one ascends to altitude, the kinetic energy of oxygen molecules entering the body is progressively reduced. The result is that they move increasingly too slowly for normal oxygen delivery. The organism must therefore compensate for the loss of external oxygen pressure by physiological means, by converting chemical energy into mechanical energy in the body. This conversion is inefficient and can compensate for loss of external pressure to a limited degree. At 10,000 ft. the loss is about 30 per cent, and many individuals can compensate efficiently. At 18,000 ft. it is 51 per cent, and from here to 23,000 ft., at which it is 60 per cent, compensatory mechanisms are of limited benefit and the individual can maintain consciousness for, at best, a few minutes. With the inefficiency that exists in the human body, physiological mechanisms ultimately become totally inadequate to compensate for extremely adverse environmental conditions, such as are encountered at still higher altitudes.

Energy is transferred from the air to the body in still another way, namely, in the form of heat. Collision of air molecules with any surface of the body results in losses in kinetic energy on the part of the air, and this energy is converted into heat in the surface tissues. The rate of absorption of such energy by the organism is optimal at sea level, where a minimal amount of biochemical energy is required for the maintenance of an essential store of heat in the body. However, metabolic activities increase, in order to supplement the heat supply, when the temperature, and therefore the kinetic energy, of air molecules is relatively low, as at altitudes. Within certain limits, as the altitude increases the extent to which body heat production is accelerated tends to be proportional to the reduction in kinetic energy of the air, assuming all other conditions to be equal.

Temperature and pressure variations with altitude are extensive, while physiological energy is limited. For this reason in the flying environment man has found it necessary to engineer appropriate means for supplying necessary energies in order to survive. Basically, this is what is done whenever efforts are made to control the environment. Heating of our houses in winter represents just such an effort, and every homeowner will agree that the cost is high even though he may not recognize that he is paying for a replacement of energy to a local environment. In the flying situation the cost of environmental control is not only high, but also the engineering difficulties become increasingly greater with each increase in speed or altitude. In actual practice sacrifices and compromises are the rule.

## Pressure Factors in the Environment

In cross-section the atmosphere may be visualized as a many-layered gaseous mass extending upward for several hundred miles. In order from lowest to highest, the layers are called *troposphere, stratosphere, ionosphere,* and *exosphere.* These are delineated in Table 2–1. Each has distinguishing physical characteristics, but from the physiological point of view only certain ones need to be considered here.

For a general understanding of the pressure variations in the atmosphere, reference is made to the United States Standard Atmosphere Table (Table 2–2), for which average values were utilized to establish the general pattern. Pressure decreases progressively with altitude, giving a straight-line relationship when plotted as a logarithmic function of altitude. Significant or limit altitudes with respect to manned flight are shown in Fig. 2–1.

**Oxygen Pressure.** Oxygen exerts approximately one-fifth the total pressure exerted by the air. To determine oxygen pressure at any particular altitude, the total barometric pressure, obtained from the U.S. Standard Table (Table 2–2), is multiplied by the factor 0.2094. The result is often referred to as *partial* pressure, although the term "oxygen pressure" is used in this chapter. For example, when the total pressure at sea level is 760 mm of mercury (mm Hg), on the average, oxygen (partial) pressure amounts to 159.

TABLE 2–1

Atmospheric Strata and Their Characteristics *

| | Spheres | Layers | Altitude in Miles | Temperatures (° C) | | |
|---|---|---|---|---|---|---|
| | | | | At Lower Boundary | At Upper Boundary | Extreme Values |
| Inner atmosphere | Bottom layer | Bottom layer | 0–.0012 | — | — | –50 to 80 |
| | | Ground layer | .0012–1.2 | — | — | –40 to 40 |
| | Troposphere | Advection layer | 1.2–5 | 10 | –40 | 20 to –45 |
| | | Tropopause layer | 5–7.5 | –40 | –55 | –35 to –80 |
| | Stratosphere | Isothermal layer | 7.5–21 | –55 | –50 | –45 to –65 |
| | | Warm layer | 21–30 | –50 | 50 | –60 to 80 |
| | | Upper mixing layer | 30–50 | 50 | –70 | –80 to 70 |
| | Ionosphere | E layer | 50–95 | –70 | 50 | 80 to 100 |
| | | F layer | 95–250 | ? | ? | 60 to 1000 |
| | | Atomic layer | 250–500 | ? | ? | 1200? |
| Outer atmosphere | Exosphere | | Above 500 | ? | ? | 2000? |

* Adapted from Haber (1), Table 21, p. 106.

Today's jet aircraft have the ability to traverse the troposphere in amazingly short times and to cruise at various altitudes in the stratosphere. The altitude of 9.5 miles (50,000 ft.) can be considered as representative of the pressure conditions encountered in advanced military jet aircraft and in space flight. From the physiological point of view, oxygen pressure reductions that occur at still higher levels are no more serious to man than those encountered at 50,000 ft. Oxygen pressure at this altitude is only 18 mm Hg, which represents a reduction of 89 per cent, as compared with that at sea level. Physiological compensation at this altitude is an impossibility, and unconsciousness will result within seconds if this air is inhaled.

## TABLE 2-2

## The United States Standard Atmosphere *

| Altitude (Feet) | Pressure mm Hg | Pressure p.s.i. | Altitude (Feet) | Pressure mm Hg | Pressure p.s.i. | Altitude (Feet) | Pressure mm Hg | Pressure lb/ft² |
|---|---|---|---|---|---|---|---|---|
| 0 | 760.0 | 14.70 | 32500 | 201.0 | 3.89 | 66000 | 40.6 | 113.2 |
| 500 | 746.4 | 14.43 | 33000 | 196.3 | 3.80 | 68000 | 36.9 | 102.9 |
| 1000 | 732.9 | 14.17 | 33500 | 191.8 | 3.71 | 70000 | 33.6 | 93.52 |
| 1500 | 719.7 | 13.92 | 34000 | 187.3 | 3.62 | 72000 | 30.4 | 85.01 |
| 2000 | 706.6 | 13.66 | 34500 | 183.0 | 3.54 | 74000 | 27.7 | 77.26 |
| 2500 | 693.8 | 13.42 | 35000 | 178.7 | 3.46 | | | |
| 3000 | 681.1 | 13.17 | 35500 | 174.4 | 3.37 | 76000 | 25.2 | 70.22 |
| 3500 | 668.6 | 12.93 | 36000 | 170.3 | 3.29 | 78000 | 22.9 | 63.8 |
| 4000 | 656.3 | 12.69 | 36500 | 166.3 | 3.22 | 80000 | 20.8 | 58.01 |
| 4500 | 644.2 | 12.46 | 37000 | 162.4 | 3.14 | 82000 | 18.9 | 52.72 |
| 5000 | 632.3 | 12.23 | 37500 | 158.6 | 3.07 | 84000 | 17.2 | 47.91 |
| 5500 | 620.6 | 12.00 | 38000 | 154.8 | 2.99 | | | |
| 6000 | 609.0 | 11.78 | 38500 | 151.2 | 2.92 | 86000 | 15.6 | 43.55 |
| 6500 | 597.6 | 11.55 | 39000 | 147.5 | 2.85 | 88000 | 14.2 | 39.59 |
| 7000 | 586.4 | 11.34 | 39500 | 144.1 | 2.79 | 90000 | 12.9 | 35.95 |
| 7500 | 575.3 | 11.12 | 40000 | 140.7 | 2.72 | 92000 | 11.7 | 32.7 |
| 8000 | 564.4 | 10.91 | 40500 | 137.4 | 2.66 | 94000 | 10.7 | 29.71 |
| 8500 | 553.7 | 10.71 | 41000 | 134.1 | 2.59 | | | |
| 9000 | 543.2 | 10.50 | 41500 | 131.0 | 2.53 | 96000 | 9.7 | 27.02 |
| 9500 | 532.8 | 10.30 | 42000 | 127.9 | 2.47 | 98000 | 8.8 | 24.55 |
| 10000 | 522.6 | 10.11 | 42500 | 124.9 | 2.42 | 100000 | 8.0 | 22.31 |
| 10500 | 512.5 | 9.91 | 43000 | 121.9 | 2.36 | 110000 | 5.0 | 13.92 |
| 11000 | 502.6 | 9.72 | 43500 | 119.0 | 2.30 | 120000 | 3.24 | 9.026 |
| 11500 | 492.8 | 9.53 | 44000 | 116.2 | 2.25 | 130000 | 2.18 | 6.071 |
| 12000 | 483.3 | 9.35 | 44500 | 113.5 | 2.19 | 140000 | 1.51 | 4.213 |
| 12500 | 473.8 | 9.16 | 45000 | 110.9 | 2.14 | 150000 | 1.08 | 3.003 |
| 13000 | 464.5 | 8.98 | 45500 | 108.2 | 2.09 | 160000 | 0.787 | 2.190 |
| 13500 | 455.4 | 8.81 | 46000 | 105.6 | 2.04 | 170000 | 0.583 | 1.624 |
| 14000 | 446.4 | 8.63 | 46500 | 103.1 | 1.99 | 180000 | 0.433 | 1.206 |
| 14500 | 437.5 | 8.46 | 47000 | 100.7 | 1.95 | | | |
| 15000 | 428.8 | 8.29 | 47500 | 98.3 | 1.90 | | | |
| 15500 | 420.2 | 8.13 | 48000 | 96.0 | 1.86 | | | |
| 16000 | 411.8 | 7.96 | 48500 | 93.7 | 1.81 | | | |
| 16500 | 403.5 | 7.80 | 49000 | 91.5 | 1.77 | | | |
| 17000 | 395.3 | 7.64 | 49500 | 89.4 | 1.73 | | | |
| 17500 | 387.3 | 7.49 | 50000 | 87.3 | 1.69 | | | |
| 18000 | 379.4 | 7.34 | 50500 | 85.2 | 1.65 | | | |
| 18500 | 371.7 | 7.19 | 51000 | 83.2 | 1.61 | | | |
| 19000 | 364.0 | 7.04 | 51500 | 81.2 | 1.57 | | | |
| 19500 | 356.5 | 6.89 | 52000 | 79.3 | 1.53 | | | |
| 20000 | 349.1 | 6.75 | 52500 | 77.4 | 1.50 | | | |
| 20500 | 341.8 | 6.61 | 53000 | 75.6 | 1.46 | | | |
| 21000 | 334.6 | 6.47 | 53500 | 73.8 | 1.43 | | | |
| 21500 | 327.6 | 6.33 | 54000 | 72.1 | 1.39 | | | |
| 22000 | 320.8 | 6.20 | 54500 | 70.4 | 1.36 | | | |
| 22500 | 314.0 | 6.07 | 55000 | 68.8 | 1.33 | | | |
| 23000 | 307.4 | 5.94 | 55500 | 67.1 | 1.30 | | | |
| 23500 | 300.8 | 5.82 | 56000 | 65.5 | 1.27 | | | |
| 24000 | 294.4 | 5.70 | 56500 | 64.0 | 1.24 | | | |
| 24500 | 288.0 | 5.57 | 57000 | 62.4 | 1.21 | | | |
| 25000 | 281.8 | 5.45 | 57500 | 61.0 | 1.18 | | | |
| 25500 | 275.8 | 5.33 | 58000 | 59.5 | 1.15 | | | |
| 26000 | 269.8 | 5.22 | 58500 | 58.1 | 1.12 | | | |
| 26500 | 263.8 | 5.10 | 59000 | 56.8 | 1.10 | | | |
| 27000 | 258.0 | 4.99 | 59500 | 55.4 | 1.07 | | | |
| 27500 | 252.4 | 4.88 | 60000 | 54.1 | 1.05 | | | |
| 28000 | 246.8 | 4.77 | 60500 | 52.8 | 1.02 | | | |
| 28500 | 241.4 | 4.67 | 61000 | 51.6 | 0.998 | | | |
| 29000 | 236.0 | 4.56 | 61500 | 50.4 | 0.975 | | | |
| 29500 | 230.6 | 4.46 | 62000 | 49.2 | 0.951 | | | |
| 30000 | 225.6 | 4.36 | 62500 | 48.0 | 0.928 | | | |
| 30500 | 220.4 | 4.26 | 63000 | 46.9 | 0.907 | | | |
| 31000 | 215.4 | 4.17 | 63500 | 45.8 | 0.886 | | | |
| 31500 | 210.4 | 4.07 | 64000 | 44.7 | 0.864 | | | |
| 32000 | 205.6 | 3.98 | 64500 | 43.6 | 0.843 | | | |

| Altitude (Feet) | Pressure Microns Hg | Pressure lb/ft² |
|---|---|---|
| 190000 | 321.6 | 0.8956 |
| 200000 | 238.6 | 0.6645 |
| 210000 | 174.9 | 0.4869 |
| 220000 | 125.9 | 0.3504 |
| 230000 | 88.69 | 0.2470 |
| 240000 | 61.02 | 0.1699 |
| 250000 | 40.9 | 0.1139 |
| 260000 | 26.65 | 0.07422 |

**Day Pressure Only Gravity Constant**

| | | |
|---|---|---|
| 270000 | 17.34 | 0.04829 |
| 280000 | 11.49 | 0.03200 |
| 290000 | 7.843 | 0.02184 |
| 300000 | 5.493 | 0.01530 |

Sources of Data:

0—80,000 Brombacher Tables
NACA Report No. 538, 1935

80,000—300,000 NACA Tech Note
No. 1200, January 1947

Conversion Factors:

1 mm Hg = 0.019339 p. s. i.
1 p. s. i. = 51.715 mm Hg

* From "Flight Surgeon's Manual," Air Force Manual 160–5, Table 1, p. 7. Department of the Air Force, October, 1954.

With atmospheric pressure at 50,000 ft. effectively equivalent to zero, engineered environmental control, i.e., energy restoration, is required. Two methods of control have been devised. These are the pressurized cabin, which can be used as high as a compressor will function adequately, and the sealed cabin above this. Full pressure

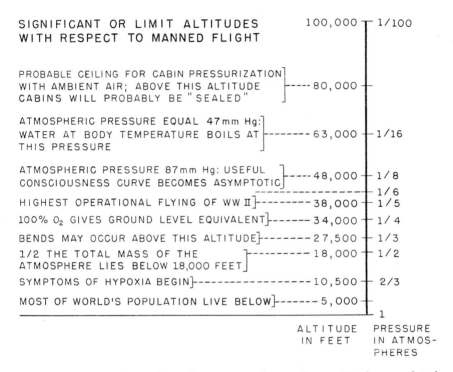

Fig. 2–1. Physiologically and aeronautically significant altitudes as related to fractions of sea-level pressures. (By A. I. Karstens from *Physical and Physiological Data for Bioastronautics*, Air University, School of Aviation Medicine, USAF, Randolph Air Force Base, 1958. Table III 1.4.1.4) (*Editors' note:* Recent data indicate that bends may occur above 22,500 ft.)

and partial pressure suits have also been developed as interim protective measures.

**Nitrogen Pressure.** Earlier it was indicated that oxygen pressure represents only a fraction of the pressure that a barometer would measure; the difference between the total pressure and the oxygen pressure is due principally to nitrogen. Although nitrogen molecules enter the body along with oxygen, they merely diffuse and become dispersed (dissolved) but do not enter into any chemical combination. Ordinarily, an equilibrium exists between the dissolved or trapped gas in the hollow organs of the body and that in the air surrounding it. Blood, tissue fluid, and cellular substance all contain nitrogen along with oxygen and carbon dioxide. The quantity of nitrogen for the body as a whole is generally 1,000 ml or slightly more.

At sea level the pressure exerted by atmospheric nitrogen amounts to 601 mm Hg. With the constant interchange of gases between the atmosphere and the body, the tendency for nitrogen to exert outward pressure is equal to the tendency for it to exert inward pressure, and the net effect is zero. However, at 50,000 ft., where atmospheric nitrogen exerts a pressure of only 69 mm Hg, nitrogen pressures cannot quickly be reduced to this level in all parts of the body.

The net effect is a condition called *dysbarism,* in which the outward force, depending upon its location, may cause pain or other symptoms. Distention of the stomach or colon, production of gas bubbles in connective tissues (initially these contain nitrogen, but water vapor, carbon dioxide, and oxygen may enter later), and disruption of cell membranes, especially in adipose tissue, represent some of the common effects of this condition, which is popularly known as *bends.*

**Engineering Control of Pressure Factors.** At an altitude of 50,000 ft., it is essential that both oxygen and nitrogen pressure factors be controlled. Cabin pressurization, which is adequate for acceptable (but not ideal) oxygen control at this altitude, would be more than adequate for nitrogen pressure control. Such an environment can be created and maintained by aircraft compressor systems, but it is not considered a safe practice in the event of sudden loss of pressure (explosive decompression). For example, consider the situation of a cabin engineered for an inside pressure equivalent to that at 10,000 ft. while flying at 50,000 ft. The oxygen pressure inside would be 109 mm Hg and that outside, 18 mm Hg. Although the physiological compensation required inside the cabin would be of only relatively minor degree, the important fact is that the pressure differential across the cockpit and cabin walls would amount to 8.4 pounds per square inch (psi). For safety reasons a pressure differential of this magnitude is not permitted in fighter aircraft.

If the pressure in the cockpit were adjusted to the level equivalent to 20,000 ft., the pressure differential would be only 5 psi, which is safer. However, while this pressure provides adequate control of the nitrogen pressure factor, it is not adequate for oxygen.

The oxygen factor can be controlled by the use of an oxygen mask and pressure regulator, using oxygen from storage cylinders rather than from air. This practice is used in military flying and by test pilots but has not been considered practicable, except for emergency, in commercial airliners, whose ceilings average about 40,000 ft. in routine flights.

Under combat conditions the pressure differential in fighter aircraft has been reduced to a still greater extent; consequently, the nitrogen pressure level may be inadequately controlled. In this situation a full pressure suit can be worn by crew members to provide control for both factors.

However, it is physiologically possible to use still another approach to the solution of the problem. This is to change the man to *fit* the environment. As unusual as this may seem, it is entirely possible and practical. This is accomplished by eliminating considerable nitrogen prior to the flight by means of breathing pure oxygen for periods of as little as 30 minutes. The "washout" of nitrogen from the lungs and circulating blood is quite rapid, but it occurs more slowly in the tissue fluid and the connective tissues. *Denitrogenation* prior to ascent to 50,000 ft. or higher must therefore be for periods of longer than 30 minutes.

The replacement of nitrogen with oxygen results in an excess oxygen supply within the body at ground level, where external and internal gaseous pressures are equalized. The excess oxygen is not harmful under these conditions. Pure oxygen induces disorders only if breathed for very prolonged periods of time (24 or more hours). Furthermore, this is the case only if the oxygen pressure exceeds 425 mm Hg. This pressure level approximates that at 15,000 ft. Since oxygen pressure in the mask can never greatly exceed ambient pressure (this is still true when pressure-breathing equipment is used), it is not possible to be exposed to toxic oxygen levels when above 15,000 ft.

The partial pressure suit is designed to control the oxygen factor but not the nitrogen. At extremely high altitude it enables the wearer to receive oxygen at physiologically satisfactory pressures, and concomitantly it applies counterpressure by mechanical means to major areas of the body. Basically, this insures that the pressure differential across the wall of the thorax especially, but elsewhere as well, is approximately zero. Denitrogenation is essential when this device is used, but with the full pressure suit there is no need for denitrogenation.

For flights to altitudes higher than 50,000 ft., cockpit pressurization becomes increasingly more difficult for the reason that compressor efficiency decreases as air density decreases. Ultimately it becomes too difficult to use methods that restore energy to atmospheric air before admitting it to the cockpit. The alternative is to transport oxygen in storage cylinders. The work of compressing oxygen in cylinders imparts a high energy content, and when this is done outside of the aircraft, there are no special problems. At altitude, through the use of appropriate equipment, it is possible to maintain precise control of oxygen pressure.

Liquid oxygen is advantageous both because it occupies little space and because it can be converted into the gaseous state and at the proper pressure level merely by supplying energy in the form of heat. With the abandonment of compressor systems that utilize atmospheric air, the entire method of control of the pressure environment becomes changed. The system that takes its place is called the "sealed cabin," which is discussed in Chapter 12. In principle the sealed cabin operates in the same manner as a submarine.

## Thermal Factors in the Environment

Air temperature is an important physiological factor, but it is not the sole thermal factor in the natural environment. Energy in the form of infrared radiations constitutes a second, and perhaps more important, thermal factor. Other physical conditions also contribute greatly to the actions of these thermal factors. These secondary factors are humidity, air density, and air movement. The net effect of these various influences is the important one to the body, and it is possible for various combinations of these factors to induce similar physiological effects.

The human body has the ability to detect and to compensate for deviations in either direction from what may be called "thermoneutrality." It must be emphasized that *thermoneutrality* does not refer to air temperature alone. However, human compensatory powers are inadequate for the extremes that may be encountered at altitude.

At ground level, where air temperature, density, movement, water-vapor content, the presence of solid objects which release infrared radiations, and solar radiations all comprise the thermal environment, the variability tends to be great. Disregarding diurnal and seasonal variations, air temperature (as seen in the idealized, or standard, atmosphere) varies with altitude. But unlike the variation in pressure with altitude, temperature falls in certain strata and rises in others.

**Conditions at Jet Altitudes.** Air temperature declines in the troposphere, on the average, at the rate of approximately 2° C per 1,000 ft. This means that, as a component of the thermal environment, air becomes progressively less of a positive force as altitude increases through the troposphere. Water vapor also decreases with altitude in the troposphere, and its value is virtually zero at all altitudes above the troposphere. The water vapor (and carbon dioxide) in the troposphere absorbs energy (infrared radiations) which comes from the sun and from the earth itself. Tropospheric air also receives heat by contact with heated objects on the earth's surface. Distribution of the heat is accomplished by convection currents.

The lowest portion of the stratosphere (the band from the altitude of from 7.5 to 21 miles) is unique in that there is essentially no variation in air temperature. The temperature tends to remain constant at $-55°$ C. It is in this *isothermal* layer that jet aircraft are being flown currently. Exposure of the unprotected body to this air would not result in heat transfer at the same rates as at ground level, assuming that other conditions were equal. This is explained by the fact that the density of the atmosphere is much lower. However, all conditions are not equal, and one which is of major importance is the windblast. Even with low density, the high air-flow rate and low temperature make this a very unsatisfactory thermal environment.

**Engineering Control of Cabin Temperature in Jet Aircraft.** Within the cockpit the conditions can be made fairly satisfactory, but the control is limited to the air temperature and air-flow rate. Air scoops and compressors, in building up pressure, also increase the temperature; expansion turbines permit sufficient expansion to bring temperature to an appropriate level. In the lowest layer of the stratosphere, referred to above, solar radiation is more intense, since the filtering action of water vapor and carbon dioxide does not exist at these altitudes or above. So-called *near infrared* radiation passes readily through the aircraft canopy and Plexiglas windows and is absorbed by the solid objects in the cockpit, including the man and his clothing. These objects all reradiate some of this energy in the form of *far infrared*, but the canopy does not transmit these radiations. Consequently, with respect to the solar radiant energy, there is a net heat gain. This may be of advantage, and cockpit air-temperature control takes this factor into account.

In the event of ejection from the aircraft, the pilot will be in direct contact with the cold air and will be subject to high windblast. Insulative clothing is the only means by which his "microclimate" can be controlled. Tests have shown that for the short time required for descent by free fall from the isothermal layer to relatively low altitudes, only moderately heavy garments are needed. Appropriate clothing assemblies have been devised and have been integrated with other garments such as the altitude protection suit.

The air forming the next higher layer in the stratosphere exhibits temperature variation; in this case temperature increases with altitude. The gain in molecular energy has been attributed to the *ozone* which is present in low concentration. This chemical constituent has the ability to absorb energy which exists in the form of solar ultraviolet radiation. Peculiarly, convection currents do not occur in this portion of the atmosphere.

**Conditions at Higher Altitudes.** Other variations in air temperature have been reported for the ionosphere and exosphere, but the air density is so low that heat-transfer properties are negligible. The air temperatures for these upper parts of the atmosphere are extremely high, but air density is so low that physiological effects would not be like those at sea level. In fact, air temperature becomes a negligible factor and radiation is the important one.

Thermal factors are expected to be extremely important for hypersonic aircraft. Air molecules that collide with the leading edges of aircraft traveling at these speeds come to complete arrest which results in the liberation of kinetic energy at a very high rate. This energy appears as heat which remains in a thin boundary layer, the *stagnant layer*. Mathematically, *stagnation temperatures* are equal to 50 times the square of the speed, when speed is in *Mach* units (designated by M, when 1M equals the speed of sound) and temperature is in degrees centigrade. For example, at Mach 10, the stagnation temperature becomes 5,000° C. A stagnant area is developed over broad surfaces also; this is due to air friction.

Air density is not a factor in these heat-generation phenomena, but it is a factor in the transfer of heat from the boundary layer to the metal structures of the aircraft, which in turn, transmit heat to the interior. Present knowledge on these matters is limited, and there is an active research program. It has been found that the air in the boundary layer fails to obey certain principles established for gases in laminar flow. Dissociation, ionization, and the formation of new chemical compounds are processes which occur in the boundary layer. The problems of control have yet to be worked out. This represents the so-called *thermal barrier.*

**Engineering Control of Cabin Temperature at Extremely High Altitudes and in Space Vehicles.** Along with thoughts of control of heat transfer or heat generation, there is the matter of protection to the occupant of such craft. Protective garments are under development. At present a "ventilated suit," which is integrated with such other garments as the partial pressure suit, anti-g suit, and anti-exposure suit, seems to have good possibilities. Comfort is not the criterion in this situation; instead, the wearer will be slightly overheated and employ his own sweating mechanism to avoid high heat storage. Obviously, time of exposure will be an important factor.

In satellite vehicles aerodynamic heating is expected to be a problem upon re-entry into the atmosphere; but while in orbit, heat gains and losses will occur entirely by radiation. Data from satellites now in orbit indicate that temperature within such structures can be kept within physiologically acceptable limits. A problem of another nature is expected to arise in occupied satellites; this is the lack of convection in the air within the sealed cabin. The satellite and its occupants will be weightless. Hence, the changes in air density, which result from warming and cooling, will not give rise to air movements of the usual type. Forced convection should solve this problem.

## Combined Control of Pressure and Temperature Factors

Thermal and pressure factors in the natural environment vary simultaneously, but experimental studies concerned with physiological responses to changes in these factors have thus far dealt with them, for the most part, separately. Relatively little effort has been made to investigate them in combination or to examine over a wide range of pressures the effects of a variety of thermal conditions or vice versa.

Degrees of hypoxia that are not serious at thermoneutrality become so when the thermal factors are altered. For example, in a moderately cold environment metabolic rate is increased considerably, thus intensifying the effects of hypoxia. Metabolic rates may also become elevated in moderately hot environments and intensify hypoxia.

On the other hand, when hypoxia is avoided, decreasing barometric pressure has a beneficial effect on the human exposed to a hot environment, because heat liberation by the evaporation of sweat becomes a more efficient mechanism. Cold environments predispose toward dysbarism, and hot environments predispose toward motion sickness and reduce tolerance to accelerative forces. While the mechanisms of action have yet to be identified, these actions of cold and heat have been adequately demonstrated.

## Gravity and Inertial Forces as Environmental Factors

Gravity is generally considered to exert its force directly upon the body. But as the force responsible for barometric pressure, gravity has indirect effects as well and should perhaps be considered the most fundamental component of the environment. In its direct action it is unlike any other known force. It is pervasive and is not diminished as it penetrates body tissues. Nor is the body shielded from it when it remains within a closed structure, such as the cockpit. Other forces cannot be transmitted through tissues without decrement; and no other force exerts its full effects when acting through some shielding structure.

The human body, both anatomically and physiologically, is gravity-controlled. In the skeletal, neuromuscular, and circulatory systems, especially, there are numerous examples of mechanisms for counteracting gravity. The ability to maintain an upright posture is a familiar example, and it involves not only skeletal development and extremely complex neuromuscular control, but also it requires special vascular structures and cardiovascular capabilities which are unusual among mammalian species.

A systematic summary of information concerning biological tolerances of gravity and inertial forces is presented in Table 2–3.

In straight and level flying the relationship of the human body to the gravitational field is the same as when on the ground. In a satellite or in a high-speed aircraft flying a particular trajectory, either *subgravity* or *zero-gravity states* can exist. These conditions, which represent the resultant sum of all forces acting on the craft, including gravity, centrifugal force, etc., occur when the sum of forces is approaching zero (subgravity) or is equal to zero (zero gravity). The zero-gravity state is also called "weightlessness." In aircraft flying within the atmosphere, the maximum duration of the zero-gravity state is limited to from 30 to 45 seconds. At extremely high altitudes, where density is lower and the vector of drag becomes altered, the duration may be longer. Outside the atmosphere the duration can be unlimited.

The state of *supergravity* is one that results from powered ascent, as in the pull-out from a dive. In supergravity states, weight is greater than normal. In aircraft maneuvers, when there are changes in velocity, direction, or in both velocity and direction, inertial forces come into being. If the motion is linear and the velocity is changing (this is acceleration in the most frequently used sense), the inertial force will be equal in magnitude and opposite in direction to the force causing the acceleration. When the motion is curvilinear, the magnitude of the force is proportional to the square of the velocity and inversely proportional to the radius.

The physiological reactions to, or the damaging effects of, inertial forces vary with their magnitude, duration, rate of increase or decrease, and their relationship to the body axes. Inertial forces acting along the longitudinal axis of the body have received considerable study. When the force is directed toward the feet, the effects are different from those resulting from headward forces of the same nature. Inertial forces acting perpendicularly to the longitudinal axis have still different effects. The forces of deceleration have also received considerable attention.

## Adverse Factors in the Environment

The point has been made repeatedly that the energy-contributing components of the natural environment serve the body best when they are at a relatively neutral point. When these external forces are other than optimal, the body must compensate. If the forces are in excess of the normal energy balance between the organism and the

## TABLE 2–3

## Biological Tolerance of Acceleration *

| Type of g | Direction of Body Movement | Aircraft Maneuver | Experimental Human Exposures (Maximum) | Physiological Limits (Human) | Activities | AMAL Centrifuge Animal Exposures | Animal Pathology |
|---|---|---|---|---|---|---|---|
| Positive | Head to foot | Pull out or tight turn | 8 g for 15 sec. | Blackout to unconsciousness | All centrifuges | 40 g for 15 sec. Chimpanzee | Slight damage with venous congestion, intravascular thrombosis, and leg muscle hemorrhage |
| | | | 4.5 g for 5 min. with g suit | Pain in legs and blackout | | | |
| | | Controlled escape deceleration | 15 g for 1.75 sec. | Unconsciousness | AMAL centrifuge | 15 g for 60 sec. Chimpanzee | Unconscious at 9 g on build-up and unconscious then confused after run |
| | | Ejection escape (upward) | 20 g for 0.1 sec. with face curtain, arm rest | Skeletal damage (spine) | AMEL and WADC ejection tower | 40 g for 30 sec. Monkey | Slight damage |
| | | Push over | 4.5 g for 5 sec. | Subjective pain | Rod Jocelyn | | |
| Negative | Foot to head | | 3 g for 32 sec. with special helmet | Fullness of neck and head, bradycardia | WADC centrifuge | 40 g for 30 sec. Monkey | Intracranial damage Subcutaneous hematomas about the head |
| | | Ejection escape (downward) | 10 g for 0.1 sec. with leg support | Pain | WADC ejection tower | 40 g for 15 sec. Chimpanzee | Severe damage with hematomas in periorbital tissues, tongue, and thyroid gland; venous congestion and intravascular thrombosis with intracranial damage |
| | | Catapult launching | 5 g for 2 sec. | No damage | Carrier take-offs and AMAL centrifuge | No exposure Chimpanzee | No damage expected up to 40 g for 15 sec. |
| Transverse supine | Chest to back | Escape deceleration or higher launching stress | 3 g for 9 min. 31 sec. Lying flat | Monotony and giddiness | WADC centrifuge | | |
| | | | 15 g for 5 sec. | Surface petechial hemorrhage and pain in chest | AMAL centrifuge | | |
| | | Crash (facing aft) | 55 g for 0.01 sec. 35 g for 0.12 sec. | Skeletal damage | WADC deceleration track | | |

| Type | Subtype | Condition | Human tolerance | Human effect | Method | Animal exposure | Animal effect |
|---|---|---|---|---|---|---|---|
| Transverse prone | Back to chest | Arrested landing | 5 g for 2 sec. | No damage | Carrier landings and AMAL centrifuge | 40 g for 15 sec. Chimpanzee | No damage |
| | | Escape deceleration or higher landing stress | 15 g for 5 sec. Special chest and leg support | Surface petechial hemorrhage and pain in chest | AMAL centrifuge | | |
| | | Crash (facing forward) | 60 g for 0.01 sec. with special harness; 38 g for 0.12 sec. with special harness | Skeletal damage | WADC deceleration track (Col. Stapp) | | |
| Fluctuating positive | Alternating positive and transverse | Uncontrolled aircraft "jostle" | 1.5 to 6.5 g for 20 sec. combined with 72° pitch and roll | Additional support required other than conventional lap belt and shoulder harness | AMAL centrifuge | No animal exposures. This type was investigated to determine pilot's ability to actuate controls | |
| Cyclic | Alternating: Positive transverse prone, Negative transverse supine | Uncontrolled escape device "tumbling" | No human experimentation due to severe damage in animal exposures | | AMAL centrifuge | 15 g and 20 rpm Chimpanzee | Fatal: cerebral hemorrhage, 3 min. exposure. Severe damage with hematoma and hemorrhage, 15 sec. exposure |
| | | | | | | 35 g and 10 to 110 rpm for 10 sec. Monkey | Fatal: severe damage with hemorrhage in lungs, spleen, and other organs; necrosis of liver cells and intravascular clotting in all organs. Increasing damage with increase in rpm |

NOTE: "g" refers to the force on the body in multiples of the body weight. Wearing g suit increases human tolerance to blackout and fatigue. The types of g, transverse-lateral and fluctuating negative, have not been studied and are not included in this table. Rod Jocelyn, stunt pilot, contracted by AMAL, for negative-g maneuvers.
AMAL, Aviation Medical Acceleration Laboratory, Johnsville, Pennsylvania; AMEL, Aviation Medical Equipment Laboratory, Philadelphia, Pennsylvania; WADC, Wright Air Development Center, Dayton, Ohio.
* From Webster, A. P., and Hunter, H. M. 1954. *Journal of Aviation Medicine 25:* 378–379.

environment, the body may be handicapped and may have to compensate in some manner to avoid too great an energy uptake. If the external forces are inadequate, physiological energy must be elicited to compensate. Either deviation is, therefore, adverse in character, but it is the quantitative difference that makes for the adversity, not the character of the factor itself.

Other factors exist in the environment which may be classified as qualitatively adverse. These are not essential for life, and any effects that they may have on the body are undesirable. Compensatory responses may be possible when such forces are at low levels of intensity or short-lasting, but high intensities or prolonged application of such forces are harmful. In this category can be included such factors as noxious gases, irritating fumes, ionizing radiations, ionized and dissociated gases, and meteorites. Some of these are never encountered at sea level, but encounters at high altitudes may be frequent.

Noxious gases (for example, carbon monoxide) and irritating fumes which may be derived from lubricating substances are associated with the aircraft and its power plant, but ozone and atomic or ionized oxygen and nitrogen appear in the atmosphere in concentrations which are of significance only at high altitudes. The peak concentration of ozone is at approximately 85,000 ft. At sea level pressure ozone in low concentration (6 ppm, by volume) causes lung *edema* if inhaled for only 30 minutes. The possibility that compressors in pressurized aircraft might increase the concentration of ozone is considered unlikely, since the high temperatures resulting from compression would tend to cause ozone decomposition. Apart from possible physiological effects, ozone is harmful in its action on plastics and rubber; thus, structures within the aircraft itself may suffer by contact with ozone.

The problem of cosmic radiation can be considered as an environmental problem. As a special and a new field of knowledge, it deserves special treatment. The topic is, therefore, reserved for Chapter 3.

## References

1. HABER, H. 1954. *The Physical Environment of the Flyer.* USAF, Air University, School of Aviation Medicine, Randolph Air Force Base, Texas.
2. WHITE, C. S., and BENSON, O. O., JR. (eds.). 1952. *Physics and Medicine of the Upper Atmosphere: A Study of the Aeropause.* University of New Mexico Press, Albuquerque.

# 3

# Radiobiology and the Environment of Flight

GERRIT L. HEKHUIS, M.D.*

The radiation hazard in high-altitude jet and space flight is one of the central problems of the advancing aerospace technology. The recent findings and related theories associated with extraterrestrial radiation surrounding the earth in its near space have brought the requirement for interpretation of the biological and medical effects of these radiations into focus. Radiobiological problems have also arisen from the increasingly large numbers of nuclear power sources, the increased industrial use of x-ray, and the extensive medical development of x-ray and radioactive isotopes in diagnosis and treatment.

The purpose of this chapter is to outline some of the basic concepts of interaction of radiation with matter, including biological tissue, and to provide guide lines for the evaluation of the hazards of radiations.

Within the wide range of radiations that are known, only a very narrow portion is readily discernible to the individual by observation, and this narrow, visible range represents but a minute portion of the entire spectrum. Most of the range of the electromagnetic spectrum can be applied to the human body without sensation or obvious effect. In addition, the existence of particulate types of radiation exemplifies different modes of interaction, and these must be compared and contrasted.

Most of the radiations of biological concern are those classed as ionizing radiation or penetrating radiation, and these are generally

* Colonel, USAF, MC, Chief, Department of Radiobiology, School of Aviation Medicine, USAF, Brooks Air Force Base, Texas.

such that they cannot be sensed in any way by the biological system, at least in terms of producing a realization that a radiation is taking place. Therefore, the determination of effect can be made only in situations in which the radiation is known to be present, in which it can be measured by instruments and then the effects observed and interpreted sometime later as a function of the measured exposure. Because of this requirement for physical measurement, the need to understand the mechanisms of radiation and their effects becomes essential, as the individual must be able to evaluate or predict the effect when an instrument reading or response is observed.

For purposes of this discussion, radiobiology is considered as the study of the biological effects of ionizing radiation. Ionizing radiation includes both electromagnetic radiations and particle radiations which can produce ionization either directly or indirectly, as discussed below in detail. It is impossible in this space to give adequate discussion of all theories concerning the mechanism of biological effects of radiation. These are covered in summary form, but a list of suggested readings for further study is provided (1–6).

Application of radiobiology to hazard evaluation depends on many uncertain factors. Among these are (1) the extrapolation of data obtained from one biological system or species to another; (2) the great problem of interpreting physical measurement of radiation dose and applying this same dose concept to the effect on the biological tissue; (3) the determination of an acceptable dose measurement for both the physicist and the biologist, the problem of measuring an energy transfer at one point and extrapolating this dose to another system at some other point; and (4) perhaps the greatest difficulty of describing a given phenomenon in a biological system as a radiation effect when the biological system is certainly a dynamic, complex, everchanging system which has the capability of receiving injury and subsequently of performing a certain degree of physiological recovery. The last consideration of the determination of effect will be discussed further as it and its misinterpretation have been reported and at times have made headlines.

## Fundamental Radiation Effects

The fundamental radiation effects which are noted in most interactions of ionizing radiation with matter are those that result from the transfer of energy from the ionizing radiation to the matter traversed. This may sound quite simple, but the difficulty lies in describing the transfer of energy from the radiation to the system in which this energy must be absorbed. It is obvious that the radiation effects observed can be the fundamental ones only if the fundamental levels of the system are also observed. In other words, the description of any given effect of radiation is in large part a reflection of the method of studying it in the experiment.

**Types of Radiation.** Radiation sources are categorized into two main types: particulate and electromagnetic. Dividing radiations into these two categories will assist in evaluating the mechanisms of action and thus pattern the approach to the effects of these radiations on tissue.

Particulate radiations are composed of high-speed particles and are further subdivided into two categories according to the presence or absence of an electrical charge. Examples of the first subcategory are alpha particles, beta particles, and protons which do carry an electric charge during the majority of their path. Neutrons are an example of a particle which has kinetic energy but no electrical charge.

Electromagnetic radiations include all those that exhibit primarily wave characteristics and are exemplified in the present discussion by x-rays, gamma rays, and secondary cosmic rays. These can in most ways be compared to our concept of light and radio waves.

**Mechanisms of Interaction.** The net result of ionizing and penetrating radiation in interaction with matter is the transfer of energy and the resulting process of ionization. In this process sufficient energy is transferred by various means to the atoms of the irradiated material to produce the removal or ejection of one or more orbital electrons from the electrically neutral atom. This produces a pair of charged particles from the previously electrically normal or neutral atom. One portion of the pair is the ejected electron which is negatively charged; the other half of the pair is the residual of the atom left after the electron has been ejected, and this residual is positively charged. The two parts, electron and residual atom, are known as an "ion pair."

The process of producing these ion pairs, or the process of ionization, requires energy which is derived from the incident ionizing radiation. Some of it may come from the particle or radiation wave by total absorption or by partial absorption in the transfer of some of its kinetic energy. Each ionization requires a certain amount of energy to accomplish the release and separation of the electrons from the atom, and in addition the effective ejection of this electron with an adequate kinetic energy to leave the immediate vicinity of the atom requires an additional energy expenditure. Each of these ionization events is thus a result of the transfer of energy from the incident radiation to the matter irradiated.

One concept of matter must be brought to mind at this point. It requires the awareness of the predominance of unoccupied space within what we call matter, whether it is in the solid, liquid, or gaseous state. The enormous amount of space in comparison with the concentration of matter occupying this space results in the possibility of predicting the interaction of radiation on the material in terms of statistics. If the radiation involved has with it an electrical charge, the major contribution of its action on matter is through the electrical and electrostatic attraction and repulsion of that charge with the electron space charge of the atom of the matter irradiated. Different energies of radiation interact with matter with different details of mechanism, but the end result is one of ionization.

This primary event of ionization also produces secondary electrons which are in themselves charged and ejected with varying amounts of energy which are apparent in their speed. These secondary electrons can additionally produce ion pairs in their passage through the surrounding matter, similarly losing their energy of motion by energy transfer. They finally slow down, come to rest, and are neutralized electrically. The initial radiation often does not stop with a single ionization event but continues on a more or less devious path to produce ionization along its entire track. If the radiation is particulate and of relatively high mass, its path may be essentially straight. If, however, it is a relatively light particle, it may be deflected repeatedly by the matter through which it travels, and thus the path may be extremely devious.

Uncharged ionizing radiation also produces ionization by transfer of energy either in a nuclear field or to the orbital electrons. The net result, as with charged particles, is the production of ion pairs. Those portions of the ion pairs with energy of motion again can produce secondary ionization and additional ion pairs until their energy is electrically transferred to the irradiated material.

**Dose.** The measurement of effective ionization is based upon energy transfer, and this provides a physical means of evaluating the dose. The measurement may be accomplished in many ways but essentially consists of measuring the effective ionization of a given radiation by detecting the ion pairs produced and equating the produced charges to a given energy transfer. If the detection and measurement is made in air, the transfer in other materials can be calculated and predicted with accuracy so far as the physical concepts are concerned, but the prediction of specific end results or effects in biological or other materials is variable.

One is always faced with the interpretation of the dose as the amount of radiation measured in one medium and by one means and then applied by secondary measurements and interpretation to another material which is to be irradiated. The measurement of the radiation is in terms of the fundamental unit of dose, the roentgen (r), which applies to x-radiation or gamma radiation. Since measurement of radiation other than x-radiation and gamma radiation is required, units equivalent to the roentgen are required, and thus the roentgen equivalent physical (rep) equates physically the ionization produced by other radiations to that produced by x-rays or gamma rays. The *rep* refers to that amount of radiation which results in the transfer of approximately 83 ergs of energy per gram of air or approximately 93 ergs of energy per gram of tissue.

Since the effective transfer of energy in rep units is variable, depending upon the type of material irradiated, *rad* (radiation absorbed dose) is used to designate that amount of radiation which results in the transfer and absorption of 100 ergs of energy per gram of the material irradiated. The rad is thus the one with the greatest common denominator of interpretation. However, the determination of the rad, particularly in the depth of any material irradiated, is still one of physical extrapolation and interpretation.

Other units have been suggested and used, and these refer to special materials or interpretations such as the *reb* (roentgen equivalent biological) which modifies the rep in terms of the biological responses to the radiation; the *rem* (roentgen equivalent mammal, or man) adds the complicated interpretation of mammalian tissue and its responses to radiation.

Having established a unit or units of measurement, the application of these units or amounts of radiation can be varied in many ways. And the resulting effects are almost as varied. The units or doses can be applied for a single dose or for many repeated doses; each dose may be small or large and may be delivered rapidly or slowly. Thus, the dose rate or the number of rads delivered in any given time unit must be multiplied by the number of radiation exposures to determine the total dose of radiation delivered and the associated energy transfer. It is usually necessary in description of doses to specify both the dose rate and the total dose. A change in either of these factors can result in biological effects which occupy almost opposite ends of the possible range.

If an effect is produced by the administration of a given dose of radiation within a specified time, this effect can be modified, and usually diminished, by extending the time over which this same total dose is delivered. This concept, called *protraction,* implies that the radiation is still given continuously but at a lower dose rate. With protraction the energy transfer per unit of time is decreased and the biological effect is decreased. To duplicate effects with different dose rates, the total time of irradiation with the lower dose rate must be increased so that the total dose delivered is actually numerically greater than the dose delivered with a shorter time of radiation.

The dose administration can be varied in another way by division of the radiation into intermittent doses, each at a higher rate than with protraction schedules. Because of the intermittent character of application, the total time of administration may not be materially different in the two programs. This concept of fractionation of dose implies that the transfer of energy may be at the same rate as with the single, rapidly delivered dose; but, because it is interrupted, the biological material is allowed interval times for recovery, and thus the end effect of successive doses is not strictly additive. In producing similar effects, fractionation and protraction require larger total dose administration to produce them than radiation doses delivered continuously at rapid rates and in a single administration.

An additional variable that must be recognized is that the units of radiation used all refer to transfer of energy per unit volume or per gram of material radiated. Since the radiation and its effect is rarely confined to a single gram or volume of tissue, it must be remembered that the application of a dose of radiation to biological material means that this dose of radiation, and thus the amount of energy transfer, is involved in each and every gram of tissue subjected to this dose. On this concept is based the differentiation of local and total body radiation.

In radiation therapy for certain diseases, high doses of radiation are administered to small, limited volumes of the body. Thus, the amount of energy transfer per gram of tissue may be exceedingly high, but the total amount of energy transferred to the individual or to the total body may be relatively small. Contrasting this in total body radiation, the dose absorbed indicates energy transfer to each volume of material irradiated. Every cubic centimeter or gram of tissue receives the same energy transfer, and the entire body with all its tissues and cells is irradiated. Thus, the total dose in a numerical value has little meaning unless the volume of irradiation is also specified.

**Radiation End Point.** To determine an effect of radiation, one must first designate the criteria for the effects to be observed. In a material as complicated as biological tissue, the effect observed is chosen by the investigator or observer; and, depending on the techniques used, the refinement of observation, and on the desired information, the end point may include chemical or physical energy changes at subcellular levels, cellular and physiological biochemical changes, and combination of cell effect, with tissue, organ, or individual changes. Each of these end points requires a specific interpretation, and obviously, because of the differences in volume, the kinetics of the energy transfers are quite different. As individual observations become more complex, it is obvious that the effects on lesser systems are contributing to these more complicated end points, and thus it becomes more difficult to determine the primary effects of radiation.

**Threshold and Recovery.** In many systems or materials subjected to radiation, there appears to be a certain level of energy transfer that must be attained before a given effect is observed. The situation is described as conforming to the threshold concept. Other changes apparently begin as soon as the energy is transferred, and the effect increases as the amount of energy applied increases either directly or in some definite relationship. This is the non-threshold concept.

In very simple systems it may be fairly easy to determine whether a threshold effect is present or not. In complicated systems in which the observed effects include the summation of the energy transfer, the recovery capability of the biological tissue, and the effect of varying the administration of the radiation, the determination of presence or absence of threshold becomes very difficult. The concept of recovery has been mentioned and is believed to be one of the major factors in the capability of biological systems to resist or overcome radiation effect.

A wide range of doses is required to produce an effect in different species of living tissues, but in any one species it appears that, if the energy is transferred at a low enough range so that the recovery or reparative capabilities of the cells are not destroyed, some of the effective damage will be overcome or diminished and thus the expected level of damage or injury is not reached. Since recovery is the result of complex physiological and metabolic changes, the rate and effectiveness are variable and difficult to predict. Thus, a physical or mathematical interpretation of biological effects of radiation is extremely dependent upon the variables of radiation administration, actual observation, and finally the evaluation of the changes in the biological system.

**Protection.** Insight into the problem of protection can be gained by realizing that ionizing or penetrating radiation loses energy and the capability of further penetration as it passes through matter. Therefore, one major factor in protection is shielding. If a shield of suitable material is placed between the source of radiation and the object under observation, the intensity and energy factors of the radiation are modified in passing through this shield, and the total dose is decreased between the source and the observed tissue. An additional factor in shielding is that of time. This involves the concept of fractionation and protraction, so that if a given effect were expected after the administration of a given dose of radiation, the effect observed in the tissue could be diminished by extending the time over which this same dose is given.

If the dose rate cannot be changed, the use of intermittent doses could accomplish a similar effect. A third means of protection follows the concept of introducing chemical medications into the biological tissues so that interaction of the radiation is with these chemicals rather than with the critical biological tissue. If this can be accomplished on a slightly preferential basis, then the biological tissue is relatively spared, and the energy transfer is selectively taken up by the biologically inert chemicals. At the present time this differentiation of selective effect is of a very small order, and thus the degree of protection provided is still quite small.

## Radiation Sources

**Natural Terrestrial Environment.** Throughout the known environment of our solar system, the presence of certain radiations is continuous. As applied to our planet, some of the radiations come from the naturally radioactive materials existing in all matter of the earth. These exist in higher concentrations in certain localities than others and are found in greater concentration in certain water samples than others. They constitute a small amount of continuous radiation to all individuals. In addition, there is continuous exposure to cosmic radiation which comes from outer space. Considerable study is being carried on at the present time to determine the magnitude of the effect of terrestrial and cosmic sources of radiation. Because of the extremely low level of this ambient radiation, the determination of specific effect requires a very long time. It depends on the use of statistically valid numbers of people and, perhaps the most difficult factor, a controlled population sample for observation.

The medical use of radiation sources in both diagnosis and treatment has increased markedly, and the emphasis on adequate radiation protection and diagnosis of effect has increased at a comparable rate. Much information is available, and fully detailed guides are provided for individuals interested in estimating radiation hazards and providing adequate protection against these sources. The exposure of individuals to diagnostic and therapeutic radiation has been subject to frequent comment, but if radiation is administered under the precept of medical control and judgment, there should be no demonstrable hazard to the population from the indicated use of medical x-ray and radioisotopes. In the case of therapeutic radiation, the application of radiation is to eradicate certain disease conditions which if untreated could be far more serious than any minor effects of radiation.

**Industrial Sources.** Numerous radiation sources have been established in industrial programs which have increased the possible exposure of personnel to ionizing radiation. The use of radioactive isotopes in sampling and counting devices, in standardization controls, in examination of metal joints and welding, and in many other ways has brought radiation sources into close proximity to working populations. These sources are usually confined to small-volume operations and can be adequately controlled.

A newer application of nuclear energy, namely, reactors for power sources, has brought larger power levels into contact with more of the population, and the associated radiations are at a higher degree of danger. However, the controls and observations required for operation of such power sources have resulted in a degree of safety which has not materially increased the hazard to any worker. The excellent record of workers in radiation as controlled by the Atomic Energy Commission is adequate evidence that, with the acceptance of recommended procedures and attention to safety details, there is no need for concern with radiation hazard so long as these practices are maintained.

**Power and Propulsion Sources.** The use of nuclear reactors for power and propulsion sources has gained much in emphasis because of the prospect of long-time operation without the necessity of refueling or excessive maintenance. Practical application has been demonstrated, and further application will be effected in future developments. Power and propulsion sources will be different from those now used in industrial power areas for electric and turbine powers in that the radiation source will be moving in relation to the population exposed. If these power sources are confined to unpopulated areas such as in the sea lanes, the hazard to personnel other than the crew need not be considered. However, the use of such mobile power sources around or over populated areas or in concentrated maintenance facilities will require a different concept of shielding and disaster handling.

**Space and Cosmic Radiation.** The recent explorations of near space by satellite probes and the continued evaluation of the radiation dosages observed in these areas have brought newer realization of the contribution of space radiation. Presently three main sources of space radiation are considered most important: cosmic radiation from other galaxies, cosmic radiation from solar flare, and magnetic trapping of particles derived from other sources of cosmic radiation.

Cosmic radiation from other galaxies is non-directional as observed from the earth and constitutes a fairly homogeneous distribution through space. These radiations consist of heavy particles with great amounts of energy measured in billions of electron volts and are heavily ionized, thus carrying a large electrical charge with them. Their main contribution to the radiation on earth is in their interaction with the atmosphere, producing secondary cosmic radiation which in the large majority of cases is in the form of protons, neutrons, and mesons.

The second type of cosmic radiation finds its origin in our own solar system and arises from the sun. This is commonly known as the solar flare effect. Associated fairly closely with the sunspot activity and traveling from the sun in a time which is commensurate with particle size and energy, these solar flares give rise to bursts of radiation intensity which travel regularly from the sun, crossing the paths of the planets in the solar system. These are associated with very severe magnetic storms and interferences. In addition they constitute an ionizing radiation hazard to a certain degree if an occupant of a vehicle were to be carried through the localized volume of one of these flares.

The third component of the extraterrestrial radiation is that which is the result of the magnetic field of various orbiting bodies such as the earth. This result is a trapping or localization of particles derived from other sources of cosmic radiation. These are held in zones of activity at certain distances and geomagnetic projections from the earth as a function of the earth's magnetic field. The auroral zone at the pole is relatively free of these zones of radiation, but the polar zone of the earth has a higher incidence of direct cosmic radiation due to the non-deflection of the cosmic particles. In the equatorial plane these particles are held in the zones which have been described as the Van Allen belts.

One important consideration of cosmic radiation is that which concerns the interaction of very high energy particles with matter. If the energy is sufficiently high, the probability of interaction is relatively low, and therefore the biological effect would be minimized. However, when the reaction does take place in a material, the interaction may result in a large release of energy in a very small volume, thus producing a high absorbed dose in this volume. The volume may be one of very near proximity to the actual event, or it may be a continuous line of energy transfer such as that described in the "thin-down" phenomenon.

An additional factor, however, should be mentioned in connection with cosmic radiation and the slowing of any high-energy electrons. This slowing results in the production of secondary x-rays. Thus, while the probability of a particle interaction with matter on its own may be relatively small in terms of expected biological effect, the resulting x-rays from the slowing of electrons may provide a source of radiation which can be far more significant in its biological effectiveness.

## Somatic Effects

In the description of somatic effects, it must be remembered that the effects described are the sum total of both the destructive or damaging effect of the radiation and the physiological reparative effect of the tissue irradiated. If the effect is observed at one given time, it may be different from the same end point measured at another time. It is dangerous to generalize on the total somatic effect of irradiation, since it must be remembered that the effect described probably is not a fundamental or basic end result of radiation.

As mentioned in the discussion of the dose concept, the delivery of a given dose of radiation implies that this energy transfer occurs in each of the volume units exposed to the radiation. The effect of radiation on a given tissue system can be described best by observing those changes produced by radiation which is limited in its application and penetration so that the effects cannot be produced in other associated systems. Thus, the effect of superficial radiation in producing an *erythema*, or reddening of the skin, can be fairly well described and in the past was used as a dose indicator of radiation.

The dose of radiation required to produce a reddening of the skin, may, however, be different when the energy of the applied radiation is changed. The effect of applying a high dose of radiation to a localized tissue volume such as to a cancer is different from the effect of applying this same amount of radiation to a larger volume of the body. As the volume irradiated to a given dose increases, the systemic effects become more and more serious. However, the effects are not adequately measurable nor is there any apparent direct relationship between the total volume exposed and the degree of effect.

Mention has been made of the concept of threshold or tolerance, and these considerations become evident when more complex results of radiation are described. If an effect is described as being due to radiation, it is necessary to establish a direct relationship between the dose administered, the time of administration, the time of appearance of the effect, and possibly an added determination of the degree of the effect. This is extremely difficult to establish in a biological system as complex as a mammal and, particularly, a man, where the control observation is impossible. It follows that the establishment of certain effects of radiation on the basis of a threshold is based mostly on extrapolation from animal experimentation and data.

It is generally believed that radiation produces some degree of damage. However, it is also believed that radiation damage is treated by the body as a non-specific injury or insult, and thus the reparative process can reduce the effective damage in the body or to the system by means of recovery and replacement of physiological tissue. Hence, the function of an organ system may not be reduced as much as might be predicted. The concept of tolerance to radiation or of permissible doses of radiation is based on the fact that a certain small amount of radiation can be received as an injury or insult, although the net effect of this radiation on the individual cannot be detected by clinical or performance studies. This tolerance concept allows operation in low levels of radiation exposure. Continued observation over the period of time since these permissible or tolerance levels were instituted has supported the concept that the effects produced are below the level of detection or observation.

**Sensitivity and Resistance.** As with drug medication on biological systems, there is a wide range of apparent sensitivity to the administration of radiation. This sensitivity again depends on the criterion chosen for evaluation, but if similar end points are chosen for different species, it appears that certain species are more resistant than others. With radiation in any given species, certain tissues fail to show radiation effects at one dose of radiation whereas other tissues show this effect with a much lower dose.

The relative sensitivity of tissue in the body can be rated in terms of the time of the first response to radiation, the apparent severity of cellular or physiological change as the result of radiation, the ability of the tissue to grow and reproduce, or according to other criteria as chosen. It appears in general that the more rapidly growing and specialized the tissue, the more sensitive it is to radiation; and, conversely, the more differentiated and mature the tissue, the more resistant it is to radiation. This is a very general rule, however, and individual exceptions have been described and reported.

The sensitivity or resistance of any tissue to radiation under one set of circumstances can be altered fairly easily by modifying the environment in which the radiation is accomplished. For example, the change of oxygen tension in a tissue markedly changes its sensitivity to radiation. The change of the metabolic activity in terms of temperature can also modify, to a certain degree, the radiation sensitivity. Other factors also will change the response of the tissue to the energy absorption, and the subsequent degree or rate of recovery will modify the observed effect of radiation on a system.

**Acute Systemic Effect.** The radiation effects from single-exposure radiation to essentially the total body of a biological system seem to fall into a pattern that can be called an acute radiation syndrome. This pattern is essentially similar for various species of animals, although individual species show characteristic modifications which are a function of their own physiology. In man and the primates a very definite pattern of radiation-injury symptomatology occurs after a certain level of radiation dosage is delivered to the entire body in a single or short-term exposure. This acute radiation syndrome has been described adequately in the literature and is believed to be effective mainly at dose levels above 200 r total-body radiation.

Under 200 r total-body radiation a very small percentage of individuals exposed will show any effect of radiation, and these effects will usually be mild and transitory. At dose levels above 200 r, the severity of the radiation effect increases, and a greater percentage of the individuals is involved until finally, on a biostatistical basis, a radiation dosage can be reached at which all individuals can be expected to show changes. Some of these changes will produce death if the doses are high enough and the number of individuals exposed is large enough. Death may be the predominant result at very high doses.

These changes, described with reference to an administration of a single dose of radiation of varying levels of dose amount, are fairly well established. However, if the total dose administered is given over a period of time extending over two or three days instead of a single dosage exposure, the expected effect may be diminished from the pattern described by as much as from 25 to 30 per cent. Some of the effects observed may be reduced to even a greater degree.

The radiation effect pattern or syndrome shows rather marked individual variation. It has been noted that the psychic effect of observing others exposed to the same radiation dose, such as has occurred in certain human population exposures, is also effective in increasing the observed effect in some individuals.

**Late Effects.** The effects of radiation may be fairly prompt or may be delayed by weeks, months, or even years. Classic examples of late effects of radiation have been reported repeatedly. Usually they are associated with degenerative changes in the tissue substance which culminate in failure of certain organ systems. The degeneration may be such that it allows the onset of an otherwise mild infection to become serious and even overwhelming. Other late effects may result in formation of tumors, alteration of life span, leukemia, and effects such as cataract formation in the lens of the eye, pigment change, hair-color change, and the like.

The evaluation of long-term effects or delayed effects of radiation is extremely difficult because of the requirement of observing significant numbers of individuals over a sufficiently long period of time and because of the necessity of having sufficient control of the population sample followed to assure that the effects noted are due to radiation rather than to other environmental factors. Since the effects noted are essentially similar, except in incidence, to those which normally may occur in the population observed, it sometimes is difficult to measure accurately the exact effect of radiation in the production of the end point noted.

An additional point of confusion arises in terminology when one describes the late or delayed effects from acute radiation exposure or the late or delayed effects from prolonged or chronic exposure to radiation. These effects are different in degree and in time of appearance and must not be confused in comparing effects and radiation-dose levels.

**Performance and Behavior.** Observations to date indicate that appreciable changes in performance or behavior as the result of radiation exposure occur only after application of high dose rate–high total doses of radiation to individuals. This has been observed experimentally in animals as well as in accidental exposure of humans. While considerable emphasis is being placed on evaluating these important factors, it appears that impairment of behavioral performance is not a problem until doses have at least exceeded those required for commoner systemic effects. Observation of performance and behavior in animals is extremely difficult, and it may be that, as criteria for determination of these responses are refined, they may reveal changes at lower-dose levels than presently demonstrated.

The possibility that a change in performance capability or behavior may be expected as a result of the reaction of a high-energy ionization particle (e.g., primary cosmic radiation) on the individual engaged in extraterrestrial space flight has been mentioned because of the high-energy transfer along the path of ionization of this heavy particle. Although no present data establish the possibility of such a major clinical crisis as a result of primary cosmic radiation interacting with a "vital volume" or "vital center" in the body (since we have no way of simulating or duplicating the cosmic radiation masses and energies), it is impossible to state that this might not happen. However, based on the experience of radiation of all portions of the body in clinical medicine, it appears unlikely that the interruption of an individual's capacity of performance by a single ionizing event could occur. The evaluation of the exact hazard must await the availability of particles with mass and energy comparable to primary cosmic particles before this can be answered with certainty.

**Estimation of Hazard.** It is evident from the previous discussion that the estimation of the radiation hazard to biological tissue depends on many variables. This estimation must also be made in terms of the operational requirement of the exposure to the radiation. In routine procedures as in industrial and laboratory operations, the requirement of exposure to radiation is such that the effects can be minimized by observing adequate and careful techniques, use of protective devices and shields, and the observation of the dose-time relationships.

When the operation of power sources becomes more prevalent, whether fixed or mobile, the requirements for handling them under circumstances other than routine may become greater. As the number of persons exposed to radiation increases, the evaluation of the effect on these larger numbers will permit statistical analyses.

The evaluation of the effect on any one individual or group of individuals is markedly modified by existing fatigue, external stimulus, associated stresses, and by motivation. Minor physiological changes in the animal that modify the perception of a given response may result in a completely distorted interpretation of the effect of radiation, since the effects noted may be the result of a combination of changes rather than primarily due to radiation. A general evaluation of expected effect following total-body exposure of humans to various doses of radiation is summarized in Table 3–1.

TABLE 3–1

The Effects on Man of Exposure to Total-Body Radiation

| Magnitude of Acute Dose (Roentgens) | Predicted Effect |
|---|---|
| 50 | No demonstrable changes |
| 100 | Minor changes detectable in laboratory |
| 150 | Minor physiological disturbances |
| 200 | Changes requiring hospital care |
| 450 | Sickness widespread; some deaths untreated |
| 700 | Early sickness; 50% deaths in treated patients |
| 1,000 and over | Lethal range |

## Genetic Effects

The effects of radiation, as described in the discussion of somatic effects, reflect a certain capability of the tissue or the individual to repair the damage. In certain tissues, however, there appears to be an anatomical circumstance in which the genetic component of a cell cannot be repaired but once damaged remains in that state for the remainder of its existence. Thus, in the radiation of genetic tissue, effects can be produced in germ cells which are permanent for those cells.

If an irradiated cell is involved in the reproduction of another individual, the effect will have full impact on this attempted reproduction. The effect produced by the radiation may be very mild or moderate, of such degree as to render genetic reproduction impossible and yet not kill the cell; or the radiation may kill the cell, at which time the genetic problem ends with that cell. If the change is mild or moderate, it may be accepted by the reproduction mechanism and be passed on to the next generation. Thus, the one category of radiation effect that may be passed on from one generation to the next is in the production of change in the genetic material of the individual.

The concept of dose effect on the individual is not applicable to the evaluation of genetic effect. As used in the evaluation of somatic effect, this concept placed emphasis on total-body radiation as related to total observed effect. In the genetic complex, however, a single ionizing event is theoretically capable of producing change in the gene or chromosome composition sufficient to be effective in the successive generation. Therefore, the concept of a threshold or a recovery in the tissue is not here applicable, and a different viewpoint must be taken in evaluating local-volume radiation as compared to the total-volume radiation in the somatic effect.

The observed genetic effects include mainly those changes that normally occur but that under the effect of applied radiation occur at a greater rate. These effects are in a majority of cases the same changes that occur in natural selection and in a large enough population over successive generations. This change rate, or mutation rate, is known to be fairly stable for each species in a normal environment. The application of a certain dose of radiation is found to increase the rate by a certain factor, and it is this rate of increase that is used as a measurement of the genetic effect.

In man it is believed that the range of radiation dose effective in doubling the normal rate of mutation is between 30 and 80 r to the gonads, with an approximate average of 50 r. It must be remembered that the doubling of mutation rate involves all types of mutations, both beneficial and harmful. The decision as to which are beneficial and which harmful is of course subject to interpretation. When marked changes are produced in a genetic component of a cell, they will probably limit the capability of the cell to reproduce, and thus the changes are self-limiting or lethal to the cell.

The evaluation of the genetic hazard can be accomplished in certain animal species by using large numbers of animals with a rapid rate of reproduction. The application of data observed in animal populations to human populations is associated with many difficulties, and the direct extrapolation is impossible. The observation of genetic change in the human population requires large numbers and many successive generations, and data have not yet been accumulated to give an accurate estimation of genetic effect.

Most genetic changes observed in animals have produced relatively minor or, at most, relatively unimportant changes in the successive generation. Major changes are usually not transmitted because of incapacity of reproduction or production of lethality in offspring. The estimation of genetic hazard becomes more important when larger proportions of the population as a whole are exposed and the resulting possibility of duplicating changes in parents increases. To this end the reduction of all unnecessary exposure to radiation of course remains of primary concern.

## Evaluation

The biological effect of radiation is no single effect nor is the effect specific for radiation. Similar effects can be produced by other agents or combinations of agents. Also the biological effect observed in any one individual is peculiar to that individual both in degree and time response. If a sufficient number of individuals are observed, a pattern can be described as the result of radiation; but this pattern can be modified by many variables in the application of the radiation in terms of its energy, its time and duration of administration, its penetration, the recovery of the individual, the specific response of the individual, the condition of the individual at the time of and following radiation, the observation of the end points collected, the refinement of the observation, and many additional biological factors well known to workers in biological experimentation. The observance of a given effect of radiation in an individual may be difficult to duplicate or evaluate except in statistical terms.

The evaluation of the radiation hazard to an individual or a population cannot be valid in terms of considering radiation as a sole source of hazard or injury. It must be realized that radiation has been present in certain amounts in our environment for a long period of time and that the increase in radiation is not providing a new hazard but a new degree of hazard. This degree of hazard must be evaluated not only in its own right but in comparison with other hazards that are also involved in the life situation and in the operational requirements. The resulting effect or damage from radiation in most cases can be fairly well estimated as it progresses, and this time relationship allows effective, corrective, and therapeutic action to be taken if the dose effect is significant. As compared with other damaging effects, this treatment of radiation provides a greater advantage to the individual in that time is provided for evaluation and effective action.

The viewpoint of persons concerned with the control and interpretation of radiation exposure must be based on education, knowledge, and experience. The hazard that can be accomplished by premature and inaccurate interpretation and publicizing of incomplete observations is often far greater than the determined effect of the radiation in itself. In many simulated cases the damage produced by the panic of the individuals believing themselves exposed to radiation far surpasses any expected effect of the radiation itself on the biological system.

Radiation must be considered as an additional factor of hazard in the field of one's daily life on the ground, in the air, or in space. By itself radiation is not the limiting factor to human participation in progress. By understanding its capabilities, its hazards, and its uses, man can apply these principles to his basic advantage and effectively use it as an investigative and therapeutic tool. Radiation can become one of the most powerful tools of mankind in his endeavor toward greater advancement both in the biological sciences and the use of radiation as a by-product in the industrial field.

## References

1. BEHRENS, C. F. 1953. *Atomic Medicine.* Williams & Wilkins Co., Baltimore.
2. GLASSTONE, SAMUEL. 1958. *Source Book on Atomic Energy.* 2d ed. D. Van Nostrand Co., Inc., Princeton, N.J.
3. HOLLAENDER, ALEXANDER (ed.). 1954. *Radiation Biology.* McGraw-Hill Book Co., Inc., New York. Vols. I, II, III.
4. LEA, D. E. 1947. *Actions of Radiations on Living Cells.* The Macmillan Co., New York.
5. LOW-BEER, B. V. A. 1950. *Clinical Use of Radioactive Isotopes.* Charles C Thomas, Publisher, Springfield, Ill.
6. NATIONAL RESEARCH COUNCIL. 1956. *The Biological Effect of Atomic Radiation: Summary Reports.* National Academy of Sciences, Washington, D.C.

# 4

# Basic Aspects of Skilled Performance

WILLIAM A. WILBANKS, PH.D.[*]

Unlike many lower animals which become adapted to their environment by genetically determined behavioral reactions, man needs to be instructed in how to survive and how to sustain adequate levels of performance under changing conditions of the environment. He can receive such instruction only if the situation has first been analyzed by scientific research.

The preceding chapters have presented a picture of the physical environment with which the human must deal during flight at the somewhat fantastic speeds and altitudes at which modern aircraft are capable of operating. Since man does not automatically and instinctively regulate his habits to the basic needs of the physiological and psychological processes, he has created a problem for himself. He has built machines that he may not be able to operate in the way intended; in fact, advanced aircraft must be operated under conditions that require even more complex bits of equipment, just to keep him alive.

A number of important factors influence man's ability to perform rapidly and accurately some of the tasks involved in operating complicated machines. These involve a number of somewhat loosely related problems which bear upon the type of human performance usually regarded as skilled. The features of human performance discussed are applicable in principle to the operation of all sorts of machine systems. However, they do not provide a concrete formula by which to determine whether or not a given machine can

[*] Associate Professor of Psychology, University of Mississippi, University, Mississippi. *Formerly,* Human Factors Engineer, Bell Helicopter Corporation, Fort Worth, Texas.

be operated with efficiency by a highly trained, highly motivated individual. Rather, they are comparable to the laws of mechanics, which set certain restrictions on the kind of machines that are physically realizable. The principles presented here call attention to certain restrictions that apply to the operation of machines by a human being.

The problems of pilot performance arising from the unique features of jet and space flight are admittedly practical. Although practical problems must be solved as quickly as possible, a narrowly practical view with respect to their solution could quickly lead to scientific mediocrity. Aircraft designers, manufacturers, and operators who seek solutions must understand the complexity of the issues and the need for information expressing the functional relationships of the multiple variables involved—and their application to a wide range of values. Too often pressure on scientists for quick answers to a problem, involving a specific combination of variables in a particular circumstance, leads to inadequate formulations which could compromise effective operation when the situation departs from the narrow conditions of the study. The scientist must also consider the broad, theoretical issues if scientific knowledge of flight is to keep pace with state-of-the-art advances in engineering and medical technology.

## General Properties of Skilled Performance

Behavior is always the result of a series of interactions between an organism and its environment. From this point of view, any activity of an individual is the result of a constant give-and-take between the capabilities he brings to a situation and the demands and limitations of the objective situation. Study of human activity and experience is essentially the study of these organism-environment relationships. Each act of the person results in the modification of the organism so that when it confronts later situations, it is in some way different from what it was before. The *plasticity* appears to be a property of the cerebral cortex. Behavior also results in modification of the environment. If the behavior is effective, it produces results. Some of the results involve changes in the organism; some involve modification of the environment.

As Bartlett (2) has pointed out, the term "skill" is not ordinarily used to describe the very simplest kinds of behavior. No one considers experiments to determine sensory thresholds or reaction-times as experiments on the measurement of skill. Nor is some marked change in a threshold or reaction-time usually taken as a change in skill. Although the functions described by these highly abstract terms may be important in the execution of a skill, they do not themselves constitute the essence of skilled performance. Much time and effort has been wasted largely because of the failure to recognize this.

Whenever a person performs a skilled task, he is faced with a constant stream of sensory information in the form of changes in the environment and changes in his own musculature, and in accordance with this information, he has to organize the responses appropriate to the objective demands of the situation. A skill of any kind involves the appropriate use of the senses. The performer knows what to look for and when to look for it; on this basis he selects the appropriate responses.

Two important principles of perception are involved in the exercise of any skill. The first is the use of information derived from sensory stimulation; the second is the use of past experience. Perception is basically an activity in which an organism engages, and not something that merely "happens" to the organism. As such perception involves mental activity and effort on the part of the observer. Although perception requires the effective stimulation of the senses, it is not a mere process of "registration" but is essentially a kind of activity in response to a situation. Thus, in perception one does not deal with ghostly, disembodied "colors," "sounds," "feels," and the like but with coherent objects. These have form and structure, they are colored, they make certain noises, they are pushed, and they push back. In a very real sense perception is dependent upon sensory stimulation; but, in just as real a sense, perception is substantially independent of the specific details of stimulation. Objects are, in an important respect, the same whether they are seen, heard, or manipulated, just as words are the same whether they are written, spoken, or printed.

In order to control any machine, the human must make correct assessments of the physical situation. He must estimate physical velocity, acceleration, and position. This capacity of the human to make correct assessments of the physical situation is one of the most important problems in the study of human performance.

The ability of a person to take account of the goings-on in the environment is to some extent the result of his hereditary constitution. This is clearly due to the capacity of the central nervous system to organize information transmitted by the sensory receptors. Hereditary factors clearly set a limit to the mechanism involved in perceiving insofar as one cannot do what he has no organic potentiality for doing.

It is necessary to recognize, however, a learned aspect of perception. Since the regulation and successful performance of a skill require the performer to take special notice of those features of the situation relevant to the task, perceiving involves the appropriate use of past training. The skilled performer must learn what to look for and what to listen to. Perception, then, is an activity of the organism that involves the application of information, gained through prior experience and training, to the incoming sensory information. Each new perceptual response leaves the observer different from what he was before, so that his "past" with which he deals with new situations is literally being constantly modified.

## Perceptual Organization in Skills

The most conspicuous aspect of skilled behavior is the motor response of the performer. However, recent research has indicated that of even more crucial importance is the perceptual ability of the operator in receiving and organizing the signals arising from the external environment and from his own musculature and nervous system (2, 9). Some of the problems of perceptual organization in skills are considered in greater detail in this section.

Whenever a person performs a task, he is faced with a stream of signals in the form of changes in the environment. He must organize the responses that are appropriate to the situation in accordance with these signals. As long as a man sees, touches, and manipulates the objects in his environment with which he must deal, he may be unaware of the importance of this sensory information in the guiding of his actions. However, as soon as direct sensory stimulation is replaced by dials, gauges, cathode-ray tubes, and loudspeakers, which provide indirect indications as to what is going on in the environment, and when the person's actions are limited to button-pushing and the like, the situation becomes unnatural. It is possible to present the operator with a task that can be done only with extreme effort or with one that cannot be done at all.

The perceptual basis of operator performance becomes of special importance in any discussion of jet and space flight. The high-altitude and high-speed nature of these operations requires the pilot to depend essentially upon his flight instruments to provide him with the sensory information required to regulate his reactions. This enforced dependence of the pilot on the flight instruments has critical implications for his perceptual organization and performance in flight. These implications can best be understood in terms of several concepts of information theory which have proved to be quite useful in the study of perception. In this discussion the operator should be thought of as an integral part of a man-machine system.

In a general way it can be said that a well-organized system is predictable: the operator knows what is going to happen before it happens. Consequently, since there is little uncertainty about the course of events, he learns very little that he did not already know when the events take place. A perfectly organized system is completely predictable and hence gives little information that the operator needs to analyze in order to react. On the other hand, a completely disorganized system might transmit an unpredictable set of signals that would, in this sense, contain a great deal of information, sometimes too much for the observer to take into account.

It is known from many recent studies (3) that the human brain is limited with respect to the amount of information with which it can deal at a given period of time. When an event is extremely uncertain, it carries much information, for its occurrence removes much uncertainty. A task in which anything might happen, that is, one in which unexpected situations might suddenly develop, is one in which much, perhaps too much, information has to be received. Tasks such as this—and the piloting of a supersonic aircraft is an outstanding example—are difficult and responsible jobs.

When information is transmitted from one place to another, it is necessary to have a channel over which it can travel. An important characteristic of all communication channels is that there is an upper limit to the amount of information that they can transmit. The upper limit is termed the "channel capacity." As the amount of information in the input is increased, this limit defines the point at which the amount of transmitted information no longer increases.

Regardless of how much the information in the input is increased, the amount of information transmitted cannot exceed the channel capacity of the system. This relationship, which is shown graphically in Fig. 4–1, is the same as that which prevails generally in human behavior between potential capacity and actual performance. A simple illustration of the principle in communication is the common experience of having too many things to take into account in too short a time. Very likely every teacher has at one time been guilty of the charge "You've given us too much information to assimilate in too short a period."

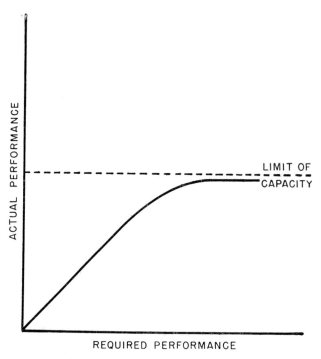

Fig. 4–1. Hypothetical relationship between required performance and actual performance with capacity as a limiting factor.

In the present context it is important to emphasize the fact that the *amount* of information with which the operator must deal, as well as the *kind*, is a crucial factor affecting operator performance. The number of signals and the speed at which they occur are two important variables that determine the amount of information. The kind of information is determined by the source. When any one of several sources might provide the next signal to which the operator must respond, the difficulty of the task confronting the operator is vastly increased.

The term "display" is a convenient one for identifying all the sources of sensory information that provide signals for action. One thing that is common to most displays is that they are continuously changing. The changing events displayed consist very largely of objects moving in a fairly predictable way. Physical objects in space or dial-pointers do not normally make frequent, sudden, and unexpected changes in course. It is also important to realize that not every signal change that occurs is of equal importance to the operator. It is of great importance, however, that the operator notice any sudden change and especially any change which necessitates that some corrective action be taken promptly. These are the "critical signals" to which responses must be made.

One problem of importance in any discussion of operator capability to respond to changes in the state of a high-performance vehicle concerns the limiting factors that determine how frequently such critical signals can be handled adequately. The work of Conrad (4) is relevant in this context. Conrad pointed out that a number of hypotheses would be possible in considering the relationship between the rate at which critical signals occur and the rate at which these signals are adequately handled. Assuming that the number of signals remains constant,

(a) the operator might respond perfectly as the critical signal rate increases, up to some critical point, after which no change in response rate would occur;

(b) performance might keep up with the demands of the situation up to some optimum point, at which responses would fall off to a level below this optimum;

(c) the response rate might increase as the critical signal speed increases, but lag further and further behind.

What actually happens is described by hypothesis (c). The faster the speed at which critical signals occur, the faster is the response rate of the operator; but responses lag further and further behind the critical signals.

Conrad also considered the case in which the operator is required to attend to signals coming from several displays. When the "load" is relatively light, the level of performance can be maintained, but there seems to be a steep fall in response rate. With heavier loads the level of performance may be severely impaired, but the rate of decline tends to level off. Hence, it is necessary to consider not only the amount of information with which the operator must deal, but also the rate at which critical signals occur and the number of sources that might provide the next signal requiring attention.

## Response Organization in Skills

Skilled performance is organized activity. Each stage in performance reflects the use of pre-existing patterns of response. Some of these may be innate, others are the obvious results of deliberate training. The muscular movements produced by the effectors have a spatial as well as a temporal organization. This is especially obvious when actions are performed in a rhythmical manner, but this organization is a characteristic of all manipulative operations.

The actual movements made on any occasion are adapted to the demands of the situation. These demands are never the same, since no situation is literally repeated. As a result the precise way in which the actual movements occur varies from one occasion to another. This variability of human performance is one of its outstanding features and deserves special consideration. The phenomenon is called *motor equivalence*. It is defined as a variability of specific muscular responses with circumstance, in such a way as to produce the same result.

There has not yet appeared a really satisfactory theoretical treatment of the basis for motor equivalence. In practice it is generally necessary to define a response in terms of its end effects. For instance, a mechanic moves a switch and starts an engine; a pilot moves a "joy-stick" and brings the nose of his plane above the horizon. Now, a person trained to do something may do it in many ways, depending upon the circumstances. A person trained to depress a lever in response to a signal may do so from any of several positions. He may grasp the lever, press it down with either or both hands, or use his elbow. About the only constant feature of the situation is that the lever gets depressed.

A second principle of response organization, which also throws light on the nature of motor equivalence, is that of *anticipation*. The performer must anticipate or predict the consequences of his responses. Consider the problem faced by a pilot in landing a large jet transport. The pilot is presented with some course or path that he must follow (defined by the sides of the runway). He has a control system which allows him to control the force that acts to propel the aircraft and to steer it in the desired direction. The same kind of problem confronts any operator whether he be the pilot of a helicopter, the X-15, or a spaceship or a man attempting to back an automobile with a trailer tied on behind.

Using the transport pilot mentioned above as an example, one may observe the movements of the aircraft. If it goes to the left when it should go to the right, the operator turns his rudder, banks, and watches to see what happens. If the aircraft corrects its course to the desired direction, he levels off and continues on his flight path. Often, and this is one of those improbable things that always seem to happen, the aircraft keeps turning to the right. The operator appears to have overcorrected because he attended only to the initial stimulus of being off course and failed to take into account the delay between turning the rudder and the final movement of the aircraft. The skillful pilot must learn not only to judge the position and direction in which the aircraft is moving but also must learn to predict the effects of his control actions as they will be summed up over a period of time.

The behaviors of a pilot, a ship captain, a truck driver, or of a person operating a cigarette machine, for that matter, all depend upon the fitting use of information. In learning to control any machine, it is doubtful that the adult learns to wiggle a stick or push a button. What he learns is to predict what effect such inputs will eventually have on the response of the machine.

The complex pattern of manipulation by which a pilot controls the propelling force and steers the vehicle in which he rides involves a number of steps. These include a continuous awareness of the present position of the vehicle, an anticipation of the point in space where he wants the vehicle to go, and a continuous prediction of where it will in fact go. The pilot can generally observe his surroundings, judge his present position, and decide where he wants to go. In order to control the vehicle, he must learn to predict his future position.

Motor learning at maturity is basically perceptual learning. True motor learning of infancy is an essential element in the adult's skilled behavior. In opening the lid of a box, the only thing that seems common to the various possible responses is a perception of the hand in final contact with the lid of the box. The movement of the hand primarily follows an eye movement that fixates the point of contact. Part of the learning of infancy must establish this ability to move either hand or foot directly from any point to the line of vision. The muscular patterns of the half-grown or adult individual are variable, not because he is learning how to make specific movements but simply because he is learning relationships, associations between perceived environmental events.

In order to operate a slot machine, the adult must make use of the results of the motor learning of infancy, the ability to bring the hand to the line of vision. What the adult learns is that a coin's moving into and falling down a slot plus the depression of a button will be followed by the appearance of a package of cigarettes. He learns that the depression of a certain lever starts the motor of his car. He learns that the movement of a control in a certain direction results in the movement of his aircraft in the desired direction. The adult does not learn to make a certain series of muscular contractions. Once the perceptual relationship between the displacement of the lever and the consequent change of direction of the vehicle is learned, an earlier infant learning is enough to provide the adult's ability to put a hand or foot—or a stick—in contact with the control and move it.

There are at least two stages in learning to operate any machine. At the first stage the learner must "interrogate" the system. He "asks the machine questions" by varying his control inputs and observing how the response of the machine follows. In short, he finds out what controls what. Eventually the learner becomes so skilled that he is able to predict the response of the machine to many combinations of inputs. At the second stage the performer can be given a set of required performance specifications (in the case of a jet pilot, a mission) and asked to select the necessary inputs to the vehicle so as to realize the required performance. When the latter stage has been reached and mastered, it is said that the person has "learned the system."

Many theorists have assumed that this variability of response is possible only because people "build up" in the course of time a vast repertoire of responses which can be put to use as the occasion demands. It is highly improbable that this is the case. The observed variability in performance, but not in achievement, is just too great to be accounted for in any neat fashion by assuming an unlimited "bag of tricks," so to speak.

The more likely situation seems to be as follows. The relating of perception to action is a process that depends upon the proper functioning of cerebral processes. These processes have been termed "mediation" by Hebb (6, 7) and "translation" by Welford (9). It would appear that the central mechanisms responsible for this translation from perception to action are capable of literally producing a response *ad hoc* on the basis of many influences derived from both present stimulation and past learning, much of which took place during infancy. How this is accomplished by the brain is an unsolved problem in *neuropsychology*. As von Neumann has emphasized, there has simply been no experience with systems of this order of complexity (8).

## Learned Aspects of Skills

It is of course true that skills are learned. The understanding of a situation and of the type of action which is appropriate is developed in the course of repeated experience. The skilled person works with speed and precision. He may give his whole attention to signals on some display or to what is going on as a result of his actions and has neither the time nor the need to pay any attention to what his hands are doing. The skilled person is notoriously unable to tell how he does what he does. The new trainee, however, may know in some abstract sense what it is that has to be accomplished without knowing how to do it or what to look for.

It is a curious paradox that before anyone can accomplish a task that requires some skill, he must first be able to accomplish the task. In order to answer a question correctly, the correct answer must be known. Herein lies one source of every teacher's frustrations. In a basic sense it is literally impossible to teach anyone to do something that he cannot do. That portion of early "radical behaviorism" that assumed that anyone can learn to do anything—provided, it was quickly added, that he has the wits and talent to do it—justly deserved C. D. Broad's quip about a theory "so preposterously silly that only very learned men could have thought of it."

The belief that flying an airplane is an exceedingly difficult task is a half-truth; it is, for those who cannot fly an airplane. Calculus is difficult for those who do not understand the basic concepts and cannot work the problems correctly. Now, is it more difficult to fly an airplane or to "discover" the physical laws governing the behavior of the airplane? Is it more difficult to fly an airplane or to drive a car? Judged in terms of accident reports, it might appear that driving an automobile is the more difficult task.

The point of this rather whimsical discussion is that many current notions of the nature of skilled performance are somewhat nebulous. It takes a certain amount of skill to keep from falling down when one walks. The infant does not display this ability. Does the baby *learn* how to walk in the same sense that he later learns that certain words are not generally employed in polite conversation? Or does he just walk when the time comes? It is very generally considered that such a basic skill as walking is not learned at all but is a result

TABLE 4–1

Classification of Factors in Behavorial Development *

| Class | Source, Mode of Action, etc. |
| --- | --- |
| Genetic | Physiological properties of the fertilized ovum |
| Chemical, prenatal | Nutritive or toxic influence in the uterine environment |
| Chemical, postnatal | Nutritive or toxic influence: food, water, oxygen, drugs, etc. |
| Sensory, constant | Prenatal and postnatal experience normally inevitable for all members of the species |
| Sensory, variable | Experience that varies from one member of the species to another |
| Traumatic | Physical events tending to alter cells: an "abnormal" class of events to which an animal might conceivably never be exposed, *unlike the other factors* |

* From Hebb (7), p. 121. W. B. Saunders Company, Philadelphia.

of maturation. Such reasoning has led to a gross oversimplification, namely, the belief that all behavior belongs to one of two types, learned or unlearned.

As a matter of fact, both maturation and learning are represented in all behavior. It has already been emphasized that the motor behavior of the adult is essentially under sensory control, being produced more or less *ad hoc* by the brain, according to the requirements of the occasion. Although genetic factors are clearly involved in behavior, the roles of early sensory experience and motor performance are too often overlooked. It has become clear that the development of behavior depends upon a number of influences.

Hebb (7) has provided a neat, although admittedly simplified, schema of significant factors in behavioral development (Table 4–1). An individual's hereditary make-up is clearly insufficient for survival in situations which demand adaptability beyond the limits provided for by purely "instinctive" mechanisms. An individual's heredity cannot produce any behavior by itself. By the same token, neither can learning by itself, for without heredity and the nutritive environment that produces a nervous system, no learning is possible. Experience may not be involved in gross reflexes, but all other behavior, including instinctive behavior in mammals at least, involves the use of early experience.

It must be remembered that the term "maturation" can be used in two different senses: physical maturation and psychological maturation. Although the learned aspect of skills is obvious, it is well to remember that other factors are involved: genetic, prenatal and postnatal chemical factors, sensory experiences common to all members of the species, individual sensory experiences, and individually traumatic factors. Although the motor learning of the adult is basically perceptual, perception in turn is dependent upon the genetic heritage of the person as well as the perceptual and motor learning of infancy.

## Deterioration of Skills

A feature of skilled behavior of great importance is that it is subject to certain limiting conditions. By this it is meant that there are conditions that set limits to the capacity of the human to perform complex skills with maximum efficiency. Some of the limits are defined in terms of environmental variables; others are defined in terms of what might be called state-of-the-organism variables. What these limits are and what changes in performance take place when they are exceeded must be accurately determined by deliberate experimental inquiry.

It is clear that one can disable the human organism, viewed as a piece of anatomical and physiological machinery, by placing it in an environment defined by variables whose values clearly exceed the limits of physiological variability. The successive changes in structure and function that take place may be quite easy to identify in extreme cases.

With the obvious exception of death, however, the effects on performance of extreme environmental conditions are not necessarily easy to determine. While it is of course clear that a man can do little by way of performing if dead, it does not follow that all performance problems will be solved merely by keeping him alive.

Nor does it follow that a man will perform his work effectively if well and happy. This may be a necessary condition for good work, but it is not sufficient. Environmental extremes undoubtedly limit the range of the organism's possible action and are likely to lead to restriction of actual accomplishment in many instances.

The nature and extent of the limits placed on behavior by any physiological disability depend upon many complex factors. One factor that merits primary emphasis is the demands of the task the person is trying to do. Another has to do with his capacity for compensation, based on the extent of his remaining capabilities. The relationship between capacity and achieved performance is certainly not simple. The general relation appears to be that suggested by Welford, namely, that achievement is probably independent of potential capacity until capacity falls to a point at which it becomes a limiting factor. It is illustrated graphically in Fig. 4–1, which was used earlier in the analysis of the effect of channel capacity on information transmission. Beyond this cutoff point achievement shows a functional dependence upon capacity. In other words, the fact that some physiological malfunctioning may result from exposure of an organism to environmental extremes does not automatically imply a corresponding decrement in performance unless the demands of the task exceed the capacity of the organism to cope with the situation.

Welford's principle should not be interpreted to imply that all performance problems can be solved by making the tasks of the human so simple that they could be adequately carried out even by a decorticated individual. It is unfortunate that certain tasks are difficult, but the fact remains that they are difficult by their very nature and cannot be simplified. Neither good intentions on the part of the performer nor sympathetic understanding on the part of the instrument-maker nor human engineering know-how can make playing a violin so simple that any fool can play like Yehudi Menuhin.

Those engineers who think that future space travelers should be placed in a state of unconsciousness during the flight and that all vehicular control should be carried out by automatic equipment fail to see that their public accomplishments in the missile field hardly make these ideas plausible to the men who must ride along. Unfortunately, at the present state of knowledge, such questions as "can a man do such-and-such under these expected conditions" must go unanswered until the necessary experimental investigations are carried out. Still, the history of science shows that experiment is the most acceptable way of answering factual questions.

The difficulties of predicting what, if any, changes in performance will result from altered physiological functioning are increased, but happily increased, by the fact that an organism, when confronted with a difficult situation, seems to make whatever use it can of the capacities it has, so that any deficiency is at least partially overcome by a change of method. If, for example, there is an impairment of foveal vision, peripheral vision may be more or less successfully employed.

The extent to which such compensatory changes in performance can occur depends upon complex factors. This may be a socially acceptable way of confessing ignorance. Yet, if the task or a portion of the task permits the use of different methods, and if the timing of the task and the method are largely under the control of the person, compensation is likely to occur. On the other hand, such compensatory changes may be virtually impossible if performance is restricted with respect to the form or timing of reactions by the demands of the objective task. However, measuring physiological deficiencies as such will seldom enable us to make accurate predictions of achievement at anything other than the simplest tasks. To this generalization there are two important, but in this context trivial, exceptions: death and loss of consciousness.

In some cases a person may not be able to do certain things at all which were formerly possible. This results from the facts that the impairment limits performance and the task does not permit changes in method or timing. However, the person may be able to achieve former levels of performance but only with the greatest personal effort. Performance at many tasks will not suffer at all if the demands of the task do not exceed the limits set by capacity or if more or less effective compensation is possible. In some cases, however, overcompensation may actually occur, with the result that achievement may actually be improved. A famous example of this is Beethoven whose most profound works were accomplished after his deafness.

In searching for the locus of changes in skill following exposure to environmental and physiological extremes, impairment of peripheral receptors and of effector organs may often be encountered. Short of total destruction of the sense organs, however, changes induced in the central mechanisms involved in the control of sensory, translatory, and response systems would be of greater importance. Such changes might produce failure to exercise adequate control over the process of bringing past experiences to bear on the present situation. In other words, an operator may forget to do something or forget how to do it. There may be a failure to keep the performance and the momentary demands of the situation in close relation to one another, so that a sequence of actions "runs itself off" with insufficient reference to the actual situation. The performer may produce "correct" responses but fail to order them in the correct sequence.

When a skill begins to show deterioration, it is wise to look for signs of partial impairment. The occurrence of a total disability of sensory, translatory, or response mechanisms is usually gradual except in the case of an unexpected, sudden calamity. As long as a person is fresh, he may be perfectly able to perform the most complicated perceptual and motor tasks accurately, even when the task makes great demands upon his attention. When the person becomes fatigued, however, his accuracy is likely to show signs of impairment.

Bartlett (1) has called attention to a distinction of great importance between the fatigue produced by hard physical labor and the fatigue produced by work that demands persistent concentration and a high degree of competence. It has generally been found that the most fatiguing tasks are those requiring some degree of attention and thought, tasks that cannot be satisfactorily performed by routine habit. A number of brilliant experiments, described by Bartlett (1) and by Davis (5), have shown clearly the far-reaching effects of this "skill" fatigue and that these effects are likely to occur without the operator's being aware of any change in his performance.

In the fatigued state, changes in displays may become quite large before they are noticed and responded to. The timing of rhythmical patterns of observation may become inaccurate. The proper events may be noticed but at the wrong time. The operator may respond to a series of display indications as if they were totally independent events rather than respond to them as an integrated pattern. The person may completely neglect those changes that need less frequent attention or require attention only when they change by a large amount. Distractions occur readily; otherwise trivial events may engage the operator's whole attention at the expense of crucial events. As flights of long duration are undertaken at altitudes and speeds that make all-instrument flight a necessity, the problem of skill fatigue may be expected to assume more and more importance. It is certainly worthy of more attention.

Skills are complex results of organization involving sensory, translatory, and response systems. Consequently, any changes in human performance will depend upon the nature of the impairment, the nature of the task, the level of competence of the performer, and the way in which these complex factors interact with one another to produce behavior. Only in the most obvious cases will any simple inference from physiological deterioration to performance deterioration be possible.

## References

1. BARTLETT, F. C. 1942. Fatigue following highly skilled work (Ferrier lecture). *Proc. Roy. Soc. (London)*, Ser. B. *131:* 247.
2. BARTLETT, F. C. 1958. *Thinking: An Experimental and Social Study.* George Allen & Unwin, London.
3. CHERRY, COLIN. 1957. *On Human Communication.* John Wiley & Sons, Inc., New York.
4. CONRAD, R. 1954. Speed stress. In FLOYD, W. F., and WELFORD, A. T. (eds.). *Human Factors in Equipment Design.* H. K. Lewis & Co., Ltd., London.
5. DAVIS, D. R. 1948. *Pilot Error.* H.M. Stationery Office, London.
6. HEBB, D. O. 1949. *The Organization of Behavior.* John Wiley & Sons, Inc., New York.
7. HEBB, D. O. 1958. *A Textbook of Psychology.* W. B. Saunders Co., Philadelphia.
8. VON NEUMANN, J. 1951. The general and logical theory of automata. In JEFFRESS, L. A. (ed.). *Cerebral Mechanisms in Behavior.* John Wiley & Sons, Inc., New York.
9. WELFORD, A. T. 1958. *Ageing and Human Skill.* Oxford University Press, London.

# 5

# Human Operator Performance Under Non-normal Environmental Operating Conditions

## W. Guy Matheny, Ph.D.*

In the deliberations on the problems that will be faced and that will need to be surmounted in sending a man into the hostile environment of outer space, the first concern has been that of protecting him against permanent or even temporary physiological damage. Many investigations have therefore been carried out with regard to man's limits of endurance or capability of withstanding marked deviations from his normal environment.

Once it became evident that it was feasible, engineeringwise, to send a man into space and that in all probability he could survive there, questions were raised as to his usefulness for effective performance of perceptual, cognitive, and motor functions, either in carrying out an explorer's function or in the control of his vehicle. Experiments designed to "stake out" man's physiological limits often reflected concern for man's ability to perform certain mental and motor functions under changed environmental conditions. A considerable amount of knowledge and understanding is beginning to accumulate about the characteristics of man's perceptual, cognitive, and motor performance under conditions now expected in the space environment. An organized effort to understand man's capabilities and limitations as a component in a man-machine system has recently been given considerable impetus, and the body of knowledge resulting therefrom should answer many questions about man's per-

* Chief, Human Factors Division, Bell Helicopter Corporation, Fort Worth, Texas.

formance in the space environment. It is not possible in one chapter to touch upon more than a few of the problems and findings, and the selection of content reflects the limitations and biases of the author.

Several streams of thought are becoming merged in the attack on this problem. In recent times aeromedical specialists, psychologists, anthropologists, physiologists, and engineers have collaborated in teams to work on the central problem and have evolved various concepts of a central unifying model for bringing their various contributions together.

A model that has proved most useful as a framework for relating the contributions of the various disciplines has been that of *servo theory*. The primary purpose of this model is to facilitate communication among the disciplines in thinking about the problems connected with man-machine operations as well as to provide a common frame of reference for formulating both the problems and their solutions.

## The Servo-Model

The central features of the servo-model can be seen in Fig. 5–1, in which outputs from the machine in the form of deviations from prescribed courses, altitudes, etc., provide inputs into displays which, in turn, are inputs to the man. The displays may be of a nature such as to provide inputs to the visual sensors of the man, or they may provide inputs to his auditory, kinesthetic, tactual, or olfactory senses. The inputs may come directly from the machine to the man, in the sense that he sees the machine depart from some prescribed course over the ground or feels its response to a gust of air. The machine output may also be modified or worked upon in such a manner that the man sees the parameter being measured as the deflection of a needle on a dial or through some other means of display.

Upon receipt of the information from the displays, the man may operate upon this information in several ways before making a response (output) to the controls. He may, for example, compare information coming from several displays; he may make computations based upon information coming from several of the displays. He may integrate or differentiate the information with respect to time before making a response. He may simply respond directly to a displayed piece of information serving merely to increase the gain or to amplify the information through the controls.

In systems in which the man exercises some control over the course of a machine, he may be said to be performing an "error-nulling" function, at any point from a very simple to a highly complex level. The model is useful to the several disciplines not only in that each will find something in its own professional vocabulary that is synonymous with *input* and *output* and with *display* and *control,* but also in that it looks at man as a component in a closed-loop system. This is to say that the perception and discrimination of

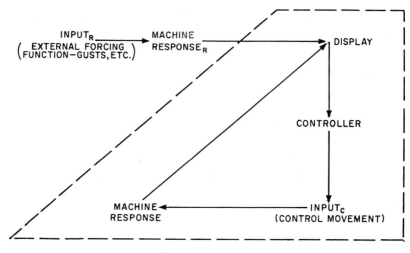

Fig. 5–1. The man-machine servo loop.

the inputs and the nature of the outputs form a closed, dependent system in which one influences the other. It is the behavior of man as an "error-nuller" or tracker that will be considered first.

## System Description

The function of a man or of any man-made assembly that is to serve as a control component within the system forces the examination of the system in one very important way. It requires that the function of the system be described in such detail that all the inputs that must be controlled and all the outputs that must be exercised by some controlling mechanism be specified. In such an analysis the machine is examined to determine which inputs it must receive and which outputs it must deliver in order to fulfill its assigned mission within the limits prescribed.

Once the input and output requirements of the system have been specified, those responsible for the engineering design of the system are faced with the problem of deciding which functions will be carried out by the human operator and which will be assigned to some electromechanical (automatic) system. It is also necessary at this point to specify the environmental operating conditions under which the system will be required to function. Just as the engineer who designs an automatic control system puts that system to test under extremes of temperature, humidity, vibration, and long periods of operation, so those who are concerned with the human in performing such a function must answer the questions as to his capability under such extremes of environment. It is at this point that the environmental extremes and the unusual and different operating conditions presented by the space vehicle come most into play and require the most serious attention.

## Input Problems—Display of Information

As a generalized way of looking at and of analyzing machines and the requirements for their control, whether it be space vehicle or submarine, the problem can be analyzed in terms of control of the machine about a set of axes and along a set of axes (Fig. 5–2). Control about the axes is sometimes called the stabilizing function, and control along a set of space axes may be referred to as the navigation or plan-position function. Further, any error-nulling device must have some point of reference or *referent* and something that it is controlling whether this "device" be man or "black-box."

In the case of the control *about* axes, if it is desired that the vehicle maintain a certain attitude, the error-nulling or control device that performs this stabilizing function must have a referent against which it compares the position of the vehicle with respect to these axes. This reference (comparison) is reflected in some index under its control. For example, in a conventional aircraft the pilot may wish to control the rotation about the lateral axis (pitch) by positioning the nose of the aircraft through line-of-sight with reference to the earth's horizon line. The earth's horizon line then becomes the referent and the nose of the aircraft the control index.

Under conditions in which there are no external real-world referents against which to place the control index, such referents are encoded into various instruments that the pilot can observe within his vehicle. In jet aircraft flying within the influence of the earth's atmosphere and depending for primary stabilization control upon aerodynamic surfaces and under the influence of the earth's gravity, this stabilization function is of primary importance, and changes in the attitude of the vehicle must precede and be integrated into

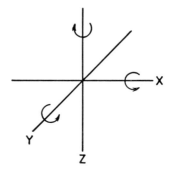

**A. DISPLACEMENT ABOUT AXES**

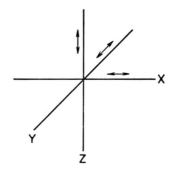

**B. DISPLACEMENT ALONG AXES**

Fig. 5–2. Reference axes for analysis of a vehicle system.

changes in its position relative to the earth's plane. Similarly, information as to the vehicle's position in some coordinate system of space, whether or not this coordinate system is oriented to or related to the earth's surface, must be encoded in an instrument so that the controlling mechanism can determine and control the vehicle's position within this coordinate system.

This principle implies a general model in the sense that it applies to the stabilization and control of the movement within $X$-$Y$-$Z$ coordinate systems of any vehicle. The major differences from vehicle to vehicle would then be in the tolerances within which control must be exercised, in the time sequence or rate of response of the controlling mechanism necessary to hold these tolerances, and in the nature of the equipment used to exercise control.

It is appropriate, then, to examine some of the ways in which the instruments and controls have been configured for the operation of vehicles within the earth's atmosphere, and especially for the high-speed jet aircraft of today, and then to look closely at the effects upon control of the vehicle of some of the major conditions of the space environment that might affect this control.

The history of instrument development for aircraft has been traced by Nicklas (16). A look at this history bears out the need for an attack on the over-all problem of how best to display to the human operator the myriad inputs requiring attention in modern aircraft. It is an overworked phrase, but bears repeating here, that instrument development has been outstripped by the aircraft. It has become abundantly clear that, if human operators are to continue to cope with the demands of the modern aircraft, their limitations and capabilities need be considered as a part of the design of the total system and that they must be provided with displays adapted to their capabilities. Further, since man has certain advantages over electromechanical modes of exercising control, a division of function can be considered between him and the electromechanical black-boxes to achieve the most efficient control.

In the face of this need, three major programs undertaken in the past ten years were aimed at evolving information-display configurations that would present all the necessary information in the most usable form for the operator. These three programs merit separate discussion since each has built a display configuration based upon an underlying principle or model which has dictated its general mode of presentation. The programs referred to are those of the Hughes Aircraft Company, of the Flight Control Laboratory, Wright Air Development Center, U.S. Air Force, and of the Army-Navy Instrumentation Program of the Office of Naval Research. It should be emphasized that behind each of these programs lies a history of the efforts of numerous individuals and laboratories whose work culminated in the formulation of the concepts and in the methods of reducing these concepts to operational pieces of equipment.

**Hughes Aircraft Company Instrumentation Program.** The work at the Hughes Aircraft Company antedated the work of the other two programs and started officially in 1950 when Hughes Aircraft Company was awarded the prime contract for an integrated all-weather interceptor aircraft and weapons-control system. The unique feature of this system was to be an integrated cockpit including flight navigation and combat displays and controls.

The first step in this program, since it involved a total system, was to state the requirements of that system in terms of the mission that it would be called upon to perform. This statement of the total requirements of the system in light of its mission is one of the aspects of these three programs that makes them worthy of discussion.

In describing the Hughes system, Roscoe (22) stated that the *systems engineering approach* was adopted. This approach, as defined by Roscoe, consists of three steps: "first, define the problem; second, determine the constraints; and third, optimize the solution within the constraints." The problem was defined as one of designing an integrated cockpit display and control system and meeting the functional mission requirements of a supersonic all-weather interceptor operating in the Semi-Automatic Ground Environment (SAGE) defense complex and having the highest possible probability of kill and survival.

The constraints, as enumerated by Roscoe, are several: first, the system had to be producible within a given time schedule and within the current state of engineering art. The system had to be reliable, maintainable, and supportable by the Air Force and one that both experienced and inexperienced pilots alike could quickly learn to use with the degree of proficiency required. Lastly, the system had to be compatible with existing systems with which it would have to work, most specifically that of the SAGE ground environment.

Recognition of the constraints laid upon the development of a system is an important step in the formulation of the problem and an attack upon it. "Optimum" solutions of *human-factor* problems which are unrealizable because of time, weight, space, or other limitations must be compromised in the interests of optimization of the solution of the total system problem. Thus, the final step in the Hughes program required the optimization of a solution of the problem within these constraints. We may note at this point that Roscoe, at the time of his formulation, did not make explicit any notions as to environmental or operational conditions that might operate to exercise a constraint upon the performance of the individual. However, it may be assumed that these considerations are implicit in his statements as to the optimization of the solution to the problem.

Faced with the task of optimizing the solution within the constraints laid down, Roscoe proceeded by examining the experimental findings relevant to the problem, in search of some general findings within the experimental literature that would serve as a guide in designing individual instruments or displays that would be most compatible with man's abilities to do the job specified. This examination of the literature (2-6, 8-9, 17-27, 33) led Roscoe to the following generalizations:

1. Pilot performance is facilitated when spatial information is presented in an undistorted spatial analog in which there is a minimum requirement to depend upon numbers. That is to say that performance would be better when the spatial dimensions of the real world are fixed so that individual indices on the display have a specific positional meaning and exact quantitative numbers do not have to be read in order to get quick approximate information.

2. Performance is facilitated when the flight task is arranged so as to be a pursuit task rather than a compensatory task. That is, the most desirable display would be one in which the index of desired performance and the index of actual performance are free to move against some fixed scale or background.

3. Performance is facilitated when the direction of movement of the index representing the particular vehicle or aircraft being controlled is compatible with the direction of movement of the aircraft itself with respect to the earth's coordinates. For example, in an altitude display the index representing the vehicle would move up on a fixed scale when the vehicle itself moves up; in a display representing the roll of the aircraft, the index would roll to the right when the actual aircraft rolls to the right.

4. Performance is facilitated when spatial displays present as much of the total situation as is consistent with scale-factor requirements. Roscoe has amplified this generalization to mean that, because of the goal-directed nature of flying, it is essential, or at least helps, to see where you are going—not just where you are but all the places you might go. He considered this important because he believed the role of the operator in this system to be more in the nature of a tactician rather than of a tracker. This point is closely related to Generalization 1, above, but is aimed more specifically at the problem of presenting the pilot with information as to his posi-

tion in *X-Y* coordinate space and as to the relation of other objects to him in that space.

Following these general conclusions from the literature, Roscoe and his co-workers evolved the configuration shown in Fig. 5–3. This configuration may now be examined more closely to point out how the generalizations are represented in specific displays.

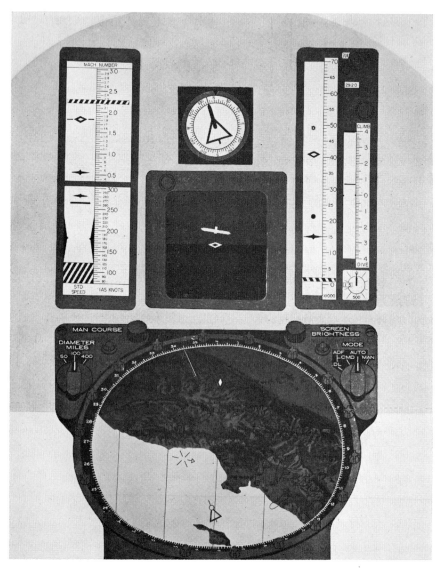

Fig. 5–3. Hughes Aircraft integrated panel.

Generalization 1 is exemplified by the left-hand scale of the instrument on the right of the panel. In this instrument altitude is displayed as a linear scale in which altitude increases from bottom to top, and therefore an approximation of altitude can be obtained at a glance by noting the position on the scale of the index being controlled.

Generalization 2 is incorporated in the horizontal situation indicator in the lower center of the configuration in that the target which the aircraft is pursuing is shown as a moving symbol corresponding to the pilot's own aircraft.

Generalization 3 is exemplified by almost all the displays in that the index being controlled represents the operator's own aircraft and moves with reference to some fixed, stable earth coordinate reference. This is particularly true of the attitude display in the very center of the picture in which the symbol represents own aircraft and rolls to the right for rolling of own aircraft to the right. The principles or generalizations underlying this configuration have been characterized as that of the "principle of the moving part." The general substance of this principle is simply that the movement of any index that represents the aircraft in a display should be compatible with the direction of movement of the aircraft proper in relation to the earth coordinates. So it appears in the Hughes display that, when the aircraft rolls to the right, the index representing the aircraft rolls to the right with respect to some fixed referent which represents the ground plane. Similarly, when the aircraft climbs higher in altitude, the symbol representing the aircraft in the altimeter goes higher or up on the scale of the altimeter.

**Air Force Integrated Instrument Panel (WADC).** The work undertaken by the Flight Control Laboratory of the Wright Air Development Center of the U.S. Air Force (29) toward the development of an integrated instrument panel proceeded from a determination of the kind of information that is required for the particular mission; that is, a systems engineering philosophy was adopted. Again, this philosophy required the examination of the mission of the system and the optimization of all the elements of the system toward the attainment of the mission within the established constraints. Within the Air Force program an analysis of the information required by the pilot for the accomplishment of a complete mission from take-off to landing revealed that this information generally falls into two categories. These categories are: (1) that which conveys to the operator knowledge as to his present or actual performance and (2) information that conveys to the operator what he should be doing or his desired performance. The design goal within this program therefore involved a means of presenting to the operator of the system his actual performance and his desired or command performance.

It also became apparent to the Air Force investigators, on close analysis of the system, that attitude control of the aircraft was a fundamental type of control. This arises from the fact that the immediate results of the pilot's input to the flight-control loop are perceived by him as changes in attitude. These attitude changes are in time integrated into changes in the magnitude and direction of the aircraft velocity vector. Basic attitude control then provides the pilot with his primary means of controlling the orientation of the aircraft's velocity vector. This basic attitude control is supplemented by the thrust control to achieve control of the vector's magnitude. Control of the velocity vector and its magnitude then eventuates in, and the pilot achieves control over, the flight path of the aircraft.

In the panel layout it was deemed desirable that the display presenting the attitude of the aircraft be primary and central to the pilot's field of vision. The displays conveying to the pilot the changes in his velocity vector and changes both in magnitude and direction were considered ancillary to this display. The priority of information having been determined, the task then remained to determine some natural frame of reference for the panel that would be consistent with external cues available to him and consistent with the control actions that he was to take.

It was concluded from considerations of the linearized equations of motion of the aircraft that the display parameters necessary to the pilot for accomplishment of his mission fell into two categories. The first of these is concerned with the forward-looking or *elevation* view, and the other is concerned with the downward-looking or *plan* view. The parameters in the forward-looking view are governed by motions of the stick, fore and aft, and include pitch, air speed or Mach, rate of climb, altitude, angle of attack, and acceleration. The parameters in the downward-looking view are controlled by motion of the stick sideways and include heading, bank, turn rate, and navigation and tactical information available in the horizontal plane.

This set the general layout for the panel and then led to consideration of the ways in which the particular parameters would be encoded within the instruments in these general categories.

In setting the design criteria for the individual instrument design, certain objectives were defined. It was desired that the panel should not only be a fully integrated one but that it should also be one in which the control action required by the pilot would be a natural and instinctive result of his interpretation of the instrument readings. A limiting requirement was, of course, that it should meet the mission requirements of new high-performance aircraft.

In dealing with the problem of the design of the attitude indicator, the problem of the relative merits of the "moving horizon-fixed aircraft" *versus* the "fixed horizon-moving aircraft" attitude presentation was faced squarely. By way of explanation, it may be noted that the moving horizon-fixed aircraft indicator displays the attitude of the aircraft in a manner analogous to the view that the pilot gets when he is seated in his aircraft looking out; i.e., the horizon line on the attitude indicator remains in physical correspondence to the actual horizon line. On the other hand, the fixed horizon-moving aircraft display presents to the pilot, as if he were outside the aircraft and observing its behavior from some position behind it, a picture representative of what his aircraft is doing. The reader will recognize the latter type of presentation as the one incorporated in the Hughes cockpit.

After consideration of the available evidence, the decision was reached to display attitude information as a type of moving horizon-fixed aircraft presentation. In the consideration of ways in which to present the velocity vector information (that is, air speed, altitude, and rates of changes of these parameters), the constraint was placed upon the design that it be one which would (1) effectively integrate command information with actual performance information and (2) facilitate instinctive control-display interpretation by the pilot. A further and important consideration was that the display design should adapt easily to the increased speed and altitude of new high-performance aircraft.

With these constraints examination of the available modes of displaying this information revealed obvious disadvantages and required consideration of new techniques. The method of presentation evolved was the use of the moving-tape instrument (Fig. 5–4) in which the referent or index of actual performance is fixed either

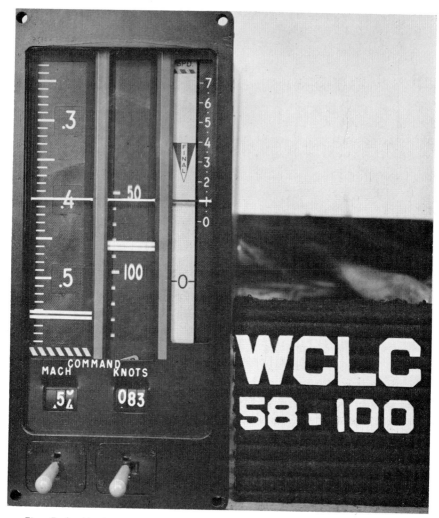

Fig. 5–4. Moving-tape instrument: Air Force integrated flight panel. (Reprinted by permission from Public Information Branch, Wright Air Development Center, Wright-Patterson Air Force Base, Ohio.)

at or near the center of the display and in which the scale moves in back of this index.

With the choice of vertical-tape displays, the natural reference line was then available for the forward-looking view. The total forward-looking panel then incorporated a horizontal reference-line concept as depicted in Fig. 5–5. In consideration of a display for presenting the horizontal situation (the plan-position information) to the pilot, the relative merits of the moving aircraft-fixed earth reference *versus* the moving earth reference-fixed aircraft philosophies were again examined.

The first step was the formulation of a suitable frame of reference. The essential question was: Should the display be referenced with

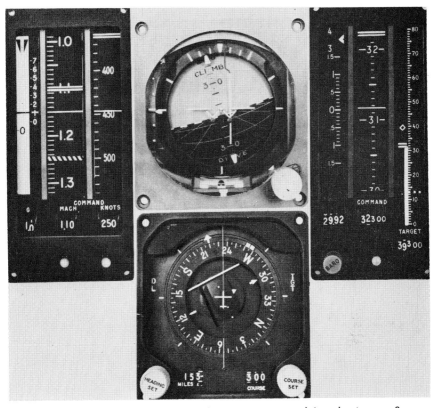

Fig. 5–5. Air Force integrated flight-instrument panel (production configuration). (Reprinted by permission from Public Information Branch, Wright Air Development Center, Wright-Patterson Air Force Base, Ohio.)

respect to geographical axes or with respect to the pilot? After review of the pilot's task, it was determined, as with the attitude display, that the natural reference is the pilot, that the total theme is one in which the pilot is an integral part of his aircraft and all displays are referenced to him. The horizontal display, therefore, is as pictured in the lower center of Fig. 5–5, in which the aircraft is fixed in the center of the dial and the round reference symbols move relative to him.  Again, the reader will note a difference between this navigation display and that of the Hughes configuration.

**Army-Navy Instrumentation Program (ANIP).**  The ANIP program was conceived as an over-all long-range approach to the problem of the display of information to the human controller of a man-machine system.  The program has been carried out with respect to three different vehicle systems.  The fixed-wing aircraft effort has been coordinated by the Douglas Aircraft Company, El Segundo Division; the helicopter effort by the Bell Helicopter Corporation; and the submarine effort by the Electric Boat Division of General Dynamics Corporation.  As with the other programs the first step was to determine the information required by the operator to control his vehicle in carrying out the mission.  These are given for fixed-wing aircraft in the Douglas Aircraft Summary Report (7) and are as follows:

1. Spatial orientation
    a. Attitude
    b. Position
    c. Heading and heading change
    d. Altitude and rate of climb
2. Speed
    a. Ground speed, forward and lateral
    b. Air speed, Mach indication
3. Course
    a. Flight path made good
    b. Flight path to fly (positions to be acquired)
    c. Best altitude and rate of climb (command)
    d. Best speed
    e. How goes it (range remaining)
    f. Endurance
    g. Point of no return
    h. V-G (envelope defining limits of safe operation)
    i. Engine power
    j. Engine condition
    k. Start (air or ground)
    l. Identification
        (1) Target
        (2) Delay
        (3) Friend
    m. Target or formation assignment
    n. Location of other aircraft in the area (position and relative altitude)

o. Friend or target rate
p. Base location and alternate base location
q. Location of target and alternate target
r. Weather (dangerous turbulence)
s. Holding position indication
t. Obstacle- and terrain-clearance information
u. Runway indication
v. Discrete command points
w. Cut or wave off
x. Wheels-off indication
y. Breakaway

Similar information requirements have been generated for the helicopter and submarine programs.

The basic tenet underlying these programs is that information displayed to the pilot should take essentially the same form as that which is perceived as being in the real world. By way of illustration, the pilot may seek to align some indicator of the axis of his aircraft (e.g., cowling, pedestal, or the like) with some referent on the earth's surface in order to control his aircraft. When these earth referents are obscured by weather or darkness and the plane of reference (earth's surface) must be generated, the basic tenet would dictate that these artificial referents be essentially those of the real-world visual experience of the pilot. This would lead, then, to the encoding of the two indices (i.e., that denoting the aircraft and that denoting the real-world ground plane) through use of symbols having a direct structural and perceptual relationship to what is perceived in the real world, rather than through the use of more abstract symbols such as needles and dials. While the variables that determine whether a human will react to an abstract display of the real world in the same way he does to the real world are not yet known, the essential problem is clear. It is that of creating the same identity relationship between the human observer and a two-dimensional picture of the real world as he has between himself and his real, observable world.

The model has an intuitive appeal since it requires that the encoding of information to the pilot be a straightforward analog of that which he perceives visually when viewing the real world. It is recognized that there may be redundancy of information, or noise, in the perceived real world which may operate against unequivocal discrimination and interpretation of pertinent stimuli. It is further recognized that the required accuracy of discrimination of changes in the pertinent areas or of absolute judgments of this value may not be possible in direct viewing of the real world. For example, judgments of altitude above the earth from direct observation of the earth's surface may be quite inaccurate at appreciable altitudes. Such information would be supplied by instruments providing precise quantitative readings.

The goal of the ANIP program can be summarized as that of providing the human controller with the necessary and sufficient cues extracted from the real world that would enable him (1) to maintain his orientation in real-world space and (2) to make the necessary decisions and exercise the necessary control to carry out an assigned mission.

This examination of the problem led to a review of current knowledge pertaining to the principles of perception of visual space and to the determination of the visual cues needed by the pilot to exercise control over his vehicle. These visual cues were outlined in the Douglas Aircraft Company (7) summary report. They are as follows:

| | |
|---|---|
| 1. Internal reference | 6. Interposition |
| 2. External reference | 7. Filled space |
| 3. Terrain texture | 8. Vertical location |
| 4. Linear perspective | 9. Size |
| 5. Motion parallax | 10. Shape |

Considerable latitude may be allowed in the manner in which these cues may be embodied in a display. For example, the principle of linear perspective might be embodied as the projection of a grid pattern, with the representation of the ground plane as in Fig. 5–6, or by means of filled circles, as in Fig. 5–7.

The presentation must convey two major items of information to the pilot. First, it must convey his orientation with respect to the earth's surface, and, second, it must allow control within specified limits of the several parameters presented. These, then, become research questions to be answered with regard to any proposed configuration. The program is oriented toward giving the operator a forward view of the situation surrounding his vehicle and a plan-position view. The forward view is illustrated in Figs. 5–6 and 5–7. A plan-positioned view is illustrated in the Hughes display, Fig. 5–3.

A central point of concern in the program is the determination of the division of function between the human controller and automatic or electromechanical devices. It is recognized that each has advantages and disadvantages in performing the necessary functions, and the optimum arrangement that will maintain system flexibility and versatility is the goal.

**Environmental Constraints upon the Inputs.** A number of forces or constraints exist in high-speed jet and space flight which may

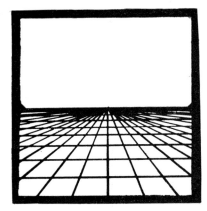

Fig. 5–6. Grid-line encoding of ground plane.

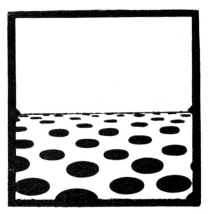

Fig. 5–7. Encodement of ground plane using filled circles.

alter man's performance in comparison with that which he exhibits within the normal, earth environment. As a general approach to this problem, it is at least conservative to assume that the man operating as a component in a jet-aircraft or space-vehicle system will face such stringent and unusual environmental conditions that predicting his behavior under these conditions from knowledge of his behavior characteristics under normal, earth conditions should be done with extreme caution. Exercising this caution, human-factors scientists have tended to place the burden upon the vehicle-design engineer for providing the human operator with an operating environment as nearly like that of his normal environment as can be obtained. As knowledge of human performance under these unusual conditions increases, perhaps many of these constraints placed upon the engineer may be relaxed. Indeed, through the concentrated and enthusiastic attack on these problems, most of the gaps in present knowledge should be eliminated within the next decade or so.

However, there are some constraints upon the operator that may be difficult, if not impossible, to "engineer" out of the system. The effect of "g" forces is an outstanding example of these. Positive accelerations, such as may be present in the initial launch of an orbital vehicle, high negative acceleration which may be associated with re-entry into the earth's atmosphere, and zero or near-zero gravity conditions of orbit are pervasive forces that cannot be restrained by barriers.

A second constraint of this type has to do with those insidious conditions in which the engineered environment fails and deviates slowly and gradually from the simulated normal, earth environment. Since it is and will be part of the operator's duty to monitor the operations of subsystems that control his environment, such insidious and gradual changes in the effectiveness of these subsystems might subtly impair his perception of these changes. It is of utmost importance to recognize and have knowledge about the effect upon the operator of changes in such subsystems as his oxygen supply and other atmospheric conditioners. In fact, it may well be that, on the first flights of man into space, one of his major problems will be the monitoring of these subsystems in order to keep himself alive. A critical aspect of the space pilot's job will involve his ability to recognize these subtle infringements on his senses which distort his perceptions and slow his responses. Consequently, learning to recognize and to correct situations before they become irreparable or even fatal must be regarded as a major training problem, however successful the design solutions.

A third constraint is that of the vibration and buffeting of the vehicle with the result that perception and response effectiveness may be seriously impaired.

SOME COMMON CONSEQUENCES OF UNUSUAL ENVIRONMENTAL CONDITIONS. Rather than look at each of these separately, let us consider some of their common consequences and effects upon the visual process, and then seek to arrive at some conclusion as to these effects upon the performance of the operator. One common consequence of high negative or positive acceleration, high-frequency vibration, certain atmospheric adulterations (such as anoxia), and wind blast is the blurring of vision or loss of visual acuity. Any vehicular system must be examined with relation to the probability of its producing conditions that might result in impairment of visual acuity of the operator. His instruments must be so designed and his tasks so arranged that this impairment does not jeopardize the vehicle in the conduct of its mission.

EFFECT ON PRECISE QUANTITATIVE READINGS. The tasks of operators of high-speed jet and space vehicles require frequent precise alignments of indices and readings of precise values of various informational parameters. If, under the normal demands of the system or under emergency conditions, visual acuity is impaired, certain safeguards must be erected so that total system failure does not occur.

Current thinking about the optimal method of presentation of precise quantitative information in situations which might involve blurred vision must be reviewed carefully. In the instrument systems discussed earlier, namely, those developed in the Hughes, WADC, and ANIP programs, two modes of presentation of this type of information were made explicit: (1) a linear scale with a moving pointer and fixed scale and (2) a linear scale with a fixed pointer and moving scale. Traditional instruments have also used a circular scale with both moving pointer–fixed scale and fixed pointer–moving scale designs. Various advantages have been stated for these different configurations. For example, the Hughes system altimeter, with fixed, linear scale and moving pointer, is configured in this fashion so as to provide an analogy between movement of the index and movement of the aircraft in space. Movement of the index upward or downward means the aircraft is moving in that direction. The linear scale with fixed pointer and moving index, as employed in the WADC cockpit, is designed to give a "natural" reference line for the forward-looking view.

When the operator of a vehicle is required to refer to a pair of indices either to determine their correct alignment or to read some precise quantitative value, he will usually wish to do so in the shortest possible time. It seems clear in these cases that the operator's task is that of finding the pointer, locating its position on the scale, and reading from the scale a precise quantitative value. One condition that is certain is that the operator must find the pointer, and the sooner that he does this the more quickly will he be able to read out the information required.

This conclusion leads to an examination of the conditions that would enable the operator to anticipate most correctly where to find the pointer. In the fixed pointer–moving card (or tape) type of instrument, the position of the pointer is always known. The problem in this case is that of reading out the scale value adjacent to or under the pointer. In moving-pointer instruments the reader may anticipate the position of the pointer on the basis of his knowledge of the system. In some systems the probability of the pointer's being in a particular area of the display may be high, as, for example, in the case of many instruments giving information as to engine conditions. Conditional probabilities may exist between instruments, so that the reading of one instrument leads to the expectation of finding the pointer on another instrument in a particular area. Finally, the operator's knowledge of the past history or progress of the system prior to the moment of reading may narrow the area in which he may expect to find the pointer, that is, certain sequential dependencies exist.

A little reflection about the situations in which instruments of this type are used leads to the conclusion that, by far in the larger proportion of cases, one or more of the above conditions exist and that a moving pointer's position may be anticipated with consequent reduction of reading time. However, these very conditions may operate against quick, precise readings under unusual or emergency conditions when the probabilities and dependencies break down. This may be particularly true under conditions of stress or anoxia in which the individual may persist in his established scanning habits at a time when they are inappropriate to the situation. The operator who has built up visual scanning habits based upon the probabilities and dependencies of a system might become the victim of these habits. He might take longer to read the instrument and read it with larger error than if he had no expectations as to what the reading would be. Thus, an instrument that directs the reader's scan to the appropriate area of the scale would seem to be highly desirable. The circular dial–moving pointer provides such direction, and, of course, with the fixed pointer–moving card or tape, the pointer position is always known as being in the fixed position.

A sometimes overlooked advantage of moving-pointer instruments lies in the fact that they convey what is sometimes called qualitative information. What may be implied from the word "qualitative" is that the information is not read out with the precision that can be realized on close scrutiny, i.e., that the intervals of measurement may be gross. For example, on a fixed-card, north-oriented heading indicator, a needle pointing to the bottom of the dial indicates in rough fashion a heading of 180°. This attribute of such instruments may prove a distinct and perhaps critical advantage in certain situations in which the reader's vision is blurred or visual acuity is lost as a function of the environmental conditions under which he is operating. The needle position may provide redundant although not as precise information, but in such critical situations it may enable the operator to ascertain the reading with enough precision to facilitate control of the system, even though he may be unable to read the number on the dial clearly.

An anecdotal yet significant instance in which this difference in display design might well have proved critical was a case in which the canopy of a high-speed jet bomber was jettisoned after an explosion. Because of an injury to one member of the crew, the copilot elected to stay with the bomber and attempt to bring it back to base. The ground station, in order to vector the aircraft to base, gave the pilot heading instructions in terms of degrees, and the pilot was required to read his heading indicator with enough accuracy as to be able, at least in rough fashion, to take up these headings. With wind blasts blurring vision, the advantages of a moving pointer–fixed card instrument in this case would seem to be obvious. With the moving pointer–fixed card the pilot could have obtained an approximation to the heading, merely by being able to see, although in a blurred fashion, the segment of the card to which the needle was pointing. With a moving card–fixed pointer, however, it would be necessary for him to be able to discern, at least at certain critical intervals, the actual value or reading of the instrument in order to be able to take up the heading.

Therefore, it seems appropriate to suggest that one of the important constraints placed upon the selection of such an instrument for high-speed jet or space flight would be that the system be adequate for those conditions under which the operator's vision might be blurred. Specifically, it should be determined that reading accuracy is sufficient to enable control of the vehicle under such conditions within the limits required. It may very well be that if, certain extreme environmental conditions are imposed upon a system, such as high g's, high vibrations, or changes in the pilot's physical capabilities due to failures of his life-supporting equipment, these characteristics of instrument display might be altered.

It would seem particularly appropriate that indices of the status of the operator's life-sustaining subsystems be indicated by moving pointers that can be read in a qualitative way, to indicate the "safe range," and do not require the operator to read precise values such as would be the case with a fixed pointer–moving scale instrument.

In summary, there may be situations induced by unusual environmental conditions in which the fixed pointer–moving scale instrument might be disadvantageous. The limitation of that type of instrument is that the visual field must be clear enough to distinguish the numerical indices on the card or tape in order to acquire the correct information. The linear scale with the moving pointer might be said to have an advantage in this respect since the position of the pointer on the scale is a rough index of value to be read. However, at any point in time in which the observer would read the scale, he must locate the pointer upon this scale. In the normal course of events, certain sequential dependencies and conditional probabilities may lead the observer to an expectation as to the area in which he might expect to find the pointer. In an emergency case in which the probabilities and dependencies may break down, the stress of the situation might lead the observer to persist in a scan of the area in which he expects to find the pointer.

A standard instrument, then, in which the moving pointer is used in conjunction with a circular dial would, in the face of many disadvantages, seem to have one advantageous characteristic. This is the fact that the angle of the pointer, from the center of the dial, leads the eye easily and naturally to the segment of the scale on which the desired value is denoted.

The general conclusion, that a moving pointer that may be visible although not clearly perceived during conditions in which the vision is blurred and that by its position upon a scale imparts a gross value or reading to the observer, would seem to apply to those instruments such as the altimeter, the heading indicator, and the newer types of plan-position or navigational displays. In the case of the navigational displays, the advantage in this respect would then appear to lie with the fixed map, north-oriented type of display in which the controlled index moves.

**Color Vision.** The practice of color coding certain segments of the scales in instruments in order to set off certain areas and attach a meaning to them has become standard practice. It is therefore important to examine this particular way of encoding information from the standpoint of the effect of extreme environmental conditions upon their interpretation. Color coding is generally used in those cases in which it is not deemed necessary for precise numerical values to be read but is primarily necessary that system states be conveyed to the operator. The information is conveyed by the pointer when it lies within any one of these areas. It has also become customary to encode information of the dichotomous or go-no-go type through the use of colored lights.

Although the evidence is not entirely conclusive, the findings of several investigators (14, 34, 35) are definite enough to indicate caution in the use of color codes when a condition of decreased oxygen supply is expected. Some experiments have shown, for example, that colored objects visible at high altitudes seem less saturated and that the reduction in saturation may even reach the point of impairment of color vision to the extent that green and blue lights appear to be absolutely colorless (34). Further, it has been found by the same authors that brief oxygen inhalation up to ten minutes does not fully restore color sensitivity. McFarland (14) also has shown that at altitudes of 15,000 and 16,500 ft. on Trans-Andean Airlines, the average time in seconds in naming the one hundred colors was not only significantly longer but also the frequency of blocking or saying the wrong color was greatly increased at these high altitudes.

It would seem most advisable in the design of instruments for space and jet aircraft that the use of color codes be avoided for those conditions in which environmental conditions might lead to a hypoxic condition, especially for the oxygen gauge and the displays that signify to the pilot the state of his life-supporting systems. No explicit consideration of this possible deleterious effect of hypoxia upon color perception appears to have been given in the design of any of the three instrument systems described earlier.

**Glare and Illumination.** Whiteside (32), in his discussion of the problems of vision in flight at high altitude, included a thorough treatment of the problem of glare. He sought to determine the conditions that make for lowered visual acuity at high altitudes and pointed out that with increasing flight altitudes certain changes in the visual surroundings occur:

1. There is a reversal in the normal distribution of light in the visual field. With an increase in altitude, the sky becomes less bright, while below the aircraft there is frequently a very bright

cloud layer. Consequently, the light distribution results in more light reaching the upper part of the cockpit and less reaching the lower part of the cockpit, which is therefore lower than it would be at the lower altitudes.

2. The external illumination is much higher at these altitudes and therefore decreases legibility. Lythgoe's experiments (13), in which he found that optimum acuity was obtained if the surroundings were of the same brightness as the test, are significant here. When the surroundings were either brighter or darker than the test, visual acuity deteriorated, the drop in acuity being most marked when the surroundings became, as in the case of high-altitude flight, brighter than the test object.

3. The blue color of the sky at a high altitude may also be a determining factor in the production of glare, since, as Whiteside pointed out, Ivanoff (12) showed that the blue sources produced more dazzle than either red, yellow, or green.

4. A factor that may contribute to difficulty in seeing at high altitude is the great sharpness of the shadows cast by sunlight. The shadows become darker on the instruments, and other shaded areas of the cockpit are darker while the sunlighted areas are more glaring. At lower altitudes there is a large particle scattering in the atmosphere. At high altitude, however, the large particle scattering is greatly reduced, and, thus, the delineation between shadow and sunlight area is much sharper than it is at low altitudes.

Overcoming the decreased legibility of cockpit instrumentation resulting from these effects requires that corrective action be taken in the design of the instrument panel to compensate for the loss of luminance. The effect of illumination on dial reading has been analyzed by Chalmers and his associates (3) and by Spragg and Rock (28). These investigators found that below a critical brightness, decreases in brightness are associated with increasingly poor performance; while above this value an increase in brightness produces little or no improvement. This particular phenomenon also interacts with the effects produced by increased g's or accelerations and the effects of hypoxia.

White and Riley (31) have shown the following results with respect to instrument-reading performance measured in terms of errors made in reading the dials: (1) at the highest brightness levels, i.e., 42 millilamberts, there are no differences in the percentage of errors among the various values of g; (2) at the three highest brightness levels for values up to 3 g's, there were no differences in the percentage of errors; (3) at the two lower brightness levels errors were inversely related to brightness and directly related to the value of g; and (4) at a 4-g condition there was a systematic increase in errors with decreasing brightness.

By way of pulling several diverse facts together, it appears that there are several conditions that may act independently or may interact to produce lowered visual acuity for the jet or space pilot. These are illumination-glare problems due to the changed conditions of high-altitude illumination, the effects of g's or positive acceleration upon visual acuity, and the effects of hypoxia upon vision. Parenthetically, the effects of accelerations, whether positive or negative, may tend to change the visual acuity if, as reported by White and Jorve (30), the conclusion may be accepted that the decrease in acuity as a function of g is a result of displacement of the lens of the eye by the g force.

**Empty Field Myopia.** One of the most interesting visual phenomena that occurs at high altitude has been characterized as empty field myopia. It has been proposed that the effect upon vision of an empty visual field is an involuntary increase in the power of accommodation in the face of any attempt on the part of the observer to relax his accommodation to infinity. This is brought about by the fact that at high altitudes the visual field outside the aircraft may contain no visible detail. Under such conditions the accommodation goes to a resting position rather than, as sometimes hypothesized, to an accommodation for infinity.

Whiteside (32) concluded that, irrespective of the brightness or darkness of the environment, an involuntary accommodation occurs if there is no visible detail that can be sharply focused. As a result of his experiments, Whiteside concluded that in the presence of an empty visual field, subjects cannot relax accommodation completely. Rather, accommodation is in a constant state of fluctuation at about a level of 0.5 to 2.0 diopters, sometimes approaching the far point but never quite reaching it. An observer with normal eyesight, then, is unable to focus at infinity if there is no detail at infinity that is capable of being sharply focused. Under these conditions the farthest he can focus is a point about 1 to 2 m away, and he becomes effectively myopic by this amount.

The implications of these findings are obvious for those tasks in which the jet pilot or space traveler is required to search outside his aircraft to locate objects in his surround. The systems designer, then, is faced with the problem of determining whether the search and location of objects in the surround might be better accomplished by means other than visual search or whether there may be some method by which he might improve the visual search capability of the human operator in the situation.

Of the three instrument systems described earlier, only one would seem to offer a solution to this particular problem. In the display system of the Army-Navy Instrumentation Program, the visual display of information would appear before the pilot on a screen on which the image was focused at virtual infinity. It seems that this would maintain the accommodation mechanism of the eye in a state more conducive to productive visual search. Also, since Whiteside has further shown that it takes approximately 60 sec. for the accommodation mechanism to reach its resting value of from 0.5 to 2.0 diopters, the alternation of visual scan viewing and the image at infinite focus might provide a means for improving man's capability in this respect.

One of the reputed great advantages that man may bring to the control of the system over that which might be done by machine is said to be that of the perception of patterns and the recognition of these patterns because of the human's peculiar propensity for stimulus generalization. The use of the human operator for this function, however, must be critically examined in the light of the effects on his visual processes of the unusual conditions which have been examined.

## Unusual Environmental Conditions and the Problem of Control

One of the problems of most concern to the designers of high-speed jet aircraft and of space vehicles has been that of the effects of certain conditions upon the human operator's ability to exercise control. The condition of most concern has been that of the effect of g forces upon control operation or manipulation, whether these forces be high-positive, high-negative, or zero-g conditions.

**Zero g or Weightlessness.** The work carried out by the Aero Medical Laboratory of the Wright Air Development Center of the U.S. Air Force, under the direction of Major E. L. Brown, has provided some interesting findings with respect to the operation of controls under zero-g conditions and tends to support earlier work in the area.

Major Brown and his collaborators found that the ability to perform certain simple motor functions, such as writing, pressing buttons, and operating toggle switches, could be performed with ease under the zero-g condition. It should be noted that in the conduct of these experiments the pilots of the aircraft, which was being flown in the Keplerian trajectory in order to produce the brief periods of zero g, were piloting the aircraft through the zero-g section of the flight with a great deal of skill and precision. They were doing this highly complex task repeatedly, and the conclusion is warranted that manipulative skills are retained and can be enacted with a high degree of skill during the zero-g condition. This conclusion seems warranted, however, only when the operator is firmly secured to his seat or to the floor.

What may happen to motor skills under long periods of zero g is unknown. The possibility has been suggested that under zero-g conditions the general muscular tonus of the body would decrease unless special exercises were engaged in and that such decrease in muscular tonus could conceivably affect the execution of certain motor skills.

**High-Positive and Negative g's.** Greater attention has been given, and perhaps greater concern shown, regarding the problem of controlling the vehicle during conditions in which it is subjected to high-positive accelerations than to other deviant gravitational conditions. During these periods the forces exerted on the body members may be seriously debilitating, even to the extent of completely inhibiting the execution of certain movements. This problem has received extensive attention in the literature (10). To summarize briefly, it has been found that: (1) at plus 2 g's (1 g incremental over normal gravity) a heaviness of hands and feet is experienced, (2) at plus 3 and 4 g's there is an exaggeration of the sensation of heaviness and movements are accomplished only with a great effort, and (3) at plus 5 g's the body is beyond the control of muscles except for slight movement of the arms and head.

**Effect of Hypoxia upon Psychomotor Performance.** It can be generally stated that the more complex a motor skill the sooner it is affected by oxygen decrement. As the extent of hypoxia increases, the simpler skills begin to be affected. Decrements in performance become greater, and the variability of performance increases. In the case of simple reaction time, it would appear that, at least until the oxygen lack is very severe, hypoxia does not lengthen the basic reaction time, but it does increase both the frequency and length of the mental blocks. When the subject does respond, he does so with his normal speed, but there is not much certainty about when or if he will respond (1).

The commonest demonstration of the effects of the lack of oxygen upon the motor processes is that of asking the subject to perform simple handwriting during the onset of hypoxia. In such cases there is a progressive deterioration in performance with increasing altitude; the letters become larger and more clumsy and lose their individual characteristics until finally the result is completely unintelligible. Subjects are typically unable to recognize that anything is wrong, and it is just this aspect of the onset of hypoxia that makes it most serious.

The high-speed jet or space pilot must be schooled to recognize the insidious onset of this condition and to train himself to react to correct the malfunction in his life-supporting equipment. A particular point of importance to the jet or space pilot is the fact that with increase in altitude his arm-hand coordination is affected as well as his arm-hand steadiness. These may be affected at oxygen-concentration conditions equivalent to from 10,000 to 12,000 ft., and complex neuromuscular control may be affected at altitudes of 10,000 ft. or lower. It cannot be emphasized too greatly that the operator must be trained to recognize the onset of this condition. Similarly, it is difficult to exaggerate the importance of proper design of informational displays for life-supporting equipment. In addition, it is well to emphasize that the controls that the pilot must manipulate to switch to alternate supplies must be designed so that they can be manipulated with gross and even unsteady movements. In some subjects bodily orientation and steadiness may be impaired under the hypoxia condition. This condition, coupled with the lack of vestibular and/or kinesthetic cues during the weightless condition, may prove more than the operator can cope with and may bring about nausea and airsickness.

**Effects of Temperature on Performance.** The expression "it isn't the heat, it's the humidity" has truth in it. In consideration of the effects of temperature upon performance, it is well to speak of the effective temperature, as defined by the *Heating Ventilating Air Conditioning Guide* (11). *Effective temperature* is "an arbitrary index which combines into a single value the effect of temperature, humidity, and air movement on the sensation of warmth or cold felt by the human body. The numerical value is that of the temperature still saturated air which would induce an identical sensation."

A scale of effective temperature was developed through a series of studies carried out by the Research Laboratory of the American Society of Heating, Refrigerating and Air Conditioning Engineers, Inc. The relationships between humidity and dry bulb temperature in degrees Fahrenheit are summarized in Fig. 5–8. In this figure the effective temperatures are given by the diagonal lines running from upper left to lower right. It will be recalled that when the wet bulb temperature is equivalent to the dry bulb temperature, the relative humidity is 100 per cent. A reference to Fig. 5–8 shows that for a relative humidity of 100 per cent (the diagonal line running from lower left to upper right), the 100 per cent humidity line is a straight line and intersects the wet bulb temperatures and dry bulb temperatures at equivalent values. Thus, the 100 per cent humidity line crosses the wet bulb temperature line at 60 and also the dry bulb temperature line at 60. It is important to note that for a given dry bulb temperature the effective temperature goes up as the humidity goes up. Thus, for a dry bulb temperature of 70° and a relative humidity of 10 per cent, the temperature is approximately 63°, while for a dry bulb temperature of 70° and a humidity of 70 per cent, the effective temperature is approximately 67°; for a dry bulb temperature of 80° and a humidity of 80 per cent, the temperature is 77.2°.

Studies thus far have indicated that the upper limits of effective temperatures for motor performance are around 90° to 95° F. In a study by Mackworth (15), for example, it was found that errors in receiving by Morse-code operators increased sharply at around 93° effective temperature. The control of humidity will be at least equal in importance in conditioning the space cabin to the control of the dry bulb temperature. If the dry bulb temperature were to be controlled at, say, 80°, then in order to maintain a suitable effective temperature in the work environment as moisture is added to the air (through the breathing and perspiration of the operator), it would be necessary either to reduce the dry bulb temperature or to decrease the humidity in the cabin.

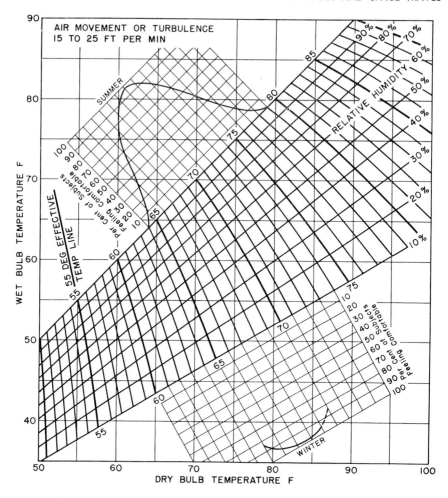

Note: Both summer and winter comfort lines apply to inhabitants of the United States only. Application of winter comfort line is further limited to room heated by central systems of the convection type. The line does not apply to rooms heated by radiant methods. Application of summer comfort line is limited to homes, offices, and the like, where the occupants become fully adapted to the artificial air conditions. The line does not apply to theaters, department stores, and the like where the exposure is less than 3 hours. The summer comfort line shown pertains to Pittsburgh and to other cities in the northern portion of the United States and southern Canada, and at elevations not in excess of 1000 ft. above sea level. An increase of one deg ET should be made approximately per 5 deg reduction in north latitude. Dotted portion of winter comfort line was extrapolated beyond test data.

Fig. 5–8. ASHAE comfort chart for still air. (Reprinted from *Heating Ventilating Air Conditioning Guide*, 37th ed., 1959. By permission from the American Society of Heating, Refrigerating and Air-Conditioning Engineers, Inc.)

**Higher Mental Processes.** When one speaks of using a human operator in a man-machine system, human engineers are fond of thinking of man as a decision-maker and tactician, and of his possessing abilities far beyond those of computers or electromechanical gadgets in performing such functions. Nevertheless, man is peculiarly susceptible to the deterioration of his complex mental processes, sometimes as a function of minor changes in the environment. This fact suggests the exercise of much more caution when thinking about the use of man in this respect. It is not advocated here that man should not be used in this way. However, it seems both necessary and appropriate to wave a red flag of warning concerning the seriousness of the impairment of these complex mental processes when certain environmental conditions occur.

The foregoing discussions of the effects of hypoxia upon the perceptual and motor processes suggested the nature of the effects of such atmospheric change upon the complex mental processes. Indeed, it is difficult to determine the extent to which the impairment of observed performance of hypoxia subjects can truly be assigned to the receptor and effector mechanisms and the extent to which it arises from some effect on the central nervous system. In studying the effect of hypoxia changes in handwriting, for example, one may observe that as the letters become larger and more clumsy and lose their individual characteristics, misspelling also increases considerably and the text changes, with irrelevant information being added until the final result is completely unintelligible. The characteristic loss of insight into the nature and extent of the subject's own deterioration under high-oxygen deprivation, noted earlier, applies to all sensory functions, mental and motor.

A number of experiments deal with the effects of anoxic conditions upon higher mental processes such as simple addition and subtraction mathematical problems, code substitutions, retention and recall, ability to change a mental set, word association, and judgment of duration of time, etc. All these are affected in a deleterious way at some equivalent altitude. One interesting observation, which may have important implications for the crews of space ships and for the interactions among crew members, is that changes in mood occur with changes in altitude. The initial change may be either in the direction of lethargy and irritability or of euphoria. As altitude increases, lassitude, irritability, slowness of reasoning, difficulty in concentrating and remembering, and the frequency of recurring ideas tend to increase. The effects of such mood changes upon interpersonal relations of the space crew can only be conjectured at present, but they must certainly be given serious consideration for space flights of any duration.

# References

1. BILLS, A. G. 1937. Blocking in mental fatigue and anoxemia compared. *J. Exp. Psychol.* 10: 437–452.
2. BRYAN, L. A., STONECIPHER, J. W., and ARON, K. 1954. *The 180-Degree Turn Experiment.* (*Aeronautics Bull. No. 11.*) University of Illinois Press, Urbana.
3. CHALMERS, E. L., GOLDSTEIN, M., and KAPPAUF, W. E. 1950. *The Effect of Illumination in Dial Reading.* (USAF Aero-Med. Lab. Technical Report No. 6021.)
4. CHERNIKOFF, R., BIRMINGHAM, H. P., and TAYLOR, F. V. 1955. A comparison of pursuit and compensatory tracking under conditions of aiding and no aiding. *J. Exp. Psychol.* 49: 55–59.
5. CHERNIKOFF, R., BIRMINGHAM, H. P., and TAYLOR, F. V. 1956. A comparison of pursuit and compensatory tracking in a simulated aircraft control loop. *J. Appl. Psychol.* 40: 47–52.
6. CHRISTENSEN, J. M. 1955. *The Importance of Certain Dial Design Variables in Quantitative Instrument Reading.* (WADC Technical Report 55–376.) USAF, Dayton, Ohio.
7. DOUGLAS AIRCRAFT COMPANY. 1959. *Long Range Feasibility Studies: A Summary Report.* (Report No. ES–26842.) Santa Monica, Calif.
8. FITTS, P. M., and JONES, R. E. 1947. *Psychological Aspects of Instrument Display: I. Analysis of 270 "Pilot-Error" Experiences in Reading and Interpreting Aircraft Instruments.* (AMC Memorandum Report TSEAA–694–12–A.) USAF, Dayton, Ohio.
9. FITTS, P. M., JONES, R. E., and MILTON, J. L. 1949. *Eye Fixations of Aircraft Pilots: II. Frequency, Duration, and Sequence of Fixations When Flying the USAF Instrument Low Approach System (ILAS).* (AMC Technical Report 5839.) USAF, Dayton, Ohio.
10. *Handbook of Human Engineering Data.* 1952. 2d ed. (rev.). (Tufts University, Medford, Mass.) Human Engineering Report No. SDC 199–1–2a.) Navy Special Devices Center.
11. *Heating Ventilating Air Conditioning Guide.* 1959. 37th ed. American Society of Heating, Refrigerating and Air-Conditioning Engineers, Inc., New York.
12. IVANOFF, A. 1947. On the Inhibitive Factor of Dazzling (Au Sujet de la Composante Inhibitive de l'Eblouissement), *Comp. Rend. Acad. Sc.* 224: 1846–1849.
13. LYTHGOE, R. J. 1932. *The Measurement of Visual Acuity.* (Medical Research Council Special Report No. 173.) H.M. Stationery Office, London.
14. McFARLAND, R. A. 1937. Psychophysiological studies at high altitudes in the Andes. I. Effects of rapid ascents by airplane and train. *J. Comp. Psychol.* 23: 191–225.
15. MACKWORTH, N. H. 1946. Effects of heat on wireless telegraphy operators hearing and recording Morse messages. *Brit. J. Ind. Med.* 3: 143–158.
16. NICKLAS, D. R. 1958. *A History of Aircraft Cockpit Instrumentation 1903–1946.* (WADC Technical Report 57–301.) USAF, Dayton, Ohio.
17. NICKLAS, D. R., ROSCOE, S. N., and WILLIAMS, A. C., JR. 1951. *A Comparison of Pilot Performance on Four Aircraft Attitude and Heading Displays: Conventional, 6N–1a, 6N–1b, and AF48–2.* (Technical Report SDC 71–16–9.) U.S. Navy Special Devices Center, Port Washington, N.Y. (Not released for distribution.)

18. ORLANSKY, J. 1955. *Pilot Performance With Two Different Attitude Displays.* Dunlap and Associates, Inc., Stamford, Conn.
19. PAYNE, T. A. 1950. *A Study of the Moving Figure and Orientation of Symbols on Pictorial Aircraft Instrument Displays for Navigation.* (Technical Report SDC 71–16–6.) U.S. Navy Special Devices Center, Port Washington, N.Y.
20. PAYNE, T. A. 1952. *A Study of the Moving Part, Heading Presentation, and Map Detail on Pictorial Air Navigation Displays.* (Report SPECDEVCEN 71–16–10.) U.S. Navy Special Devices Center, Port Washington, N.Y.
21. POULTON, E. C. 1952. Perceptual anticipation in tracking with two-pointer and one-pointer displays. *Brit. J. Psychol. 43:* 222–229.
22. ROSCOE, S. N. 1957. The development of integrated display panels at Hughes Aircraft Company. In RITCHIE, M. L., and BAKER, C. A. (eds.). *Psychological Aspects of Cockpit Design: A Symposium Report.* (WADC Technical Report 57–117.) Wright Air Development Center. Pp. 28–40.
23. ROSCOE, S. N., SMITH, J. F., JOHNSON, B. E., DITTMAN, P. E., and WILLIAMS, A. C., JR. 1950. *Comparative Evaluation of Pictorial and Symbolic VOR Navigation Displays in the 1–CA–1 Link Trainer.* (Report No. 91.) C.A.A., Division of Research, Washington, D.C.
24. ST. CLAIR, R. S. 1956. *Evaluation of Flight Attitude Indicator Model Number 1035, Summers Gyroscope Company.* (ES 26322.) Douglas Aircraft Company, Inc., El Segundo, Calif.
25. SENDERS, J. W., and CRUZEN, N. 1952. *Tracking Performance on Combined Compensatory and Pursuit Tasks.* (WADC Technical Report 52–39.) USAF, Dayton, Ohio.
26. SIMON, C. W., and ROSCOE, S. N. 1956. *Altimetry Studies: II. A Comparison of Integrated Versus Separated, Linear Versus Circular, and Spatial Versus Numerical Displays.* (Technical Memorandum 435.) Hughes Aircraft Company, Culver City, Calif.
27. SIMON, C. W., SLOCUM, G. K., HOPKINS, C. O., and ROSCOE, S. N. 1956. *Altimetry Studies: I. An Experimental Comparison of Three Pictorial and Three Symbolic Displays of Altitude, Vertical Speed, and Altitude Commands.* (Technical Memorandum 425.) Hughes Aircraft Company, Culver City, Calif.
28. SPRAGG, S. D., and ROCK, M. L. 1948. *Dial Reading as Related to Lumination Variables: 1. Intensity.* (USAF Memorandum Report No. MCREXD–694–21.)
29. SVIMONOFF, CONSTANTINE. 1958. *The Air Force Integrated Flight Instrument Panel.* (WADC Technical Report 58–431.) USAF, Dayton, Ohio.
30. WHITE, W. J., and JORVE, W. R. 1955. *Gravitational Stress of Visual Acuity.* (WADC Technical Report 53–469.) USAF, Dayton, Ohio.
31. WHITE, W. J., and RILEY, M. B. 1956. *The Effect of Positive Acceleration (G) on the Relation Between Illumination and Dial Reading, in Air Force Human Engineering, Personnel, and Training Research.* (Technical Report 56–8, 306–310.) Air Research and Development Command.
32. WHITESIDE, T. C. D. 1957. *The Problems of Vision in Flight at High Altitudes.* Butterworth & Co., Ltd., London.
33. WILLIAMS, A. C., JR., and ROSCOE, S. N. 1949. *Evaluation of Aircraft Instrument Displays for Use with the Omni-Directional Radio Range.* (Division of Research, Report No. 84.) C.A.A., Washington, D.C.
34. WISCHNEWSKY, N. A., and ZIRLIN, B. A. 1935. Effect of lowering barometric pressure on dark adaptation, color vision and the electric excitability of the eye. (Wirkung des herabgestzen Barometerdrucks auf die Dunkeladaptation, das Farbensehen und die Elektroerregbarkeit des auges.) *Fiziol. Zhur. S.S.S.R. 18:* 237–249.
35. WISCHNEWSKY, N. A., and ZIRLIN, B. A. 1936. Physiology of vision in nocturnal high altitude flying. *Vo.-sanit. Dyelo 2–3:* 58–65. (Abstract: *J. Aviation Med. 7:* 215, 1936.)

# 6

# Group Behavior Problems in Flight

## S. B. SELLS, PH.D.*

The importance of group behavior factors in aircrew effectiveness is so great that this area merits profound consideration. Both military and civilian programs could benefit by immediate application of presently known group behavior principles; nevertheless, continued support of research is strongly indicated. With the rapid advance of flight technology to higher-performance multiplace and passenger-carrying jet and space craft, it is virtually mandatory that a comparable technical capability be maintained with relation to human organization and methods of control. Otherwise a condition may prevail in which man produces machines that he is unable to operate.

An intrinsic aspect of human behavior in flight is that it involves the behavior of persons as members of organized groups, in which there is some division of labor and differentiation of roles. As a result each individual must depend on other individuals, to some extent, for the over-all accomplishment of his tasks. The in-flight interdependence of the crew members of bombardment, refueling, and transport aircraft is readily apparent. Similarly the coordination required among the solo-flying pilots of fighter-interceptor flights with each other and with control stations on the ground is

* Professor of Psychology, Texas Christian University, Fort Worth, Texas. *Formerly,* Chief, Department of Medical Psychology, School of Aviation Medicine, USAF, Randolph Air Force Base, Texas. This chapter is based on a paper presented at the meeting of the Aeromedical Association, Washington, D.C., March 25, 1958, and published in the *United States Armed Forces Medical Journal 10:* 926–944, (August) 1959.

easily recognized. The coordination network is greatly extended, however, by the participation of many specialized support agencies, such as maintenance, weather, airways and air-traffic control, and others, when the operation is viewed in its totality. This thought was neatly expressed by an Air National Guard jet pilot (25) in the words "You can't set a record by yourself," after a record-shattering F-86-F flight from Los Angeles to New York in 1954.

In recognition of the interdependence of human behavior in organized, group situations, terms such as *team work, leadership, morale,* and *coordination* have high status as desired values in human affairs. However, systematic understanding of the behavior processes by which they may be achieved has been slowly acquired and is as yet meager. It is gratifying that a vast amount of research effort has been directed at these problems and that some substantial results can be reported. This chapter is concerned with research related directly to the behavior of flight personnel in flight operations. As a result it makes only a few other references to the substantial and growing research literature on group behavior or to the broader aspects of coordination involved in the operation of the over-all flight organization. General reviews of these fields are presented by Cartwright and Zander (4), Lindzey (23), and McFarland (24). A comprehensive bibliography is also available (26).

## Semantic Problems

A great deal of confusion has resulted from the imprecise and often misleading use of terms related to group behavior, as, for example, *leadership* and *morale.* One problem is related to their functional purposes. Such terms can have systematic explanatory meaning only when they refer to dimensions of group functioning, but they are often used to describe specific behaviors of individual group members.

*Leadership,* in an organized group, is the general function of facilitating the movement of the group toward the accomplishment of its designated goals, that is, of expediting group effectiveness. The behaviors of various designated individuals in this respect must depend on the nature of the task and the people involved and the goals. Thus, the leadership behaviors required of an aircraft commander, a squadron commander, and, say, a hospital commander may be quite different and may also vary under different task conditions.

Similarly, *morale* represents attitudes associated with membership in a group which reflect the cumulative satisfaction of group members derived from their participation in the group. It should not be confused with other concepts, such as general level of individual adjustment, although these are related. And, it cannot be specified by a particular list of behaviors, but rather depends on the relation of individual behaviors to the status of functioning of the group. Thus, people in an organization might be either happy or unhappy, while at the same time either mission orientated and effective or not; and evaluation of their morale would be different in each of these cases.

If a recent report by Fruchter, Blake, and Mouton (11) was taken at face value, one would conclude that leadership is highly, but negatively, related to B-47-crew effectiveness as rated by superiors and wing standardization boards. It is of interest that in this study the ratings of leadership were based on specific behaviors, principally of aircraft commanders, such as putting other crew members at their ease, making crew membership more enjoyable, and accepting responsibility. The authors themselves questioned the appropriateness of such behavior by a bomber commander to his military mission and cited similar results of a study of B-29 crews in combat by Halpin (13). However, Halpin used the more appropriate term "consideration" for the same behavior which he, too, found to be negatively related to effectiveness ratings of aircraft commanders by their superiors. Halpin properly referred to this finding as a "dilemma of leadership" since the more the commander pleased his crew, the lower he tended to be rated in effectiveness by his superiors.

A similar finding was reported by Smith (36) in a study of B-17 groups based in England during World War II, whose mission involved the bombardment of heavily defended targets in Germany. Smith compared groups selected as highly effective and highly ineffective in terms of bombing results and found that morale, defined as feelings of well-being and cohesion reflecting enjoyment of group participation, was low in the effective groups and high in the ineffective groups. On the other hand, in the most successful groups cohesion was found, but it was centered around the mission, emphasizing military combat duties, rather than social and recreational activities. They were welded together with a common purpose, but this was to get their job done and get home. Group cohesion did not appear as an end in itself, and other purposes incompatible with the mission, such as safety and survival, were kept in check.

Smith concluded that superior performance in a combat bombardment group is more likely to be achieved if the designated leader (1) stresses mission objective over all other considerations, (2) is not himself overly identified with the personnel of the group to the point at which this identification interferes with the mission, and (3) achieves a high degree of cohesion, confidence, and cooperation but not necessarily "morale" in the sense of well-being. This ruthless emphasis on the mission was truly a "dilemma of leadership" which many combat commanders found too difficult to accept. It was dramatically portrayed in the play *Command Decision*.

The work of Fiedler (8), supported by the Office of Naval Research, throws further light on these problems. Fiedler's research, based on groups as diverse as high school basketball teams, student engineer surveying crews, and B-29-bomber crews, produced a number of consistent results. One of them related the group's perception of its mission to the attitudes of group members toward each other. For example, high school basketball teams that were high in league standing and competing for top honors tended to prize competency ahead of social participation, while low-standing teams placed more emphasis on "being a good fellow." These variations, which correspond with those observed by Smith with respect to morale attitudes of B-17 groups, illustrate the importance of situational specifications in the study of morale.

With respect to superior-subordinate relationships, Fiedler emphasized the importance of interaction between the two in relation to effectiveness. If the superior is outgoing and approachable and tends to get too friendly with his subordinates (i.e., identify with them too much), he may find himself unable to make clear-cut decisions. However, if the organization has rigid barriers between ranks and is part of a highly disciplined system, such a superior may be more effective. In contrast, an aloof superior who isolates himself from his subordinates may lose touch with the group. Such a superior, however, may be more effective in a situation in which rank barriers are relaxed. Hence, the relation of consideration, as a variable describing superiors' behavior, to group effectiveness should be expected to depend not only on the requirements of the mission but also on the nature of the group membership and group structure as reflected in attitudes of group members toward each other.

The principal lesson in semantics that can be drawn from this discussion is that in the study of group behavior a distinction must be made between terms used to describe human behavior, such as "consideration," "identification," and "cooperation," and terms used to describe group functions, which are essentially abstractions, such as "leadership," "morale," and "group effectiveness." The systematic task with reference to the goal of clarifying the principles of group behavior is to relate behavioral concepts to the abstractions of group function. Since the problem is to explain group function in terms of behavioral data, it is essential that concepts of group function, such as leadership, morale and group effectiveness, be employed to define criteria, while the predictions are based entirely on behavioral data.

Another important semantic point concerns the use of words to represent particular aspects of behavior. Throughout the literature in the field, terms are assigned to represent particular attitude, role, and behavior scales which are necessary for communication purposes but are often imperfect symbols of the behavior described. Until a standardized taxonomy of behavior description is achieved, caution must be exercised in the comparison of results of different studies on the basis of the verbal symbols only, without reference to the supporting behavior descriptions.

## A Frame of Reference for the Study of Group Behavior

All behavior represents the interaction of the individual and the environment, in which significant variance can be attributed both to the abilities, habits, and dispositions of the individual and to the pressures and forces exercised on him by the environment. In group behavior many of the significant environmental forces are derived from the structure of the group as it channels communication of information to various individuals, defines prestige, power, and influence, and determines the roles that individuals play in the concerted effort of the group.

The practical application of psychological principles of group behavior in flying activities lies in the understanding of factors in organization and interpersonal relations which may be used to increase group effectiveness. From this point of view it becomes necessary to consider not only the characteristics of the individuals who participate in flight and support crews and organizations but also to consider the various aspects of group structure and the purpose, goals, or mission of the group on which the concept of effectiveness depends.

There are, then, three dimensions of group functioning which interact and must be considered in interrelation in the study of human behavior in organized groups. Keeping in mind the practical application aspect, these dimensions may be regarded as subject to external control by top management, and this is reflected in the following terms, which will organize the remainder of this discussion: (1) *Group goals* define the mission in terms of the task objective set for the group and the priorities and cost limitations under which they are to be accomplished. (2) *Group staffing* defines the constitution of group personnel, and therefore the upper and lower limits of their potentiality, in terms of the abilities and capabilities of the individual members. (3) *Group utilization of personnel* refers to the nature of the work environment provided for the group and hence defines the extent to which the potentiality of the group may be realized.

The interrelation of these factors is illustrated in an impressive report by Paterson (27) who, although a radar control officer, was assigned by his station commander to attack the problem of a dreadful and destructive accident rate at an RAF fighter station during World War II. Available evidence suggested that the accidents represented careless errors of judgment rather than accident proneness. Paterson approached the problem by efforts to increase group cohesion and to achieve a group norm of "good flying" for pressure to conform. After observing and analyzing conversations among pilots and other personnel, he decided that it was frustration of the desire to get into battle that was responsible for the prevalent irritability, carelessness, and lack of team spirit and that this might be overcome by giving the pilots something to fight, symbolic of the enemy. Since constant bad weather prevented the pilots from engaging the enemy in battle, the weather was on the side of the enemy and could be made symbolic of the enemy. The station might fight the enemy by fighting the weather.

The account of how he identified the respected, influential members of each group, whom he called *exemplars,* and, working tactfully and unobtrusively through them, set in motion group interactions that gradually affected everyone on the station with a common purpose, is one of the thrilling anecdotes of the war. In addition, in discussing his successful efforts to reduce aircraft accidents, which have since been tested as well in industrial situations, Paterson made a number of important theoretical observations. With reference to team spirit and teamwork, he emphasized the importance of morale based on appreciation of the common purpose and knowledge that everyone in his role is "doing his bit." Teamwork, the coordination of the various functions, depends on the development of such morale, although "leaders" or "experts" are necessary to that coordination. But it is not sufficient to have one person tell others how to perform their functions. They must also know something of the way in which their functions are coordinated, which is the background to the popular interest in *communication* and *liaison*.

On *group structure* and *roles* he pointed out that:

. . . not only was appreciation of functional co-ordination necessary, but also appreciation of the persons performing these functions; that is estimation of role . . . Function, hence role, has no meaning unless it is one of a structure of functions necessary to achieve the purpose of a group . . . If a man performs no function of significance to a group, he cannot be a member of that group . . . Thus at Bogfield, there could be no room for one who did not perform a function which helped in some way to put an aircraft and its pilot into battle with the enemy . . . If the word "work" is taken to be synonymous with "job," then work may be said to refer to what a man does when what he does has functional significance, his contribution to the group activity. A man working fills a role. He and his role are identified and in this he becomes a meaning to society . . . Unless there is a structure of functions work is not meaningful . . . For a sense of belongingness, role, hence structure, is essential . . . Belongingness gives security.

Thus, behavior of individuals as members of groups and their collective behavior in groups reflect the complex interaction of many variables. These are grouped logically in the three categories: group goals, staffing, and utilization. The remainder of this chapter illustrates a number of important issues related to staffing and utilization. However, in each case the results must be interpreted with reference to the established goals of the particular group and the particular perceptions of them found among the members of the group, as well as with reference to all other conditions of staffing and utilization not specifically isolated for study. The fact that relevant variables are not always taken into account by investigators does not alter their relevance or effectiveness.

## Measurement of Group Performance: The Problem of Criteria

One of the most baffling and elusive problems in personnel research has been the development of appropriate, reliable criteria of performance. Measurement of group performance is necessary to evaluate the effects of various factors presumed to account for group performance.

Research, primarily with B-29 crews by the Combat Crew Training Research Laboratory at Randolph Air Force Base, has given a rather discouraging picture of a number of *objective* indicators of bomber-crew performance. For example, Forgays and Irwin (9) who studied 600 B-29 student crews in training, reported results such as the following:

(a) Radar bombing circular errors obtained by the Radar Bomb System (RBS) showed a corrected odd-even mission reliability of .33. Attempts to increase reliability by correcting for target and mission differences, presence of instructors and condition of radar set were unsuccessful.

(b) Mean circular errors on the ultrasonic (ground) trainer had a reliability of .47, and questionable validity in relation to radar bombing scores in flight.

(c) Target identification scores on simulated visual bombing missions ("visual camera" scores) had a reliability of .20, which was believed to be inflated by instructor estimates in scoring. Circular errors in actual visual bomb drops had a reliability of .18.

(d) Average errors in making good control times showed a reliability of .49, with some indications requiring verification, that these errors relate meaningfully to mission difficulty and stage of training.

(e) Ground school written examinations had relatively high Kuder-Richardson reliabilities (.60 to .91) in the cases examined, but these failed to correlate meaningfully with objective in-flight measures.

These results are representative of efforts to obtain satisfactory objective measures of flight-crew performance. On the other hand, ratings of crews by superior officers and by standardization boards have proved reliable in a number of studies, although not related to objective measures. Knoell, French, and Stice (20), for example, obtained several types of ratings on combat performance in the Far East for 108 B-29 crews which had trained initially at Randolph Air Force Base. Their results showed:

(a) that ratings by squadron commanders and, in some cases, wing officers, were satisfactory as to inter-rater agreement; however, although nine dimensions were rated, factor analysis revealed that they were accounted for by one general factor;

(b) that similar ratings of individual performance were most satisfactory for aircraft commanders, navigators, radar operators and flight engineers; ratings of copilots, bombardiers, radio operators and gunners, did not reach satisfactory levels of agreement;

(c) that ratings of flight crews by ground crews assigned to their aircraft offer a reliable source of rating information, although these ratings did not correlate significantly with anything else.

In view of their demonstrated reliability and authoritative status in the operating affairs of the organization, *superiors' ratings* have in one or another form been used in most of the research known. However, this is probably more expedient than satisfactory, and the criterion problem remains an important and challenging area for continuing investigation.

## Staffing Problems in Flight Situations

**Technical Competence.** The most important single factor controlling the assignment of personnel to any flight crew is technical competence. Although, from the standpoint of crew effectiveness, the possession of a minimum standard of technical competence may be regarded as a necessary rather than sufficient requirement, the study of Fruchter, Blake, and Mouton (11) reported a positive, linear correlation of 0.43 between crew members' ratings of each other on this factor and the superiors' rating criterion. These ratings were based on such items as frequency of errors in the air, competence and interest in technical specialty, satisfaction with performance in both air and ground activities, and consistency of performance.

There is some impressive evidence, from another study of B-47 crews, that crew members' approval of the technical competence of other crew members is not entirely a matter of individual proficiency but depends also to a substantial degree on their experience in working together. Hood and his associates (18) found that crew agreement on "who does what when" in flight, which is highly correlated with superiors' ratings, is a direct function of crew members' experience in flying *together;* the important factor is neither individual flying experience nor even multi-jet time per se but is experience together as a team. The importance of operational training to supplement initial crew assembly is clearly indicated and illustrates neatly the interdependence of staffing and utilization measures.

**Crew Assembly.** The problem of rational crew assembly has received considerable research attention and yielded useful results. Rational approaches imply that some combinations of personalities, backgrounds, skills, and other individual characteristics may be more compatible and adaptable to effective task performance than others. The general literature on interpersonal attraction and selection of mates and work partners is relevant to this problem and has contributed to approaches which have been investigated. A comprehensive review by Haythorn (16) cited a number of generalizations as well supported by experimental evidence:

(a) Research on crew composition and efforts to assemble crews for optimal performance has confirmed that variations in crew effectiveness can be accounted for by variations in the particular combinations of individuals composing the groups (32).

(b) The most successful method of assembling crews thus far has been that of self-selection, in which crew members express their own choices of preferred crew mates. The improved effectiveness obtained by such methods is apparently a result of increased crew compatibility observed in crews composed by these methods. A limitation of self-selection methods has been their feasibility, but this is less of a problem with smaller crews such as in the B-47 and B-52 type aircraft, as compared with the much larger B-29 and B-36 crews. To accomplish self-selection, it is necessary to give potential crew members an opportunity to become acquainted with those from whom they are expected to choose. The more extensive this acquaintance, the more effective the assembly procedure is likely to be. Practical procedures for setting up contact situations have been described by Roby and Rosenberg (29, 33).

(c) One of the most important determiners of compatibility among crew members is similarity of values regarding issues relevant to group performance. Hence, compatibility and resulting efficiency can be improved by assembling in the same crews individuals whose values and attitudes on mission and work-related issues are alike. The more relevant the issue, the more important this sharing of values becomes.

An unpublished study by Sells and Templeton (34), on compatible matching of primary training students with flight instructors, showed also how individual needs may influence choice. When asked for preferences with reference to their choices of students, the instructors' replies included such statements as "I prefer to have no students taller than 5 feet 6" and "I would prefer non-college graduates." Among the students' replies were preferences for "older, more patient and fatherly" instructors and for instructors "who don't chew you out on the radio."

In a related study using basic airmen as subjects, French (10) studied the influence of needs for achievement and for affiliation with others, measured by psychological tests, on work-partner selection. She assumed that the behavior of a person making a choice between a work partner who was a competent non-friend and one who was a less competent friend could be predicted by the relative strength of these two kinds of motivation. The results were in accordance with the hypothesis, although subjects low in both achievement and affiliation showed no patterning. In addition, the achievement-motivation mean scores showed a significant increase and the affiliation a significant decrease from subjects who chose a friend, through those who chose both the friend and the competent person, to those who chose the competent person only.

The accomplishments of research on crew-assembly problems warrant further support of effort in this direction as well as practical application of techniques already available. The refinement of techniques using proficiency measures and personality-test profiles, following up promising beginnings referred to above, and the use of mathematical models (6, 7) need to be investigated. The methods developed in this field will also have application to the development of other significant work groups in aircraft, missile, and space-flight operations.

## Research on Utilization Problems in Flight Situations

The challenge to top levels of control in an organization is not only to obtain the best talent for the required tasks but also to make the most effective use of it. This is the strategy of the term "utilization," which implies the exploitation of all possible relevant factors in the work environment that may contribute to group effectiveness. Of course, there must be a balance between goals, capabilities, and facilities. If the goals are unrealistically high or low in relation to the other two, one set of problems may arise. If either the personnel or facilities are inappropriate to the goals, other problems may be expected. However, a commonly overlooked problem is that of a crew or other organization in being, with qualified personnel and generally reasonable goals, that falls short of optimal effectiveness and has room for considerable improvement.

**Three Approaches to Utilization Problems.** Aircrews and other organizations have been approached by different investigators in terms of several different conceptual viewpoints. One approach, which has been used more in relation to larger groups, such as squadron, wing, and the larger administrative units, is concerned with organizational structure, lines of authority, communication channels, span of control, pay, promotions, and other formal, structural aspects of the system. This may be called the *structural approach*. A second approach views a crew or other group as a social group, which is part of a social system. The sociocultural background provides a common set of symbols to which the members respond. The members are differentiated in terms of roles, status, power, and various patterns of interrelation, which affect and are affected by each others' attitudes, interindividual compatibility, cooperation, and performance. The emphasis here is on *group dynamics*. Finally, the third approach looks at an aircrew as a *man-machine system*. It is task-oriented and involves a flow of communications in relation to group (actually system) work output.

Although each of these approaches has been productive, individually none is sufficient to the total problem. Indeed, there is no reason to expect that the picture of an organization from the viewpoint of group dynamics, the analysis of formal structure, and the man-machine system need be consistent. Whether the effects of different aspects are complementary or contradictory may be important in many cases. The interplay of various factors can only be evaluated through comprehensive and integrated experimental study. However, at present one must be content to consider the contributions of the separate approaches.

**The Structural Approach.** Important contributions from this approach have come from the Ohio State leadership studies, which have received support from the Office of Naval Research and the Air Force. The profound importance of the formal structure and its implications for the behavior of organized groups was graphically analyzed by Stogdill (38). The act of organization involves specification of jobs and their functions in the over-all division of labor. The specification of a job constitutes definition of *responsibility to whom, for what function*, and incidentally *at what level* of prestige, status, and power. Thus, the official lines of authority and communication, power and status hierarchies, and the basic prescriptions of

roles in the group are specified by the formal structure of the organization. They may contribute positively to effective operations or
interfere with it.

However, responsibility can never be spelled out in complete
detail nor is this desirable. A proper balance must be struck between
the dangers of ambiguity at one extreme and of excessive restraint
and red tape at the other. Behavior within the organization occurs
according to *expectations,* resulting partly from custom and tradition
and partly from interactions between superiors and subordinates
within the organization. *Conforming expectations* reflect favorable
goals, formal structure, and personnel capabilities, reinforced by
effective discipline and exemplary behavior by superiors; while
*deviant expectations* and *non-conformity,* which impede and may
undermine the organization, may result from unfavorable conditions
or lax discipline and deviant examples by superiors and high-status
persons. To the extent that superiors are conscientious about influencing conformity with organizational patterns, their own freedom
of behavior is sharply restricted.

Conformity with expected behavior of a particular job, or *assumption of expected role* in accordance with the prescribed formal structure, often produces unintended behavioral results of far-reaching
significance. The traditional unpopularity of the inspector and of
the comptroller in large organizations is virtually written into their
job descriptions and is intensified when conscientiously followed.
Departmental rivalries, "empire building," budget padding, and
similar bureaucratic institutions can be shown, to a large extent, to
be inherent in the basic formal structure of an organization.

Research on role behavior of members of aircrews (2, 12, 14, 15)
has generally confirmed these principles in both student and operational B-29 crews, both with respect to the interaction of aircraft
commander behavior with crew interpersonal relations and expectations and with relation to crew proficiency and combat-effectiveness
ratings. Torrance (40) has shown the influence of power position
on group-decision making in B-26 crews, and his results, like those
of Hood and his associates (18) in the B-47 study mentioned earlier,
have emphasized the importance of training together in supporting
and solidifying a "crew norm" of operating procedure.

Another important contribution from the Ohio State group is
Hemphill's development (17) of a taxonomy of situational factors in
group situations which have behavioral implications and which can

be measured by his "Group Dimensions Description Questionnaire." Examples of his dimensions are *group autonomy, control* over activities of members, *flexibility* of procedures, *stratification* by rank, authority, and prestige, *stability* of personnel, assignments, and organizational structure, *affect* associated with membership, and a number of others.

**The Group Dynamics Approach.** Although the formal structure of an organization has a profound influence on roles, attitudes, and behavior, this influence is exercised through the reactions and interactions of members of the group. In addition, many interactions occur in the form of group pressures and group standards, reflecting patterns of cohesiveness and communication among group members, which are not directly related to the formal structure. Actually, the formal structure may be considered as a plan, whether spelled out in detail or implied, and an organization in operation seldom corresponds with the organization model as charted (4, 38).

Group dynamics is reflected by the intervention of human social factors interacting with the formal plans and other influences in the situation. The resulting work performance, attitudes, and relationships among members reflect the organization in operation. In his efforts to make the actual organization conform to the formal plan, the appointed leader is continually confronted with the task of reconciling discrepancies between what should be done and what is done, between the needs of the organization and the needs of individual members, and between prescribed and actual lines of communication. Many of the most important decisions he faces involve compromises between maximum goal achievement and the costs they imply in terms of risks of jeopardizing the organization by impairment of the welfare, motivation, and capabilities of its members.

In their introduction to the problems of group pressures and group standards, Cartwright and Zander (4) quoted Bill Mauldin's book *Up Front* in which he stated that combat outfits "have a sort of family complex." That is, the men know what is expected of them and readily accept group pressures to behave in a certain way while they are group members. Mauldin stated:

Combat people are an exclusive set, and if they want to be that way it is their privilege. They certainly earn it. New men in outfits have to work their way in slowly, but they are eventually accepted. Sometimes they have to change their way of living. An introvert or a recluse is not going to last long in combat without friends, so he learns to come out of his shell. Once he has "arrived" he is pretty proud of his clique, and he in turn is chilly to outsiders.*

This quotation illustrates *identification*. One of the concomitants of identification involves acceptance of group norms which function as pressures to conform. This is part of the explanation of the importance of communality of values in a cohesive group. However, except in the relative isolation and intensified stress of a combat group or a space crew, where situational pressures and survival needs may obscure other affiliations, most people affiliate with many groups, which exercise various pressures on those who identify with them. Religious, social, political, and other group memberships not only represent basic values but also styles of living, likes and dislikes concerning a wide range of activities, and prestige, status, and resulting power and influence among associates.

Some of these, which have equally important civilian counterparts, are illustrated by military status categories, such as rank (flag, field grade, company grade, warrant, and NCO), type of aircraft rating, regular *versus* reserve, and Academy graduate *versus* other. The importance of such status categories is clearly shown by the many symbols of status that are displayed and coveted, such as insignia, distinctive wings, flags, badges, parking spaces, office furniture, rugs, desk sets, private dining rooms, cars, clubs, and the like. These not merely utilitarian conveniences but are also means of reinforcing and displaying evidence of power, prestige, and status, which have implications for the behavior of their owners and their associates.

In a formal organization in which authority is hierarchical, cooperation is enhanced when the various dimensions of status are consistent throughout the organization. Top management of an organization might well investigate many of its existing status conventions if it is desired to exploit fully these informal forces within the group. For example, Lanzetta and Haythorn (21) in a study of B-29 instructor-crew influence on student attitudes and performance found a decided lack of prestige attached to instructor status. In view of the well-known influence of prestige persons on attitudes of their associates, and of the demonstrated relations of crew attitudes to crew effectiveness (5, 14, 19), the possibility of positively

---

* Published by Holt, Rinehart & Winston, Inc., New York, 1945, and quoted by permission from the publisher.

affecting attitude development among student crews by improving the prestige status of instructors appears as a worthwhile problem.

The effects of various forms of *interaction among aircrew members* have been studied in relation to crew effectiveness. DeGaugh and Knoell (5) found a significant relation between a factor that they called "pride-in-work-group" and superiors' ratings of 89 B-29 groups in combat. The items that identified this factor were chiefly related to liking for the members of one's crew, satisfaction with the accomplishments of the crew, and a sense of safety in flying with the crew.

Haythorn (14) reported significant correlations for 103 B-29 crews which indicated that crew mean sociometric scores covary with crew mean attitude scores, particularly on the same dimension of pride-in-crew, and with combat ratings of the crew by superior officers. In a later study of 42 B-29 crews which remained together from training into combat in the Korean War, Knoell (19) reported that crew attitudes measured in training and also in combat are significantly correlated with the crew's rated combat performance. The same interpersonal factors reported in earlier studies, namely, pride-in-crew, acceptance of Air Force goals, and sense of well-being in the Air Force, which reflect group acceptance of the same task-oriented values, were reported by Knoell as criterion related.

The relations between superiors and subordinates, particularly between the aircraft commander and the combat crew, which have been studied most in the flight situation, are significant in achieving the attitudes most compatible with effective performance. These relations are subtly dependent on the nature of the task and the mission. Although no empirical data are available, it is likely that the negative relation to effectiveness of *consideration* and *nurturance* by the aircraft commander, among combat crews, as reported by Fruchter, Halpin, and others, might be positive among commercial aircrews whose duties are relatively less hazardous and stressful. In his role in the crew, the aircraft commander is the source of information that affects the performance and sense of individual security on the job of his subordinates. He must keep his crew informed, but the nature and purposes of his communications will be conditioned by the requirements of the situation.

Research on group dynamics has repeatedly emphasized the importance of *communication of information* necessary to the group for feelings of individual well-being and effective performance (3,

35). For example, Riecken (28) described a work-camp group in which the behavior code prohibited criticism or aggression of any kind. As a result the usual minor antagonisms and conflicts enlarged, since they could not be discussed, until the entire group lost its cohesiveness and effectiveness. Cartwright and Zander (4) pointed out that international conferences and workers at noisy jobs both suffer the loss of effectiveness and cohesiveness due to communication difficulties unless compensatory mechanisms for communication can be obtained. Taylor (39) found a highly effective functioning communication system in an Air Force squadron which was independently rated outstanding.

In an extensive study of a mental hospital, Stanton and Schwartz (37) noted the formal organization structure and from it constructed a chart of the "formal expectation of the transmission of information," which carried a small but vital part of the communications among the staff to higher administrative levels. They repeatedly observed the causes and effects of the "blocking" of this type of information. Blocking was usually due to the overloading of these formal channels or to changes desired or not desired in hospital procedures. The effect was the emergence of informal channels to carry needed facts. The informal channels were usually slower, less accurate, and more misleading, but eventually a needed bit of information reached the person who needed it, although frequently too late or too inaccurately for effective action.

Stanton and Schwartz also found that the informal channels could be roughly predicted from a chart of the formal expectation of communication, once the location of the block of formal channels was known. Furthermore, the informal channels were unstable due to their excessive length and unreliability. They would form, then break up, then re-form repeatedly until the blocked formal channel was reopened. The persons used as intermediates in the informal channels became noticeably tense without realizing why, while the two primary persons concerned were constantly seeking newer and better informal channels. Whenever a block in the formally expected line of communication between staff members was removed, considerably improved behavior was noted in patients dependent upon the persons involved, although these patients had not been greatly concerned.

Stanton and Schwartz caution against confusing lines of formal authority with the formally expected channels of communication.

Forcing the use of the former for all formal communication quickly leads to blocking due to channel overloading, and this in turn leads to the establishment of informal or even *sub rosa* channels, which are much less effective methods of communication. Thus, communication should not follow but actually reinforce the formal organization through a network of expected communication derived from formal job descriptions. This conclusion is supported by centuries of combat history; men in actual combat must communicate not only with their superiors to the rear but also with the groups on their flanks.

To the degree that existing channels of information support the formal organization, the more they reinforce the positions of the leaders and decision-makers, and the less likely will there be discrepancies between formal and informal power structure.

**The Man-Machine System Approach.** It is possible, as some investigators have shown, to ignore structure, status, roles, and interpersonal problems and to regard an aircrew or other task group as a system in which crew members and equipment are linked and information must flow efficiently to enable decisions and responses in appropriate sequence and timing. This approach is concerned with discovering the most efficient arrangements for information flow for various types of group and task.

A simple model illustrating this problem is given in a study by Bavelas (1) who demonstrated experimentally that different forms of communication structure have differential effectiveness in group performance. He arranged five cubicles into each of several geometric configurations, such as a star, fork, circle, and straight line, and placed a person in each cubicle. Each was given a bit of information, which together with the other four bits of information given the others constituted solution of the problem. The geometric pattern markedly affected the assembling of the bits of information; highly centralized figures, such as the star and fork, organized faster, were more stable from problem to problem and from test group to test group, solved problems faster, and evolved as leaders the centrally placed persons. The flow of information could thus be seen to be an important resultant and determinant of how well a group functions.

Roby and Lanzetta (22, 30, 31) investigated task performance in the laboratory under four different conditions of communication structure roughly simulating aircrew problems. The experimental conditions ranged from that in which control agents had direct access to none of the information required to operate their own controls to that in which control agents had direct access to information for all but one of their controls. They found that differences in team performance are associated with task communication structures even within the comparatively narrow range of the structure studied. Performance efficiency increased as the structure permitted more direct transmission of information and less dispersion. Learning was more rapid with an easy communication system than with a difficult one, and replacing an interphone circuit with a telephone circuit resulted in wider differences in performance and an increase in errors.

These and related studies have suggested three principles of job structure to maximize group performance in a man-machine system:[*] (1) *load-balancing*, wherein each member of a team is equally occupied in attaining the goal, regardless of the importance or magnitude of the contribution or of variations in type of activity; (2) *autonomy of function*, which implies that jobs are self-contained with reference to information necessary for their performance; and (3) *homogeneity of function*, wherein the functions performed by each job have a high degree of homogeneity with respect to information handled.

These principles have implications for technical competence and, therefore, for the content of selection and training programs as well as structure of the organization. The Roby and Lanzetta studies have shown that, when they are violated to various degrees by varying the proportions of information-giving and relaying requirements, decrements of performance resulted.

In a study by Voiers (41) of factors involved in bombing accuracy of B-29 crews, it was found that the aircraft commander and radar observer were directly dependent on one another for effective expression of their respective proficiencies. The proficiency of each member, as measured in ground school, correlated most highly with the bombing criteria under conditions of higher-than-average-proficiency in the other member. High proficiency in the navigator appeared to compensate in some degree for lack of proficiency in

[*] Appreciation is expressed to Dr. Bryce O. Hartmann, Department of Medical Psychology, School of Aviation Medicine, USAF, Brooks Air Force Base, for his help in formulating these principles and for his helpful criticism of the manuscript.

the aircraft commander and radar observer, in that the navigator's proficiency appeared most highly correlated with the criteria under conditions of low proficiency in these members. The results for bombardiers were inconclusive.

Voiers interpreted the relationship between bombing accuracy and the proficiency structure of the bomb team by means of a crude electrical analogy in which the proficiencies and performances of the aircraft commander and radar observer were represented as being "in series" with one another and collectively "in parallel" with the proficiency performance of the navigator. These observations fit in nicely with the principles of load-balancing, autonomy, and homogeneity of function.

# References

1. BAVELAS, A. 1953. Communication patterns in task-oriented groups. In CART-WRIGHT, D., and ZANDER, A. (eds.). *Group Dynamics*. Row, Peterson & Company, Evanston, Ill.
2. BERKOWITZ, L. 1953. An exploratory study of the roles of aircraft commanders. ARDC, Human Resources Res. Center, Res. Bull. 53–65.
3. CARTWRIGHT, D. 1957. Social psychology and group processes. In FARNS-WORTH, P. R., and McNEMAR, Q. (eds.). *Annual Review of Psychology*. Annual Reviews, Inc., Palo Alto, Calif. Vol. 8, pp. 211–236.
4. CARTWRIGHT, D., and ZANDER, A. (eds.). 1953. *Group Dynamics*. Row, Peterson & Co., Evanston, Ill. Pp. 73–91.
5. DeGAUGH, R. A., and KNOELL, D. M. 1954. *Attitudes Relevant to Bomber Crew Performance in Combat*. (Res. Bull. AFPTRC–TR–54–18.) AF Personnel Train. Res. Center.
6. DWYER, P. S. 1956. *The Problem of Optimum Group Assembly*. (Res. Rept. AFPTRC–TN–56–18.) AF Personnel Train. Res. Center.
7. DWYER, P. S. 1956. *Development of Generalized Mathematical Procedures for Optimal Assembly of Potentially Effective Crews*. (Res. Rept. AFPTRC–TN–56–139.) AF Personnel Train. Res. Center.
8. FIEDLER, F. 1955. *The Influence of Leader-Key Man Relations on Combat Crew Effectiveness*. (Tech. Rept. No. 9.) ONR Contract NS–ori–07135. *J. Abnorm. & Soc. Psychol. 51:* 227–235.
9. FORGAYS, D. G., and IRWIN, I. A. 1952. Measures of combat crew performance used in B-29 training. ARDC, Human Resources Res. Center, Tech. Rept. 52–14.
10. FRENCH, E. G. 1957. *Motivation as a Variable in Work-Partner Selection*. (Res. Rept. AFPTRC–TN–57–63.) AF Personnel Train. Res. Center.
11. FRUCHTER, B., BLAKE, R. R., and MOUTON, J. S. 1957. Some dimensions of interpersonal relations in three-man aircraft crews. *Psychol. Monogr. 71:* No. 19.
12. HALL, R. L. 1956. *Predicting Bomber Crew Performance from the Aircraft Commander's Role*. (Res. Rept. AFPTRC–TN–56–28.) AF Personnel Train. Res. Center.
13. HALPIN, A. W. 1955. *The Leadership Ideology of Aircraft Commanders*. (Res. Rept. AFPTRC–TN–55–57.) AF Personnel Train. Res. Center.
14. HAYTHORN, W. W. 1954. *An Analysis of Role Distribution in B-29 Crews*. (Res. Bull. AFPTRC–TR–54–104.) AF Personnel Train. Res. Center.

15. HAYTHORN, W. W. 1954. *Relations between Sociometric Measures and Performance in Medium Bomber Crews in Combat.* (Res. Rept. AFPTRC–TR–54–101.) AF Personnel Train. Res. Center.

16. HAYTHORN, W. W. 1957. *A Review of Research on Group Assembly.* (Res. Rept. AFPTRC–TN–57–62.) AF Personnel Train. Res. Center.

17. HEMPHILL, J. K. 1956. *Group Dimensions: A Manual for Their Measurement.* (Res. Monogr. No. 87.) Bureau of Business Research, The Ohio State University, Columbus.

18. HOOD, P. D., HALPIN, A. W., HANITCHOK, J. J., SIEGEL, L., and HEMPHILL, J. K. 1957. *Crew Member Agreement on RB–47 Crew Operating Procedure.* (Res. Rept. AFPTRC–TN–57–64.) AF Personnel Train. Res. Center.

19. KNOELL, D. M. 1956. *Relationships Between Attitudes of Bomber Crews in Training and Their Attitudes and Performance in Combat.* (Res. Rept. AFPTRC–TN–56–49.) AF Personnel Train. Res. Center.

20. KNOELL, D. M., FRENCH, R. L., and STICE, G. 1953. Criteria of B-29 crew performance in Far Eastern combat: I. Ratings. ARDC, Human Resources Res. Center, Tech. Rept. 53–32.

21. LANZETTA, J. T., and HAYTHORN, W. W. 1954. *Instructor-Crew Influence on Attitude Formation in Student Crews.* (Res. Bull. AFPTRC–TR–54–79.) AF Personnel Train. Res. Center.

22. LANZETTA, J. T., and ROBY, T. B. 1957. *Effects of Work-Group Structure and Certain Task Variables on Group Performance.* (Res. Rept. AFPTRC–TN–57–45.) AF Personnel Train. Res. Center.

23. LINDZEY, G. (ed.). 1954. *Handbook of Social Psychology.* Addison-Wesley, Cambridge. Vol. II.

24. MCFARLAND, R. A. 1953. *Human Factors in Air Transportation.* McGraw-Hill Book Co., Inc., New York.

25. MILLIKEN, W. W. 1954. You can't set a record by yourself. *Air Force,* Feb. 1954.

26. OFFICE OF NAVAL RESEARCH. 1957. *Bibliography of Unclassified Research Reports in Group Psychology.* (ONR-Rept. ACR–22.)

27. PATERSON, T. T. 1955. *Morale in War and Work: An Experiment in the Management of Men.* Max Parrish, London.

28. RIECKEN, H. W. 1952. Some problems of consensus development. *Rur. Sociol.* 17: 245–252.

29. ROBY, T. B. 1953. Problems of rational group assembly exemplified in the medium bomber crew. ARDC, Human Resources Res. Center, Res. Bull. 53–18.

30. ROBY, T. B., and LANZETTA, J. T. 1956. *An Investigation of Task Performance as a Function of Certain Aspects of Work-Group Structure.* (Res. Rept. AFPTRC–TN–56–74.) AF Personnel Train. Res. Center.

31. ROBY, T. B., and LANZETTA, J. T. 1957. *A Replication Study of Work Group Structure and Task Performance.* (Res. Rept. AFPTRC–TN–57–85.) AF Personnel Train. Res. Center.

32. ROSENBERG, S., ERLICK, D. E., and BERKOWITZ, L. 1955. *Some Effects of Varying Combinations of Group Members on Group Performance Measures and Leadership Behaviors.* (Res. Rept. AFPTRC–TN–55–83.) AF Personnel Train. Res. Center.

33. ROSENBERG, S., and ROBY, T. B. 1956. *Experimental Assembly of B-29 Crews by Self-selection Procedures: A Description and Validation of the Method.* (Res. Rept. AFPTRC–TN–56–104.) AF Personnel Train. Res. Center.

34. SELLS, S. B., and TEMPLETON, R. C. An experiment in matching students and instructors in primary pilot training. Unpublished paper. USAF, School of Aviation Medicine, Randolph Air Force Base, Tex.

35. SELLS, S. B., and TRITES, D. K. 1960. Attitudes. In HARRIS, C. W. (ed.). *Encyclopedia of Educational Research.* The Macmillan Co., New York.

36. SMITH, D. L. 1951. *A Criterion for the Study of Leadership in Certain Combat Air Groups.* Stanford University, Calif. (Copies available in Air University Library, Maxwell Air Force Base, Ala.)

37. STANTON, A. H., and SCHWARTZ, M. S. 1954. *The Mental Hospital: A Study of Institutional Participation in Psychiatric Illness and Treatment.* Basic Books, Inc., New York.

38. STOGDILL, R. 1953. Leadership, membership and organization. In CARTWRIGHT, D., and ZANDER, A. (eds.). *Group Dynamics.* Row, Peterson & Co., Evanston, Ill.

39. TAYLOR, E. R. 1957. A case study of squadron communication and its aeromedical aspects. Unpublished paper, 1957. (Copies available in Library, School of Aviation Medicine, USAF, Randolph Air Force Base, Tex.)

40. TORRANCE, P. E. 1954. *Some Consequences of Power Differences on Decisions in B-26 Crews.* (Res. Bull. AFPTRC–TR–54–128.) AF Personnel Train. Res. Center.

41. VOIERS, W. D. 1956. *Bombing Accuracy as a Function of the Ground School Proficiency Structure of the B-29 Bomb Team.* (Res. Rept. AFPTRC–TN–56–4.) AF Personnel Train. Res. Center.

# 7

# *Human Qualifications for and Reactions to Jet Flight*

CHARLES A. BERRY, M.D., M.P.H.*

The human problems peculiar to jet flight, in comparison with those that have become familiar in reciprocating engine aircraft, are related directly to the altitudes and speeds involved. Jets are not really new to military aviation, since they have been flown since World War II. However, the widespread international and domestic use of jet airliners is a recent development in civil air operations. There are a number of important differences between the military and civilian jet operations, affecting both crew and passengers, that must be considered. The following discussion is divided into two major sections, dealing with aircrew problems first and then with problems related to passengers.

## Aircrew Problems

**Qualifications of Flying Personnel.** Only minor changes have been made in the psychological and physical bases of initial aircrew selection since World War II. This state of affairs does not mean that crew requirements are the same for high-performance jet fighters and bombers and for the new jet airliners as they were for the P-38, P-40, B-25, B-17, DC-3, and DC-4. On the contrary, the evidence is that crew-performance demands for such jet aircraft as the F-100 series, the B-47, B-52, and B-58, and the jet airliners such as the Boeing 707, Douglas DC-8, and Convair 880 are considerably more stringent.

* Lieutenant Colonel, USAF, MC, Chief, Flight Medicine Branch, Aerospace Medicine Division, Office of the Surgeon General, USAF, Washington, D.C.

The nature of the changes in crew requirements imposed by the jet cockpit and by jet altitudes and speeds has not received adequate study. Since crews have been assigned to such aircraft by up-grading of experienced personnel, the selection problem has not been acute. Nevertheless, such study could contribute not only to improvement of the effectiveness of personnel selection for up-grading to high-performance aircraft but also to the improvement of crew accommodations and cockpit arrangements for safer and more effective performance. As Moseley (25) stated: "It is apparent from accident data that we do not have at present adequate objective measurements of the task imposed upon the pilot in high performance aircraft."

Several trends in aircraft design have had obvious effects on jet-crew requirements. The transition of jet bombers from the ten-man B-36 to the three-man B-58 illustrates one source of increased complexity. The new jet bomber flies higher, faster, farther, and on more difficult missions. The smaller crew size requires expansion of the duties of individual crew members and cross-training for greater versatility and coordination. Higher altitudes and speeds on military missions impose not only new patterns of duties but also the added stress of protective gear for survival which must be worn in flight.

Civilian airlines have continued to use three-man crews on the Boeing 707 and Douglas DC-8 but now require that the position of flight engineer be filled by an engineer who is also a pilot. The trend has been away from the use of a flight engineer in the military as well (e.g., in the B-47 and B-52 aircraft), and there is a critical need to define the functions and qualifications of the third man in the jet airliner cockpit.

The desired characteristics of jet airline pilots were discussed by the Medical Director of the British Overseas Airways Corporation (5) on the basis of early experience with Comet-type aircraft. His report emphasized adaptability, mental alertness, methodical work habits, ability to plan ahead and anticipate, quick reaction time, thorough knowledge of instrument flying, and ability to work as a member of a closely coordinated team. More applicants were reported to be rejected for inability to function as a team member than for any other reason.

The navigator's role has become more important and more complicated in jet aircraft. The speed with which terrain is traversed keeps the navigator constantly busy even on long flights and in spite of the myriad electronic aids at his disposal. His traditional requirement for intelligence and ability to read dials and tables and to calculate must be exercised under vastly more stressful circumstances.

The selection problems of military and civil air operations have traditionally been considered fundamentally different, in that the military have found it necessary to select *trainees* with potentiality to become pilots, while the airlines have hired experienced pilots. With reference to jet operations, however, which are comparatively recent, this difference is slight. The military air services, as well as the airlines, have recruited their jet crews from the ranks of experienced airmen. However, as noted above, inadequate research has as yet been done on this *advanced selection* problem.

**Physical Standards.** Early in World War I there were no formal physical standards for aviators. The man with "nerve" was allowed to fly, and even those no longer fit for ground duty were assigned to the Air Service. Inevitably, as with other skilled activities and unselected operators, the result was wastage of personnel and funds. This was later remedied by the adoption of a set of physical requirements for pilots (8).

The authors of the *Air Service Medical Manual* (1), however, disdained as "utterly absurd" the concept that a combat pilot must be a "superman." Picking the "birdman" seemed to have so many contradictory requirements that Patten (3) described the ideal fighting pilot as a "tall, short, slim, blond, brunette, quiet, nervous, languid, alert, reckless, and conservative individual." Much of this contradiction exists today.

Aviation has rapidly outgrown the period when all that a pilot needed to qualify was "nerve." The physical standards for flying have reflected several purposes, which are summarized by the terms *safety, proficiency,* and *longevity.* Safety implies that qualification standards must be based not only on considerations of whether or not the man would be able to operate an aircraft but also on his ability to do so at peak proficiency under stressful conditions, such as insufficient oxygen, high-g forces, and in-flight emergencies. Proficiency in relation to physical standards is not so much a matter of flying skill but rather is expressed by the policy of the U.S. Air Medical Service in World War I that "No aviator shall fail in his mission because of discoverable physical defect." The same attitude of responsibility prevails today. Longevity refers to the exclusion of latent or potential physical defect that might reduce the expected period of active flying service of a crew member.

These multiple purposes of physical standards for the initial selection and periodic qualification of flying personnel have been widely misunderstood by crew members and even by flight surgeons, who have been constantly harassed by individuals demanding waivers of disqualification for physical defects as defined by the standards. The number of cases of persons wanting to fly with one good eye, one leg, a "little coronary," and the like have been amazingly large. Many instances have been cited of individuals who have flown numerous accident-free hours with disqualifying conditions under routine circumstances. However, the physical standards are designed necessarily with reference to emergency and maximum-effort situations, which cannot always be anticipated and hence must apply to all personnel who operate aircraft. In high-performance flight the margin of safety is reduced, and standards must be high for all.

Traditionally standards have tended to fluctuate with supply and demand for flying manpower. The reduction of the need for large numbers of new pilots and observers in present aircraft favors the concept that there should be no compromise with required standards of quality on initial selection. After the pilot is accepted and trained, different standards may function as "selection-in-depth" or continuing selection devices. The standards should serve as a guide, and the training and experience of the pilot should be weighed against the risk and waivers considered. Any relaxation of standards affecting either flying safety or safety of the individual must be avoided. In the final analysis the standards must be high enough to eliminate the medically unfit, although reasonable enough to insure adequate numbers to accomplish the mission (28).

The validity of instruments or tests used in the physical examination depends on their relevance to appropriate performance measures with reference to each of the purposes that the standards are intended to serve. Cutting scores must also be established for each test; these are actually the physical standards. The efficiency of the standards, thus defined, to discriminate successful from unsuccessful pilots must still be ascertained as a consideration separate from the validity of the instruments. The question of the validity of physical standards for aircrew has always been a difficult one.

Closely related to the validity of selection tests and standards is the question of the reliability of the measurements. Physical examinations for flying are often performed by physicians with varying backgrounds, training, and motivation; varying amounts of time and effort are expended on the actual examination. It is essential that the examiner be trained in aviation medicine and be aware of the problems. A routine physical examination will *never* suffice. It is realized that many factors altering the time spent are not always under the control of the examiner. Many defects are found during the course of thorough history-taking and physical examinations by consultants on persons who have had many previous flying-type examinations. More time and effort must be spent on these examinations, because in the continual selection process it is becoming increasingly important for the flight surgeon to detect significant variations within the range that in routine medical practice would be considered "normal." Unfortunately the average physician's training has been biased toward recognition of pathology (27), and he finds himself somewhat at a loss in trying to categorize normal.

To validate physical standards empirically, large numbers of applicants need to be examined and all entered into training regardless of findings. Naturally, any defect representing an obvious hazard to flight safety would require elimination; this in itself represents a compromise. Follow-up studies should be conducted to check the outcome of the test group as to safety, longevity, and proficiency in actual flight experience over a given period (29).

The radical type of acceptance study, referred to above, would provide normative data allowing the construction of tables useful in predicting the risk in returning an individual with such a condition to flying status. It is doubtful that such a program could ever be initiated, but there are numerous opportunities for follow-up studies under the present system of examination, selection, and classification. These opportunities should be exploited by all flight surgeons, for there is a great need for additional information on the natural course of certain medical conditions in the flying population.

The environment of the pilot of jet and rocket aircraft imposes a large number of stresses. These include reduced total and partial barometric pressures, temperature alterations, accelerations, disorientation, anxiety, and fatigue. The difference between civilian and military missions may cause the civilian situation to be regarded as less hazardous, but the environment at 35,000 ft. is no less hostile for the unprotected civilian than for the unprotected military aircrewman.

An obvious method of reducing the effects of these stresses is to select pilots and other crewmen who have superior tolerances. However, superior tolerances to single stresses may be overcome by the synergic action of multiple stresses (27). Hence, in spite of arguments concerning differences in tolerance acquired by the use of personal protective equipment, the physical standards must be high enough to insure some resistance to the hazards of unexpected events and resultant unprotected states.

Various agencies concerned with physical standards are still coping with the problem of developing reasonable standards for fliers. Physical standards for aircrew have recently undergone a critical appraisal by both military and civilian agencies and will continue to be periodically reviewed. As far as the Air Force appraisal is concerned, the most significant fact is that only a small number of actual major changes have been suggested by reviewers of present standards.

**Recent Additions to Physical Standards for Flying.** The detailed physical standards for flying may be found in *Air Force Manual 160-1* (USAF); *Army Regulation 40-501A* (USA); Chapter 15, Section V, *Manual of the Medical Department* (USN); and Part 29, *Civil Air Regulations*. The Air Force revision attempts to clarify the definition of questionable areas and to place the standards in a more functional order by arranging chapters by body systems.

The following discussion includes recent additions and proposals for changes in various physical standards believed to be of greatest interest and importance for jet flight.

WEIGHT. Obesity is of particular concern to the flight surgeon entrusted with the care of jet or rocket pilots. It has been shown to have some relationship to coronary artery disease and to dysbarism. The present Air Force weight tables are lenient in the maximal values allowed. Many pilots remain grossly overweight until a few weeks before their annual physical when they reduce to within one pound of their maximum allowable weight. They are still overweight! It is proposed to reduce the maximum allowable weight to a figure equal to the standard weight plus 15 per cent. This is a more reasonable figure, but still short of the ideal of lean body mass plus 10 per cent.

EYE. Inability to pass visual acuity standards has been the commonest cause of physical rejection in pilot selection. There has been no true validation of visual standards, but studies indicate that present visual standards could not be called standards of flying fitness. In determining standards for the trained pilot, true unfitness should be the criterion for grounding. Nevertheless, the speed and performance characteristics of jet and rocket aircraft require superior visual acuity and will do so until an enclosed cockpit with adequate instrument presentation is a reality. Distant visual acuity of 20/15 has been suggested as a requirement for high-performance aircraft. Byrnes (14) suggests requiring at least 0.5 diopter of hyperopia in all meridians for initial selection.

The present depth-perception examinations actually test binocular parallax, and this has been shown to have no relation to ability to land a fixed-wing aircraft. Motion parallax is related to this ability. The only value of binocular-parallax testing is the verification of the visual acuity and of the fact that two eyes are used simultaneously. A portable motion-parallax tester is in use at Lackland Air Force Base, Texas, for validation studies, but the high cost of the machine makes it impractical for use at smaller installations.

Color-vision requirements could be engineered out of the flying environment, but the test must be kept until this is done. The new standards will allow qualification by a passing score on the School of Aviation Medicine Color Threshold Tester if the standard plates are failed.

LUNG. No routine pulmonary-function tests are advised, but normal function is the important criterion. Segmental resections and total lobectomy should not be disqualifying per se, but function should determine the qualification.

EAR, NOSE, AND THROAT. A more stringent view has been taken concerning *allergic rhinitis*, for it has proved to be an in-flight problem. Emphasis is placed on the in-flight evaluation of hearing losses.

CARDIOVASCULAR SYSTEM. Speed and altitude and their effects exert adverse influences on the cardiovascular system, and thus a normally reacting cardiovascular system is a prime prerequisite to flying high-performance aircraft. The electrocardiogram (ECG) has proved to be a valuable tool in assessing cardiac integrity. Baseline ECG's on all flying personnel followed by repeated tests if over age forty are now required. The School of Aviation Medicine,

Brooks Air Force Base, Texas, has studied some 70,000 baseline ECG's on flying personnel as a basis for formulating more definitive ECG standards.

RETICULOENDOTHELIAL SYSTEM. In 1949 peculiarities in the arrangement of the hemoglobin molecule were blamed for the sickling phenomenon. The particular type of hemoglobin responsible was termed "S," or sickle, hemoglobin. Some nine inherited types of hemoglobin have now been identified by electrophoretic methods. These include "A" (normal), "F" (fetal), "C," etc. The abnormal hemoglobins may occur in homozygous form or in heterozygous combinations with either normal (A) hemoglobin or with another abnormal hemoglobin as S-C, etc. Homozygosity for an abnormal hemoglobin usually results in a disease state as sickle-cell disease or anemia (S-S). Heterozygous combinations of an abnormal and a normal hemoglobin are termed "traits" and usually do not result in an overt disease state. The frequent reports of *splenic infarction* following exposure of persons with A-S, S-S, and particularly S-C hemoglobins to altitude make rejection of such individuals for flying an important preventive-medicine measure.

STANDARDS FOR CIVIL AIRMEN. The Federal Aviation Agency changed its standards for civil airmen after study by the Flight Safety Foundation, Inc. Changes involved rejection for flying of those with: (1) established diagnosis of diabetes requiring insulin or other hypoglycemic agents for treatment, (2) a history of *myocardial infarction* or other evidence of coronary artery disease, and (3) a history of an established diagnosis of psychosis, severe psychoneurosis, severe personality abnormality, epilepsy, chronic alcoholism, and drug addiction (15).

**Physiological Training of Crew Members.** The tremendous financial investment in jet aircraft and personnel has led to increased use of simulators in the training of aircrews. Much effort has been expended in making simulators as nearly like the actual vehicle in design and reaction as is engineeringly possible. The use of these devices saves money, fuel, and training time, to say nothing of the reduction of the accident risk always present in training flights. The military services and the airlines have assigned large blocks of their transition and proficiency-training hours to simulator time. For example, a representative airline has its captains receive 20 hours of simulator experience and from 10 to 30 hours of in-flight transition.

First officers and flight engineers receive more simulator training and less in-flight training.

An important aspect of crew training, and one of primary concern here, is of a medical nature—physiological training. The problems of loss of cabin pressure and hypoxia as they concern the passengers will be discussed later.

The U.S. Air Force and the U.S. Navy by regulation require crews of high-altitude aircraft to undergo classroom and altitude chamber training at regular intervals. *Air Force Regulation 50-27* requires that personnel flying aircraft that normally operate in excess of 10,000 ft. or at high Mach numbers will remain proficient in aviation physiology. Refresher training is mandatory at least every three years and emphasizes new methods and equipment. The training consists of a series of lectures on the physiological effects of altitude, speed and acceleration, night vision, sensory illusions of flight, and oxygen equipment and of an altitude-chamber "flight" to 43,000 ft. with a rapid decompression from 8,000 to 22,000 ft. This training is of great value in preparing aircrews for emergencies. They are made aware of the hazards and develop a healthy respect for hypoxia, dysbarism, and related problems. In addition, crew members obtain the personal experience of exposure to altitude, both slowly and after a rapid decompression, and thus gain the opportunity to know their own reactions and the value of their protective equipment.

Crews assigned to aircraft operating at altitudes in excess of 50,000 ft. are required to wear partial or full pressure suits. At the time of fitting and issue of these protective garments, they are given a closely monitored chamber flight tailored usually to the mission profile of the particular aircraft. It instills confidence in their equipment to have personal assurance of its competence to protect at altitudes equal to or higher than that usually flown in the mission aircraft. Every effort is usually made to expose the crewmen to an altitude in excess of that anticipated on the mission and in a manner inspiring confidence and ease with a "routine type" operation.

The airlines are now facing the problem of high-altitude operations and are thus considering training. Some unfortunate incidents in chamber training of BOAC jet crews tended to cast some early doubts on the desirability or necessity of physiological training for commercial jet crews (34). The increased incidence of decreased-pressure phenomena (dysbarism) with age has also caused the airlines to worry, for with the seniority system it seems inevitable that the older pilots will fly the more lucrative "jet jobs."

The writer feels very strongly that physiological training including low-pressure chamber flights and rapid decompression should be mandatory for jet crews. These can be made innocuous and still be valuable training for emergencies. If there are crewmen who for age or other physical reasons should not be, or feel they should not be, exposed to altitudes in excess of 30,000 ft., then they should *not* be flying jet aircraft regardless of the number of arguments raised concerning the improbability of decompression of a jet airliner.

**Crew Oxygen Requirements.** Two interesting studies bearing on this topic have been completed. Barron and his associates (4) studied a group of 154 subjects decompressed from 8,000 to 30,000 ft. in 12 seconds. The time of useful consciousness (TUC) at 30,000 ft. with subjects at rest in an ideal environment is from 40 to 74 seconds. A factor that can never be duplicated in tests is the susceptibility of the individual crew member, which tends to vary greatly. Though 40 per cent of these subjects had used oxygen equipment previously, their mask-donning time increased with the delay in descent from altitude (usually 20 seconds) until at 60 seconds they were unable to don their masks at all. Even with the 20 seconds delay at 30,000 ft., 88 subjects had mild hypoxia symptoms (lightheadedness, dizziness, faintness), and 11 became confused and disoriented. All could apply masks by the time 15,000 ft. was reached, and all recovered completely within 30 seconds after the mask was applied.

Bryan (13) studied an experienced aircrew being indoctrinated to fly the RCAF Comet. They were given a 30,000-ft. chamber flight with hypoxia demonstration and then a decompression from 8,000 to 40,000 ft. in 15 seconds. Three subjects out of 26 were unable to don their masks. It was impossible to determine exact TUC's and was deemed wiser to assume that a delay of 5 seconds meant hypoxia. The conclusion from both these studies is that commercial jet aircrews should be indoctrinated in the altitude chamber.

These studies also support the conclusion that one pilot should wear his oxygen mask at all times. Until an adequate quick-donning mask is developed, the pilot in control of the aircraft should wear his oxygen mask during the entire flight above 25,000 ft. Each additional crew member should have a regulator and mask easily available for instant use. Ample oxygen should be available for the total flight time at cabin altitudes greater than 10,000 ft.

Either cabin attendants should carry portable oxygen equipment, or the aircraft should have ample extra outlets at each seat row and in galley, latrines, and other areas. It is most important that these attendants be thoroughly briefed and tested for their knowledge of both the physiology of hypoxia and the equipment available.

The Society of Automotive Engineers (SAE) subcommittee A-10 has drafted a set of recommendations for the altitude indoctrination of commercial jet transport crews. As proposed the indoctrination is to be required of pilots, flight crews, and stewardesses or cabin attendants and is similar to the Air Force program in requiring rein-doctrination every three years. It includes a comprehensive lecture and demonstration course, to be followed by an altitude-chamber flight and rapid decompression, with peak altitude equal to the pressure ambient altitude at which the indoctrinees are expected to fly.

**Aircrew Maintenance.** The selected and trained aircrewman must also receive proper maintenance, just as his aircraft, if both are to continue active flying careers. In the ideal program the crew would receive a great deal of aviation preventive-medicine support in the form of frequent "on the line" and "in the air" visits by the flight surgeon. Such frequent close observation in the working environment maintains flyer-flight surgeon rapport and enables early recognition of problem areas (mental or physical) before they become serious. Small warning signs, such as in-flight omissions or near misses, are observed and followed up by interviews with the crew member and his family to forestall any serious emotional problem.

Even with such an ideal program, however, the annual physical evaluation is an essential and important tool in proper crew maintenance. The objective of the examination is the prevention of serious illness by early detection and prompt treatment and the maintenance of a full-strength flying force—military or civilian. This will be successful only if the examination is viewed properly by both patient and physician. The patient (aircrewman) must be persuaded that the objective is to keep him flying and not to remove him from flying unless he is shown to be a safety hazard. He must cooperate in furnishing all pertinent details and in discussing his condition freely and fully. The flight surgeon on the other hand must realize his responsibility in trying to maintain operational effectiveness and also in doing a thorough and competent physical examination.

The flight surgeon frequently finds himself in conflict in deciding whether to think in the traditional manner (What is best for my patient?) or in a cold "man-machine complex" manner (Is this vital-link man capable of peak performance?). In actuality what is best from the latter concept is also best for the patient, for he may be spared a fatal accident.

In many instances, both military and civilian, the annual physical examination is looked upon as a necessary evil, as something the "healthy" aircrewman must go through for routine's sake and as something to take the busy flight surgeon away from more important patients. This examination, if properly conducted, may well be a lifesaving measure on occasion and is one of the most important acts the flight surgeon can perform. It should never be routine, hurried, or accomplished by a group of examiners on an assembly-line basis. The individual doctor-patient relationship should be utilized to the fullest extent in order to have a true understanding of the crewman's physical and mental status.

In the ideal relationship, when the flight surgeon conducts a thorough and painstaking initial examination followed by frequent "on the line" and in-flight visits, the aircrewman may feel free to consult the flight surgeon at the onset of any medical difficulty. In such a system it would be possible to reduce the frequency of examinations. Every attempt should be made to free the flight surgeon from non-productive and non-essential routine and to enable him to practice operational and aviation medicine.

Further, the conscientious performance of the examination is only part of the flight surgeon's responsibility in relation to the physical examination. In addition, the findings must be recorded properly and in detail. Attention should be directed to the fact that in both civilian and military situations the recorded results of the physical examination will often constitute the only source of information to decide whether or not a crewman may fly. The recording physician should attempt to think critically of the information needed to make a decision concerning any finding and record every pertinent detail.

Even an annual physical examination and frequent line visits will not assure perfect crew maintenance. The aircrewman has an individual responsibility to "keep in training" for his job and to use common sense and judgment in his exposure to stresses such as fatigue, alcohol, drugs, anxiety, and the like. The addition of these stresses to the stress of flying a high-performance aircraft can be deadly.

In recent years there has been an increasing interest in "executive physicals." These are detailed examinations of key personnel with the objective of recognizing stress, strain, and disease and of treating it effectively. The pilot population should always be treated as "executives," for the investment is great; but the number of special examination procedures done should be dictated by thorough history and not merely by routine.

The question of aging, that is, how long airmen can continue to fly actively, has been reopened in relation to jet flying. Is a man of sixty-five or seventy as capable of carrying out his pilot duties as a man of fifty or fifty-five, or, more simply, is he a "safe" crew member? There is no good medical evidence to answer these questions. However, the airlines are piling up experience by using many pilots in their fifties and even in the sixties. It is known that reaction times and dark adaptation decline with age, but the extent to which experience may compensate for any physiological deficiencies and for how long are still matters of conjecture. One crewman of sixty may have the physiological and mental function of a man of age twenty, while the reverse may also be true. Unfortunately there is no good yardstick by which to measure physiological age.

Kidera (22) has followed a group of 100 airline pilots for twenty years in the hope of observing some effects of their job on routine measurements. The age range was from forty-five to fifty-nine years. Some 20 per cent needed glasses to correct to 20/20, and 90 per cent were presbyopic. The average weight gain was only 10 lbs., and there was no increase in blood pressure. There was no evidence of premature deterioration or of any predilection to particular medical or surgical conditions. The airlines and the Federal Aviation Agency have attempted to meet this problem in the only manner possible at present, by setting an arbitrary age limit for retirement at sixty.

## Passengers

The "job" of the jet airliner passenger is generally only that of sitting and enjoying the flight. The majority of those flying as passengers, however, are on some business trip and must function effectively on arrival at their destinations. In the civil airlines and on some military passenger aircraft, every attempt is made to keep the passenger as comfortable as though he were sitting in his living room. Most of the stresses are potential or only threatened, such as hypoxia, dysbarism, acceleration, and cold. The modern jet airliners are pressurized and would expose passengers to these stresses only in the event of loss of cabin pressure. This is a possibility to be considered regardless of its remoteness, for unintentional decompressions occur in spite of the best engineering efforts. Intentional decompressions also occur at times.

Some stresses or effects of flight are not dependent on loss of pressurization. Apprehension may be caused by exposure to a new form of travel, loss of contact with Mother Earth, an engine sputter, or by a recent story in the headlines of an airliner crash. Fatigue may occur from excitement and planning, packing, and finally traveling. Jet aircraft cover great distances and cross many time zones in a few hours' flight, thus further deranging usual schedules and adding to fatigue. These factors also may disrupt the normal diurnal rhythm and interfere with social or business accomplishment. Allowance for these effects should be made by passengers in arranging their schedules.

**Pressure Changes.** TOTAL PRESSURE. The decrease in atmospheric pressure with increasing altitude has been covered earlier. Even though the jet cabin may be pressurized to simulated altitude of from 5,000 to 8,000 ft., the same pressure changes in the ears and sinuses will be noted as in conventional aircraft. Care should be taken to swallow or otherwise exert pressure on the eustachian-tube orifice to insure equalization of air pressure in the middle ear on descent.

DYSBARISM. Dysbarism has been mentioned briefly in an earlier chapter; but it is necessary here to analyze carefully the symptoms resulting from evolved gas as contrasted with those due to trapped gas. The various symptom complexes making up the dysbarism family tree are shown in Fig. 7–1.

An estimate of the incidence of dysbarism is very difficult to obtain, and there are no absolutely accurate figures. The only systematic data available have been obtained for altitude-chamber experience. These data reflect extensive variation, resulting from lack of control of many factors that have substantial effects, such as peak altitude, rate of ascent, time at altitude, and amount of exercise.

An arbitrary grading system is used in the USAF Physiological

Training Program, and these chamber flights are fairly well stand-ardized as to procedure, exposure, and other factors (17). Grade I is any slight unnatural sensation, Grade II is slight to moderate pain not requiring removal from or interruption of the chamber flight, Grade III is moderate to severe pain or other reactions requiring removal from the chamber, and Grade IV is any chamber reaction requiring admission to a hospital.

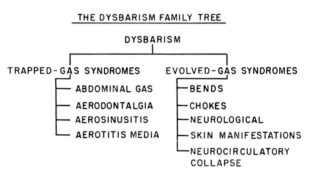

Fig. 7–1. The dysbarism family tree.

The occurrence of various symptom grades in 51,580 chamber trainees in the USAF Physiological Training Program in 1955 is shown in Table 7–1. Similar data for the year 1954 show that 17 per cent of individuals exposed developed some grade of dysbarism. Of these, 69 per cent were classified as Grade I; 26 per cent, Grade II; 4.7 per cent, Grade III; and 0.3 per cent, Grade IV. Of the small percentage of Grade IV cases, 62.3 per cent were mild, 36 per cent serious, and 1.7 per cent resulted in death (9).

TABLE 7–1

Symptoms by Grade in 51,580 Man-Chamber Flights, USAF, 1955
(Number per 100,000 Man-Flights)

| Symptom | Grade | | | |
|---|---|---|---|---|
| | I | II | III | IV |
| Ear | 6,650 | 2,347 | 514 | — |
| Abdominal pain | 2,738 | 1,187 | 322 | 12 |
| Bends | 1,594 | 642 | 155 | 21 |
| Sinus | 1,516 | 723 | 176 | — |
| Tooth | 285 | 142 | 118 | — |
| Chokes | 47 | 19 | — | 2 |
| Central nervous system | 12 | 6 | 6 | 4 |
| Other | 432 | 167 | 178 | 54 |

There have been several recent reports of severe in-flight dysbarism resulting in death and an increasing number of reports of
in-flight dysbarism in which the victims recovered (11). The majority of these have occurred in jet trainer aircraft (T-33). Recent
emphasis on this subject has uncovered more in-flight cases as flight
surgeons watch for and report them. The actual number of such
cases remains unknown, but at present they represent an extremely
small percentage when compared to the total hours of exposure
flown each year. As the civil jet airliners frequent higher altitudes,
it is possible that passengers also may encounter this hazard if pressurization is lost.

The symptoms noted include *bends*, a deep, aching bone pain
usually near the joints and similar to the pain experienced when one
is struck in the testicles; *chokes*, a burning substernal sensation,
and non-productive cough; any number of *neurological symptoms*
ranging from paresthesias to paralysis and loss of visual fields; *skin
manifestations* ranging from prickling sensations to a bluish-red mot-
tling or rash; and, lastly, a combination of neurological and circulatory symptoms frequently resulting in collapse and thus called *neurocirculatory collapse* or severe dysbarism.

Most cases of severe dysbarism have the other symptoms before
they develop neurocirculatory collapse. Consequently, this latter
condition is discussed in the remainder of this section. In a recent
study of the records of 125 Grade IV chamber reactors, an attempt
was made to divide the reactors into groups based on the symptomatology (12). The two largest groups noted were: (1) 52 per
cent who experienced bends, chokes, gas, etc., as initial symptoms
followed by syncope or signs of impending syncope with recovery
by the time ground level was reached or within a few minutes thereafter and (2) 37.6 per cent with any of numerous neurological signs
and symptoms who either proceed to recovery or have residual
defect. Bends was the most frequently reported first symptom in
both groups, and loss of consciousness was the most frequent in the
chamber. Severe skin reactions occurred five times more frequently
in the neurological group than in the others. They should be considered a serious sign.

The following brief report of an in-flight case of severe dysbarism
may be helpful in elucidating this syndrome.

This forty-five-year-old USAF pilot departed Randolph Air Force Base at
0850 hours on January 15, 1959, in a T-33. He had eaten a breakfast consist-

ing of dry toast, black coffee, and grapefruit. He was flying from the rear cockpit. A rapid climb was made as the aircraft reached an ambient altitude of 35,000 ft. over the San Antonio omnirange. Cabin altitude for the entire flight ranged between 26,000 and 28,000 ft.

The patient flew the aircraft for one hour and twenty-five minutes after take-off when he complained of tingling of the arms, lightheadedness, and incoordination of the left hand. He asked the other pilot to take the controls and asked that the cabin heat be turned up. He then turned his oxygen regulator to 100 per cent as he felt his oxygen mask was leaking over his nose. Five minutes later they descended to 28,000 ft. where the cabin altitude was from 16,000 to 18,000 ft. The other pilot landed at Biggs Air Force Base at 1110 hours. (The oxygen system of the T-33 was checked and found to be in satisfactory operating condition.)

Immediately on landing the patient was noted to be ashen in color, perspiring, and breathing heavily. He was unable to get out of the cockpit unaided due to weakness of his left arm and left leg. He was assisted to a litter, started on 100 per cent oxygen, and immediately examined. He seemed to be well oriented and could answer questions. His pulse was 80 and blood pressure 130/85, and the only abnormal finding on cursory examination was a positive Hoffman reflex on the left. An electrocardiogram revealed T-wave inversion in leads I, V5, and V6.

On admission to the hospital approximately three and a half hours after take-off his blood pressure was 114/66, pulse 84, respiratory rate 22, and temperature 101° F (R). His speech was slurred, but he could sit upright and was coherent. A left facial paralysis and weakness and paresthesia of the left arm were noted. His height was recorded as 75 inches and his weight as 212 lbs.

One and one-half hours later his temperature was still 101° F (R), pulse 88, and blood pressure 128/70. He was very lethargic and restless with a very short span of attention. The left pupil was larger than the right, and both reacted sluggishly to light. The visual fields were decreased and showed bitemporal hemianopia. The Hoffman sign was negative.

Two hours later the vital signs were still stable, and a lumbar puncture was done. Pressure and fluid were normal, and the only fluid removed was for the necessary laboratory studies.

That evening the patient complained of severe aching and discomfort "all over his body," and he still had a left-arm weakness. A repeat electrocardiogram confirmed the previous findings. At 2000 hours the patient developed incontinence of urine and feces and then became disoriented, confused, semistuporous, and began to thrash about the bed. He was found to have a left hemiparesis and a temperature of 102° F (R), but vital signs all remained in normal range throughout his course.

The following day he continued lethargic, drowsy, and restless, and the left hemiplegia was unchanged. The hematocrit and white-blood count were elevated. As the case was neurological in type, he was only treated supportively. That evening he developed a right-foot drop and the following day a right facial and ninth nerve paresis. The left-sided findings improved, and the right-sided ones progressed in the next twenty-four hours. During the next few days he improved rapidly, but thirteen days after the incident he still needed assistance to walk and was unable to dorsiflex the right foot. There was residual weakness of the left arm and hand, and the Babinskis were bilaterally positive.

The white-blood count and hematocrit returned to normal, as did the ECG. Serial EEG's showed abnormal paroxysmal rhythms and generalized non-specific dominance of slow activity compatible with cerebral hypoxia—diffuse organic brain syndrome.

Two months after the incident the EEG was still abnormal, and there was weakness of the left arm and hand and a right-foot drop. Such residual is not common in this condition but is seen.

Many factors have been studied for their effect on the development of dysbarism, but the most definite ones are age and weight (6). An increase in either of these has been shown to increase the incidence of dysbarism. Exercise at altitude also will produce more symptoms. Some investigators have stated that old fractures are predisposed to the development of dysbarism, but it seems that recent sprains and contusions are more potent in this regard, probably due to poor circulation in the area.

Residence at altitude has been shown to have a preventive action. Doctor Bruno Balke of the Air Force School of Aviation Medicine found that bends following exercise at 38,000 ft. could be prevented by residing at an altitude of 14,800 ft. for forty-eight hours prior to the exposure. Other host factors such as inherent susceptibility, apprehension, fatigue, and the like await further study.

The following environmental factors have been shown to increase the occurrence of dysbarism: increasing altitude of flight above 30,000 ft., increasing time at altitude, rapid rate of ascent, cold, and vibration. In the study of 125 reactors, it was noted that a long exposure time above 30,000 ft. is not necessary, for 90 per cent of the reactors had less than ten minutes over 30,000 ft. before developing severe dysbarism. An altitude of 30,000 ft. is generally used as a round figure to remember as the starting altitude for dysbarism. Recent reports have shown several in-flight cases and even deaths to have occurred at altitudes as low as 22,000 ft. Therefore, we should lower our sights at least to 25,000 ft. in looking for this condition.

The clinical course of these cases of neurocirculatory collapse may progress to primary shock and then recovery, or it may progress directly to secondary shock with or without unconsciousness. There may be a period of compensated normality between the two shock periods. Recovery is the rule, but deaths do occur, and residua of neurological abnormality have persisted (11).

The therapy of these cases is still largely supportive and symptomatic. Early recognition is most important. As these cases are rather rare and scattered, no one individual has seen a large number, and thus therapy has been extremely varied. The Royal Air Force has formed a team which is called to see all such cases, whether fatal or not. Thought has been given to doing the same in the United States Air Force. The time lag is important, however, and most of these cases are severe enough to frighten the average physician into either bothering the patient as little as possible or trying a number of drugs in the hope of improving his status.

Any person with well-defined evolved-gas symptoms should be hospitalized for observation. Intravenous-fluid therapy should be initiated early in order to assure an open vein in case of rapid shock development. Initial use of a mixture of 95 per cent oxygen and 5 per cent carbon dioxide is indicated to combat cerebral vasospasm. There are arguments concerning the use of vasoconstrictors or vasodilators. If the patient is in shock, it would be difficult to keep from using the usual vasoconstrictors. Stellate block, intravenous procaine, cortisone, and ACTH might also be considered. In the writer's estimation spinal tap should be used as a diagnostic procedure if indicated, but its therapeutic use is questionable. The availability of chambers capable of compression to greater than atmospheric pressure as well as decompression will allow study of this theoretically indicated measure. A recent Air Force report described the first successful use of compression in the treatment of a severe case of dysbarism.

The disposition of these cases still poses a problem for the military. Individuals who have residual defects are no problem for they cannot return to flying. Are those who have recovered from a serious episode more susceptible? We believe so and thus in the military services cannot return them to flying duty. As civilian passengers, however, the only limitation would be to insist on pressurized aircraft, and then the risk is the same as for the other passengers until decompression.

The development of this condition may then be prevented by maintaining the passengers and crew at a pressure equivalent below

25,000 ft. through cabin pressurization. If it is necessary to go above this as in some military aircraft, the individual may be protected by proper denitrogenation prior to or during the early stages of the flight. Attempts to select dysbarism-resistant individuals have had little success, for there are too many factors involved.

The etiology of dysbarism is generally conceded to be the release of nitrogen bubbles from body fluids and tissues, principally fat, when decompressed. There is still a great deal of argument as to whether these bubbles are intravascular or extravascular. There seems little doubt that other mechanisms are also involved, probably initiated by the nitrogen bubbles, for the symptoms do not always clear on recompression to sea level. Vasospasm, blood sludging, *fat emboli*, and fatty livers have all been implicated in theories of etiology. The finding of fatty emboli and *patent foramens ovale* in many of the fatal cases lends interest to this study.

PARTIAL PRESSURE. The partial pressure of oxygen is of primary concern. Again this is an acute problem only in the event of loss of pressurization in the commercial airliners. In military aircraft oxygen is used by crew and passengers alike when flying above 10,000 ft.

Many of the military transport-type aircraft which might carry passengers are unpressurized and must depend on flight profiles below 10,000 ft. or on the availability of proper oxygen equipment to maintain adequate oxygen partial pressures. A recent amendment to *Air Force Regulation 50–27* requires that "All passengers and maintenance personnel who fly in jet aircraft, other than transport aircraft with C-designation, at or above 18,000 feet mean sea level must have received training within the last three years." This training must include the classes and the chamber flight. Care should be taken to avoid prolonged exposure of unprotected passengers to borderline altitudes of from 10,000 to 14,000 ft.

There has been a great deal of controversy about the use of oxygen in the jet airliners. As there is no proof available that a jet liner cannot decompress and every indication that it might, some rules concerning the availability of oxygen are mandatory. Those evolved by the Committee on Aircraft Oxygen Equipment of the Society of Automotive Engineers as Aircrew Recommended Practice (ARP)-505 are based upon sound principle and are reasonable (2).

The new Federal Aviation Agency regulations concerning oxygen equipment in jet aircraft became effective on November 30, 1959.

In essence they embody the SAE recommendations. Aircraft manufacturers had anticipated these requirements and attempted to reduce the retrofit problems by including the required equipment in the jets.

After a great deal of discussion, it was agreed that the individual passenger should be oxygenated with a mask which would be automatically presented in case of decompression and which would also be easily donned. Oxygen would then be available to all passengers for a limited period and in high concentrations to a few passengers (who may require it for physiological reasons). Both American- and foreign-built jet transports have adopted these fundamentals.

In the Boeing 707, the oxygen masks are stowed in closed pods arranged transversely above each seat row. In the event of decompression, an automatic sensing device responds to the drop in cabin pressure and automatically turns on the oxygen system, whereupon the pods are automatically opened and oxygen masks dropped within reach of the passengers. No oxygen is delivered to the mask until such time as the passenger grasps it and pulls it downward to his face. When this is done, the traction on the mask tube trips an oxygen-flow control valve which causes oxygen to be delivered to the mask. Thus, the oxygen is not wasted, because none is consumed unless the mask is actually in use.

In the Comet IV, the same principle is used except that the mask compartments, instead of being transversely arranged, are placed longitudinally along the bottom of the hatrack. In the event of cabin decompression, the change in cabin pressure is sensed by a barometrically controlled trigger valve which activates the oxygen system, causing the compartments to open and drop the masks within reach of the passengers. The action of the passenger in pulling the mask to his face trips the oxygen-flow control valve, allowing oxygen to be delivered to the mask (24).

This same basic system is being installed in the Sud Caravelle and in the Bristol Britannia.

In the Douglas DC-8 the general arrangement is the same except that the masks instead of being located in overhead compartments are located in the seatback. The mask compartment is normally closed, but in the event of decompression, an altitude pressure-sensing device turns on the oxygen-system pressure which causes each compartment to open, exposing the masks to view and within reach of the user. When the mask is picked up from the tray and applied to the face, the traction on the mask tube actuates an oxygen valve controlling the flow of oxygen to each mask (24).

In the Convair 880 the mask compartments are transversely arranged and recessed into the bottom of the hatrack. Loss of cabin pressure triggers a barometric control which activates the oxygen system, causing the compartment to open and the masks to drop. Oxygen flows to each mask when the mask is grasped and pulled downward to the passenger's face (24).

A great deal has been said about crew indoctrination, but it is obvious also that the passengers will need some briefing. If carefully and thoroughly done, the passengers need not be frightened any more than they are by Mae West demonstrations for overwater flights. It is essential that they realize that this knowledge is of importance to them in case of emergency.

The briefings observed to date by the writer (on the Boeing 707) have not been thorough and did not mention and emphasize that the passengers must pull on the mask and hose to initiate oxygen flow. Further, it is necessary to exert suction to open the mask inlet valves. There have also been complaints that the hose from the overhead container to the mask slips off the C-lever, and thus pull does not initiate oxygen flow to the mask. This connection is only designed to withstand a 20-lb. pull, and in the excitement of decompression, it may be pulled off.

The United States Air Force has purchased some Boeing 707 aircraft to be designated CV-137's. The oxygen equipment delivered in these aircraft lacks many of the features supplied in the commercial versions.

**Turbulence.** In the civilian jet aircraft turbulence is a minor problem, due to aircraft characteristics and altitudes flown. In the military fighter-type jets nausea is sometimes experienced on the pitch-out landing approach and, of course, during acrobatic maneuvers.

**Physical Requirements for Passengers.** The jet airliners, in general, have provided greater passenger comfort, for they shorten the travel time and so reduce fatigue, provide excellent food and drink, and have a comfortably air-conditioned, pressurized cabin. Thus, it would certainly appear that anyone who can travel should be able to do so by air. This is true of the healthy passenger unless he has an abiding fear of flying. It is also almost true for the passenger-patient.

The expanding airline network and the many advantages of jet aircraft mean that inevitably more ambulatory patients will become, or will try to become, passengers. Indeed, many patients fly to and from the larger medical centers in many stages of illness and disease. The military services have established air evacuation as the method to be used in transporting patients either overseas or in the continental United States. In our air-minded world the physician, general practitioner, and specialist alike must be aware of the forms of aerial transportation and their problems if he is to answer his patient's needs. There are large numbers of air ambulances available for private hire, and these are generally equipped for in-flight care. Here, however, attention is directed to the large group of patient-passengers who may purchase jet airliner tickets.

The differences, or in most cases potential differences, between the environment of the patient traveling by air and that of the patient traveling by surface transportation have been discussed previously. Any effects of such travel on the patient must be considered in the light of these environmental changes.

It is the job of the physician to understand these changes and to evaluate his patient in the light of the resulting stresses. He must then make a knowledgeable decision concerning travel by air. The physician must understand the things that can cause apprehension and relieve this apprehension by timely explanation. He also must be aware of the relevant characteristics of the aircraft to be used and of the provisions made for coping with the atmospheric changes noted previously.

Most airliners are pressurized and are thus able to maintain a maximum cabin altitude of 8,000 ft. during any portion of the flight. The pressure differentials of the various airliners are available and should be considered in evaluating air travel; see Table 7–2. The pressure in pounds per square inch (psi) at the flight altitude must be added to the pressure differential of the aircraft in order to determine cabin altitude. For example, a jet liner flying at 35,000 ft. would have a simulated cabin altitude of 6,250 ft. The pressure at 35,000 ft. is 3.46 psi; the pressure differential of a typical jet is 8.2; the total is then 11.66 psi, which is the pressure at approximately 6,250 ft.

TABLE 7–2

Cabin-Pressure Differentials for Various Aircraft

| Type of Aircraft | Normal Pressure Differential (psi) | Maximum Pressure Differential (psi) * |
|---|---|---|
| DC-6 | 4.16 | — |
| Viscount | 5.41 | — |
| DC-7 | 5.46 | — |
| Boeing 707 | 8.60 | 9.40 |
| Douglas DC-8 | 8.77 | 9.27 |
| Convair 880 | 8.20 | 8.50 |

* Pressure differential at which the relief valve is activated.

**Patient Selection** (10). The military services have set up an elaborate aeromedical evacuation system with some broad criteria for patient selection (16). The following types of cases are ordinarily not acceptable for air transportation by the Military Air Transport Service (MATS):

1. Patients in infectious stages of a quarantinable disease
2. Patients with a fatal prognosis, in a moribund or semimoribund state, unless lifesaving measures are available at the destination hospital which are not available at the point of origin
3. Patients with permanently fixed tie wires between the jaws.

Other cases require special consideration before acceptance:

1. Conditions involving cardiac failure
2. Severe anemias
3. Respiratory embarrassment
4. Conditions in which quantities of gas are confined in body cavities, such as pneumothorax.

In order to allow better scheduling and handling of patients, a patient classification system is utilized. All neuropsychiatric patients are placed in Class I, which is subdivided into categories for locked-ward patients requiring restraints and sedation (Class IA), locked-ward patients not requiring restraints but who do require watching (Class IB), and open-ward patients (Class IC). All other litter patients are placed in Class II which has immobile (IIA) and mobile (IIB) subdivisions. Class III is made up of walking patients requiring medical care, and Class IV consists of walking patients requiring no care.

It should be emphasized that the selection and classification procedures mentioned are for use in a very formalized air transport system operated by the Military Air Transport Service. Whereas these same selection and classification procedures apply in general to all aeromedical evacuation, in the air rescue and tactical aeromedical evacuation system they are frequently ignored in order to provide more rapid definitive medical care to the seriously injured. Indeed, it has been found that any patient who is transportable by any means can be transported by air if the proper facilities are available. Some evidence confirming this statement may be found in a summary of 41 air-rescue missions in the Caribbean area (7). These cases included numerous acute abdomens, burns, fractures, and head injuries, and only one in-flight death occurred. This death involved a patient with third-degree burns over approximately 80 per cent of his body.

Though the severity of illness is not the same, the airlines and air-rescue or front-line (tactical) aeromedical evacuation have much in common in that there is little selection of patients. Almost anyone can purchase an airline ticket, and a medical history or physical examination is not a prerequisite to such a purchase. The Air Transport Association regulations direct carriers to refuse to carry any passenger whose status, age, and physical or mental condition are such as to (1) render him incapable of caring for himself unless he is accompanied by an attendant, (2) render him objectionable to other passengers, and (3) involve hazard or risk to himself or other persons or property. As the only selection is done by the airline agent, very few passengers are rejected unless they are obviously intoxicated or show overt signs of an infectious disease.

Therefore, any screening requires the patient's cooperation by volunteering information or his exhibiting illness easily recognizable by non-medical personnel. Any attempt at further screening is impractical. It is of importance for the physician to discuss the possible modes of travel with his patient. After evaluation of the probable effect of altitude on the patient's condition, if air travel is elected, the patient should be given a letter notifying the airline of his condition and clearing him for such travel.

**Specific Problems in Air Transport of Patients.** Travel by air requires special consideration in some cases because of the mild hypoxia involved. Smoking and use of alcoholic beverages may add to the hypoxia produced by altitude.

CARDIAC CASES. Hypoxia increases cardiac output and therefore increases the workload of the heart. Any patient whose heart is in a borderline or frankly overworked state would be harmed by exposure to low-oxygen tensions. Patients with congestive failure should fly only if oxygen is available for their continuous use; those with recent myocardial infarction (within six weeks) should not fly. If ambulatory, they may fly with oxygen available.

Patients with *angina* brought on by slight exertion should be rejected for air travel according to recommendations of the Air Transport Association Medical Committee (21). *Hypertensives* with diastolic pressures above 110 should be carefully evaluated before flight, and mild preflight sedation is recommended.

A committee of the American College of Chest Physicians has recommended a more detailed and complicated system based upon cabin altitudes of 6,000 and 8,000 ft. Patients with major cardiac disorders with adequate functional reserve at sea level could go to an 8,000-ft. cabin altitude, and those with cardiac conditions in which myocardial oxygen is marginal should not go over a 6,000-ft. cabin altitude.

Graybiel (20) has prepared a table which is useful in determining the severity of flight stress by evaluating such factors as distance to the airport, number of steps in ramp, duration of flight, weather, and the like. He then classified various cardiac conditions as to their ability to withstand three different degrees of flight stress.

PULMONARY CASES. Asthmatic and other pulmonary conditions have received special study because of the possibility of patients with these conditions being more likely to develop symptomatic hypoxia. In a study of cardiopulmonary patients transported on MATS air-evacuation aircraft (non-pressurized) flying below 10,000 ft., only 6 of some 215 patients with asthmatic conditions manifested symptoms. Three of these had acute attacks of asthma. This shows there is no contraindication to an asthmatic patient's being flown if he is under control with medication and oxygen is available. Patients with *pneumonia, atelectasis, lung neoplasm,* and *pleural effusions* were also flown with few symptoms reported (30).

Poliomyelitis cases should be flown only in an air ambulance or in a military (MATS) aircraft. The airlines will not accept a patient in a respirator. A patient with acute poliomyelitis should not be flown, for physical activity has been shown to have an adverse effect on such cases. The National Foundation has made arrangements with the Department of Defense and the Air Force to transport poliomyelitis patients via MATS air-evacuation aircraft. Special teams and the School of Aviation Medicine portable respirator are used.

Certain precautions are necessary before transporting such a patient. Adequate ventilation must be assured by use of a device such as the Bennett ventilometer to obtain the actual tidal air. This actual value is then compared with the required value found on the Radford nomogram. A *tracheotomy* should be done if there is bulbar involvement producing difficulty in swallowing or if secretions are excessive. A chest roentgenogram should be taken twenty-four hours prior to flight to rule out atelectasis. Constant in-flight care is necessary with particular regard for removing secretions that tend to thicken in the dry air at altitude and for maintaining adequate respiratory function in the less dense air in which the respirator is less efficient (18).

Pulmonary function and reserve must be evaluated in order to decide the propriety of transporting persons with such conditions as *pneumonia, asthma, cancer,* and *emphysema.* The American College of Chest Physicians' recommendations again are more detailed and restrict patients with severe emphysema to altitudes below 4,000 ft. *Acidosis* or severely limited ventilation by *fibrosis* should contraindicate flying. Patients with tuberculosis, both active and arrested, have been flown. The only contraindications are the usual ones of communicability in the active cases and of caution in those treated by pneumothorax.

ANEMIAS. Severe anemia of any type interferes with oxygen transport, thereby producing an anemic type of hypoxia which can only be made more severe by the addition of altitude hypoxia. The Air Transport Association states that persons with hemoglobins down to 60 per cent may be flown, but oxygen should be available.

In 1947 Sullivan (31) reported the case of an eighteen-year-old Negro soldier who developed nausea, vomiting, and left upper quadrant pain during a flight from the East Coast to California at an altitude of from 10,000 to 16,000 ft. These complaints occurred on the return flight and persisted. Sickling was found on examination of his blood. Since that time more than 30 cases exhibiting the triad of *splenic infarction, sicklemia,* and *aerial-flight disturbances* have been reported. It is interesting that sickle-cell disease (all S hemoglobin) is not necessary, for many of the patients have had only sickle-cell trait. Electrophoretic analysis of hemoglobin has been helpful in studying these cases. Some cases of splenic infarction have been reported in Negroes who flew in commercial airliners at cabin altitudes of only 4,000 to 6,000 ft. All these cases have had sickle-cell–C-hemoglobin disease, which indicates that patients whose hemoglobin analysis shows S and C hemoglobin should be advised not to fly at all or only with supplementary oxygen being used. If current investigations demonstrate that pressure diminution alone may produce sickling in those individuals with S-C hemoglobin, then they should not fly at all.

EYE CONDITIONS. The importance of minimizing or avoiding the effects of both hypoxia and gas expansion in eye cases must be stressed if vision and even the globe itself are to be preserved. The injured or postsurgical eye may have air injected in the anterior chamber to re-form it. Flight at low altitudes or in pressure cabins is necessary to prevent gas expansion. Above cabin altitudes of 10,000 ft., hypoxia produces measurable dilation of the retinal and choroid vessels, a rise in intraocular tension, and a decrease in pupil diameter. All these changes produce adverse effects in the injured or postsurgical eye case. The retina has the highest oxygen demand of any body tissue. Therefore, patients with eye conditions should have oxygen or cabin pressurization above 4,000 ft. (10).

GASTROINTESTINAL SURGERY. The intestine always harbors some gas and ordinarily can handle its expansion by elimination, either orally or rectally. Occasionally spasm or other abnormality may render this elimination difficult or impossible, and the intestine will be distended. This is not desirable in acute abdominal or post-surgical cases. A ten-day delay between surgery and air transportation is suggested. Gas expansion will cause more peritoneal soiling in a ruptured ulcer, although such cases have been transported successfully. Patients who have had a *colostomy* should be warned of the expansion problem and advised that their colostomy bags should be slightly larger than usual.

PNEUMOTHORAX. Although patients with pneumothorax have been flown with little difficulty, these cases are still cause for careful evaluation in regard to size and expected expansion. Dowd (19) has reported the death of a patient flying aboard a Canadian airliner after a pneumothorax refill. If such patients are to be flown, emergency equipment for needling the chest and individuals experienced in its use should be available.

NEUROSURGICAL COMPLICATIONS. Patients who have had air studies (ventriculograms and the like) should not be flown until the air has been replaced by fluid.

PREGNANCY. Most airlines feel that the only contraindication to air transport of the pregnant woman is the danger of delivery during flight. A pregnant woman is accepted for flight without question through the eighth month. During the ninth month of pregnancy, she will be accepted if she furnishes a certificate from her physician dated within seventy-two hours of departure indicating that he has examined her and found her to be physically fit for transportation from one given place to another on a certain date and estimating the date for the birth. Such patients should select rearward facing seats to allow use of only a loosely fastened lap belt across the legs. The patient should be warned of possible gas expansion in the gut and the possibility of *dyspnea*. False labor contractions following flight in the last month of pregnancy are not uncommon. In many cases travel by air may be less traumatic than ordinary surface means of transportation.

FRACTURES OF THE MANDIBLE. The basic problem in transporting patients with fractures of the mandible is the possibility of their developing airsickness. Any patient with permanent wiring between jaws should not travel by air, because, with the onset of airsickness, he may vomit before such tie wires could be removed. Either a cotter or ripcord mechanism for quick release should be employed with elastic bands (32). The incidence of motion sickness can be reduced by the use of Bonamine, Benadryl, or 'Marezine' (50 mg three times a day); Phenergan (25 mg three times a day); or Dramamine (100 mg three times a day). Medication should be started one hour prior to flight and continued during the flight pattern.

NEUROPSYCHIATRIC CONDITIONS. Epilepsy tends to manifest itself at altitude due to apprehension, hyperventilation, and hypoxia. Consideration of sedation, reassurance, and oxygen may prevent such difficulty. In advising a psychiatric patient to fly, the safety of the other passengers should be considered. Certainly if the patient requires sedation and restraint, he must be transported in an air ambulance. Recent studies (33) have shown such patients do as well continuing on the *ataractic* drugs as being given 7.5 grains of Amytal preflight. Further studies are under way on the transport of patients with head injuries and on the use of drugs.

COMMUNICABLE DISEASE. Patients with a communicable disease are not accepted for flight because of the danger to others. Particular care is taken to avoid transportation of one of the internationally quarantinable diseases (cholera, plague, typhus, relapsing fever, yellow fever, and smallpox). The contraindications to flight are not engendered by the danger to the patient but by the public health import of such movement. The cooperation of the public and the medical profession is vital if such patients are to be excluded from air travel, for the airline ticket agent will be unable to diagnose the prospective passenger at the time of ticket purchase.

INFANTS AND THE AGED. Infants are accepted by most airlines as soon as they leave the hospital. The Air Transport Association believes infants should not be transported great distances by air until they reach seven days of age because of their lack of ability to stand a respiratory disease (23). Some airlines have reported a higher incidence of ear trouble in infants, but the anatomy indicates there should be less. The nursing infant should be given bottle or breast during descent in order to keep the eustachian tubes open by the swallowing movements. There are no contraindications to flight based on age alone.

BURNS. Recent experience indicates that even patients with extensive burns involving nearly 100 per cent of the body surface may be safely transported by air in the first twenty-four to thirty-six hours after the burn. The burn is unique in that it is one of the few injuries that early transportation not only will do no harm but is often mandatory for safety of the patient (26).

## References

1. *Air Service Medical Manual*, U.S. Army Air Corps. Government Printing Office, Washington, D.C., 1918. P. 11.
2. *Aircrew Recommended Practice* (*ARP*)-505. Oxygen Equipment, Provisioning and Use in High Altitude Commercial Transport Aircraft. Society of Automotive Engineers Committee A-9, November, 1957.
3. *Aviation Medicine in the AEF*. Government Printing Office, Washington, D.C., 1920. P. 9.

4. BARRON, C. I., COLLIER, D. I., and COOK, T. J. 1958. Observations on simulated 12-second decompressions to 32,000 feet. *J. Aviation Med.* 29: 563.
5. BERGIN, K. G. 1959. Medical aspects of civil jet air transport operations. *J. Aviation Med.* 30: 22.
6. BERRY, C. A. 1956. Dysbarism—An Epidemiological Analysis. Harvard School of Public Health master's thesis.
7. BERRY, C. A. 1958. Medical problems of air rescue. *J. Aviation Med.* 29: 316.
8. BERRY, C. A. 1958. The role of physical standards in jet and rocket aircraft flight. *J. Aviation Med.* 29: 631.
9. BERRY, C. A. 1958. Severe dysbarism in air force operations and training. *U.S. Armed Forces Med. J.* 9: 937.
10. BERRY, C. A. 1958. Transport of patients by air. *Texas State J. Med.* 54: 11.
11. BERRY, C. A., and KING, A. H. 1959. Severe dysbarism in actual and simulated flight. *U.S. Armed Forces Med. J.* 10: 1.
12. BERRY, C. A., and WAYNE, H. H. 1958. *Grade IV Chamber Reactions or Instances of Neurocirculatory Collapse Occurring in the U.S. Air Force, 1950–1955.* (Report 58–85.) USAF, Air University, School of Aviation Medicine, Randolph Air Force Base, Tex.
13. BRYAN, A. C. 1958. *Rapid Decompression in Transport Aircraft.* (RCAF Report IAM 58/3.) Institute of Aviation Medicine, Royal Canadian Air Force, Toronto, Canada.
14. BYRNES, V. A. 1957. Discussion of papers by Major J. J. Claro and Doctor H. W. Rose. In *Symposium: Physical Standards and Selection.* USAF, Air University, School of Aviation Medicine, Randolph Air Force Base, Tex. Pp. 66–70.
15. *Civil Air Regulations Amendment 29–2.* Physical Standards for Airmen; Medical Certificates. Federal Register, 24 F.R. 7309, 11 September 1959.
16. DEPARTMENT OF THE AIR FORCE. *Air Force Regulation 160–52.* Aeromedical Evacuation. Washington, D.C. 28 October 1955.
17. DEPARTMENT OF THE AIR FORCE. *Air Force Regulation 50–27.* Air Force Physiological Training Program. Washington, D.C. 23 September 1958.
18. DEPARTMENT OF THE AIR FORCE. *Air Force Pamphlet 160–5–15.* Poliomyelitis. Washington, D.C. 8 August 1956.
19. DOWD, K. E. 1945. Report of death of passenger under treatment by pneumothorax. *J. Aviation Med.* 16: 346–349.
20. GRAYBIEL, A. 1954. Air travel and heart disease. *Modern Concepts Cardiovascular Disease* 23: 217.
21. KIDERA, G. J. 1958. Medical and surgical considerations in selecting airline passengers. *N.Y. State J. Med.* 58: 853.
22. KIDERA, G. J. 1958. Twenty-year study of physiological measurements in one hundred senior airline pilots. *J. Am. Med. Assoc.* 168: 1188.
23. McFARLAND, R. A. 1953. *Human Factors in Air Transportation: Occupational Health and Safety.* McGraw-Hill Book Co., Inc., New York.
24. MILLER, A. E. 1959. Final philosophy and design of oxygen equipment for jet transports. Paper presented at 30th Annual Meeting Aero Medical Assoc., Los Angeles, Calif., April, 1959.
25. MOSELEY, H. G. 1957. Aero Medical Research in Cockpit Factors. Memorandum for the Surgeon General, USAF.
26. PILLSBURY, R. D., MACMILLAN, BRUCE D., and ARTZ, CURTIS, P. 1957. Experiences in air evacuation of severely burned patients. *Military Med.* 120: 349.
27. POWELL, T. J. 1957. Medical selection for high performance aircraft. *Can. Serv. Med. J.* 13: 349.
28. POWELL, W. H. 1957. The philosophy of physical standards for military service. In *Symposium: Physical Standards and Selection.* USAF, Air University, School of Aviation Medicine, Randolph Air Force Base, Tex. Pp. 5–14.

29. SELLS, S. B., and BURWELL, R. R. 1957. The establishment of norms. In *Symposium: Physical Standards and Selection.* USAF, Air University, School of Aviation Medicine, Randolph Air Force Base, Tex. Pp. 77–90.
30. STRICKLAND, B., and DOWNEY, V. 1954. *Effects of Aeromedical Evacuation on Various Clinical Conditions: In-Flight Symptoms of Cardio-pulmonary Patients.* (Project 21–40–002, Report 3.) USAF, Air University, School of Aviation Medicine, Randolph Air Force Base, Tex.
31. SULLIVAN, B. H., JR. 1950. Danger of airplane flight to persons with sicklemia. *Ann. Internal Med.* 32: 338.
32. SZMYD, L., McCALL, C. M., HARTLEY, J. L., SHANNON, I. L., and GIBILISCO, J. C. 1957. *Emergency Oral Medicine.* USAF, Air University, School of Aviation Medicine, Randolph Air Force Base, Tex.
33. WARD, J. 1957. *Trip Report on Research Task 7759–4: Improvement in Care and Handling of Neuropsychiatric Patients Evacuated by Air.* USAF, Air University, School of Aviation Medicine, Randolph Air Force Base, Tex.
34. WHITTINGHAM, H. E. 1954. *Aero medical problems of jet passenger aircraft.* *J. Aviation Med.* 25: 440–450.

# 8

# Human Requirements for Space Travel

S. B. SELLS, PH.D.*

AND

CHARLES A. BERRY, M.D., M.P.H.†

The successful transportation of man at extremely high altitudes and in space reflects scientific and engineering accomplishments with reference to human requirements as well as to those of vehicle construction, propulsion, and control. Human requirements include two related but quite different phases of research and development. The first phase involves the critical information concerning environmental-protection and crew-compartment features that must be furnished to engineers as requirements for incorporation in the vehicle design. Its purpose is to enable survival and to maximize effective performance by the human operators. The second phase involves the men who will adventure to space in this vehicle. It consists of the specification of necessary and desirable operator characteristics and the development of selection, indoctrination, and training procedures to achieve them. The second phase is the principal concern of this chapter.

At present space travel is in the larval, undifferentiated stage of its evolution. The scientists and technicians who work on a development project usually follow it through most stages of progress and

* Professor of Psychology, Texas Christian University, Fort Worth, Texas. *Formerly*, Chief, Department of Medical Psychology, School of Aviation Medicine, USAF, Randolph Air Force Base, Texas.
† Lieutenant Colonel, USAF, MC, Chief, Flight Medicine Branch, Aerospace Medicine Division, Office of the Surgeon General, USAF, Washington, D.C.
This chapter was originally prepared for an Air Force symposium on "The Human Factor in Space Travel" and appeared in slightly modified form in the *Air University Quarterly Review*, Summer 1958.

participate in the functions of maintenance, countdown, launch, and flight monitoring. Such informal arrangements are at best temporary, however, and must ultimately give way to organization and management as the field advances and expands. These developments will first be seen among civilian manufacturers and the using military organizations but will eventually follow in the creation of a civilian space transport industry. Parallel with these technological changes, we may expect profound social, economic, and political developments throughout the world.

Although these problems are beyond the scope of this book, it is desired to emphasize the importance of staffing the entire supporting organization, in addition to the space crews. Every aspect of space travel depends on the complex, coordinated team effort of many specialists. For example, should the need arise during launch to abandon ship and escape, it is possible that only the range-control officer of the ground crew might be able to actuate the mechanism. His actions, in turn, would be coordinated with other members of the team. The various occupational specialties that will comprise the teams will need to be studied. Finally, the mission and group structure of the new teams that will be required are problems that should begin to receive careful attention. The success of the program and the safety of personnel will depend to a significant degree on these factors.

## Human Requirements for Engineering Design

Adaptation of engineering design to human survival requirements has received most attention in research and development thus far. Since man could not survive either the strenuous flight through the atmosphere nor the unfriendly environment of space without protection, the development of a feasible spacecraft has had the first priority.

Most of the *requirements for environmental protection* have been identified, and engineering solutions have either been developed or are considered feasible by responsible workers in the field at the time of this writing (4). These requirements are summarized briefly in the following discussion.

*Sealed Cabin.* Simulation of a life-sustaining environment by control of oxygen, pressure, temperature, humidity, gases, and gravitational force, if necessary; provision for food and water, removal of waste, and sanitation. The duration of missions may be limited, first, by the capacity of the system used to provide necessary materials and controls and, second, by its efficiency. As efficiency progresses, from pressure suits to sealed cabin, from containers of supplies to reconversion and recycling systems for gases, food, and water, the life-sustaining capacity of the cabin environment will be extended. As such improvements remove the need for fatiguing harnesses and restraints from the body of the operator and increase his comfort, his endurance and stamina will also be prolonged.

*Decompression.* Protection against meteor particles and against leakage and the loss of pressure in the crew compartment. This involves both the structure of the cabin shell and supplementary equipment, such as pressure suits.

*Radiation.* Protection against radiation, both cosmic and solar. Mayo (5) has reported that no practical solution has yet been found to provide adequate shielding against the very high energy cosmic particles which can penetrate even a foot of solid lead.

*Escape.* Provision of reliable means of emergency escape, particularly during the boost and re-entry phases of the mission. Escape in orbital and space travel has generally been regarded as really no problem, since the escape capsule would be no safer than the primary vehicle under those conditions.

*Acceleration.* Protection against high-g forces during take-off and re-entry acceleration.

*Weightlessness.* Protection against psychological and physiological problems attributable to weightlessness. At this time the available knowledge concerning effects of weightlessness is based on exposures in experimental situations of very brief duration, and effects of longer or prolonged exposure must be extrapolated speculatively. From such information as is available, this problem is regarded by the authors as probably minor and one involving the development of new habits and procedures, comparable to the adjustments involved in pressure breathing. It is likely that indoctrination may be feasible through a graduated schedule of training missions, providing progressively longer exposure to weightlessness during which personnel will practice prescribed maneuvers and the use of special equipment and procedures. However, if difficulties not now expected should be encountered, aeronautical engineers (5) have expressed confidence that artificial weight can be produced by rotating the craft around its own center of gravity.

A number of the problems of environmental protection are discussed elsewhere in this book. Until a solution for cosmic-ray protection is found, this will have to be regarded as one of the hazards of initial space travel. Research will be continued to calculate the extent of this hazard. With the exception of this problem, it appears that the remaining survival problems have either been solved (at least in a preliminary fashion) or are capable of solution. The duration of missions will, however, depend on the further adaptation of equipment to human requirements.

With reference to the feasibility of extended missions in space, attention in the design of crew compartments must next focus not only on survival requirements but on requirements for comfortable living and efficient performance as well. The development of habitability programs in nuclear submarines, capable of sustained submersed operation, was found to be a necessary condition of their effective operation. It is mandatory that the same trend follow in the design of manned spacecraft; otherwise human fatigue may prove to be a limiting factor in the duration of missions. Of equal importance is the requirement that, at every point linking the human operator to the control system of the vehicle, equipment should be designed for optimal human performance.

It can be concluded that the means have been developed, with certain calculated risks and error tolerances, to transport a man for a brief period through the environment of earth into space and back through the environment to earth (4). In this limited sense the basis for human space travel appears to be a practical reality. Even allowing for the known shortcomings of present designs, they represent a triumphant breakthrough in the efforts to get man into space. Thus, phase one of the human-requirements research and development efforts has reached the prototype stage for manned spacecraft. The limits of future refinement and development will probably exceed present expectation.

Although space is limitless, present manned spacecraft are sharply limited by the payload they can allot to human requirements and by the adequacy of equipment available within these limitations. A number of space scientists and engineers, enthused by the eventual prospects of round trips to the moon, Mars, and even more distant goals, have written with such elation that erroneous opinions have been created and widely circulated. In fact, many recent statements in standard news-reporting media appear to have been fantasies based on carelessly worded official releases. For example, one authority (10) wrote of a two-and-one-half-year round-trip voyage to Mars on an interplanetary ship in which the crew "will have more comfort and more space in which to move around than the crew on a modern submarine." He stated: "They will be in constant contact with the earth by means of radio and television."

Such comforts would be excellent to offset the monotony, isolation, and stress of life and work on a two-and-one-half-year space voyage. No doubt they will eventually be developed, in view of the incredible progress already made. However, "shirt-sleeves missions" with "first-class accommodations" and missions in excess of, at most, a few hours are not yet in actual sight.

In addition to payload, there are still unsolved and partially solved problems of protection. Some of the present solutions are untested and may not be improved until tried out, probably at the cost of some lives. Further, some of the present solutions are compromises which fall short of optimal protection and require special equipment, such as the full pressure suit developed for Crossfield's work with the X-15. These are at best bulky and restrictive.

The conclusion that *space travel* is a practical reality must be regarded with restraint and with insight into the present limitations and remaining problems. It will be many years before operations in space will be as reliable and free of hazard as even high-performance jet flying of today.

## Human Requirements for Staffing Space Operations

The ultimate goal of human-factors contributions to the engineering design of spacecraft is to adapt the equipment optimally to human requirements for environmental protection, comfort, and functioning efficiency. To the extent that this goal is fully realized, demands on the individual with reference to task performance and adaptability will be reduced. Nevertheless, there remain requirements for crew performance, involving application of highly complex and technical knowledge and skills under extremely hazardous and stressful circumstances. These additional human requirements for optimal staffing of space operations are at least of importance equal to those of engineering of the spacecraft.

The analysis of staffing requirements presented here assumes that the space crewman will be an operator of the ship, linked with its control system as a crucial part of a man-machine complex. If he were only a passive occupant, perhaps as a collector of scientific data on an automatically guided ballistic missile, the problem would be somewhat different. However, the difference would be primarily one of emphasis within the same general frame of reference. In either case it must be assumed that the occupant has been placed on board to perform necessary and useful functions. It seems unlikely that men will be shipped aboard ballistic missiles merely as subjects for physiological and psychological experiments in which animals might be used as well.

The requirements for selection, indoctrination, and training of crew personnel must be initially inferred with reference to the task requirements and environmental conditions under which these functions are expected to be performed. Establishment of standards and procedures to implement these requirements will first depend on the judgment of experienced and responsible leaders, supported by the advice of experienced flight surgeons and aviation psychologists. Of necessity these must be used prior to validation against actual performance criteria, and they will undoubtedly be modified as experience accumulates.

**General Perspective.** Manned space operations may be expected to evolve through a progressive and roughly predictable series of stages. Some of the problems that have caused greatest concern to aviation-medicine scientists are not expected to arise critically during the early developmental stage of space operation. It may therefore be clarifying to outline the principal stages of progress, as these are presently contemplated, in order to place the various personnel problems in perspective.

STAGE 1: EXPERIMENTAL-DEVELOPMENTAL MISSIONS. This is the initial stage which was entered from about 1957 to 1959 with high-altitude balloon and rocket flights. Early attempts involve maximum stress and require matching individual capability in testing the reliability of the vehicles and of component equipment. During this stage compromises with total protection have to be endured as boost and re-entry techniques are tested, weightlessness is explored, and data are collected on radiation absorption, meteor-particle penetration, and countless other known and unknown hazards. The early missions must initially be solo and of relatively short duration, with emphasis on technical and scientific aspects of experimental spacecraft operation.

The crewman has highly responsible duties involving control of the ship at least at some critical points, monitoring of flight and cabin-environment instruments and controls, making and recording observations, and the like. Even if boost and glide are automatically controlled, observation and corrective action at his discretion will be required. The re-entry glide and landing may also be under pilot control. With the exception that it is dropped from a mother ship at altitude before the rocket engine is ignited by the pilot, the X-15 is probably in other respects a representative prototype of the manned spacecraft of this period.

STAGE 2: ASTRONAUTICAL-EXPLORATORY MISSIONS. Voyages to the vicinity of the moon, Mars, and other planets as well as orbital missions of longer duration can be foreseen by the time that men and equipment have been tested and "checked out." Spacecraft of this stage may be expected to be larger, roomier, better equipped, and more reliable than their earlier prototypes. Their crews will consist of two or more experienced spacemen and will possibly include one or more observers. Their longer missions, voyages to greater distances and unexplored areas of space, and multiplace crew arrangements will introduce serious new problems not experienced in the earlier stage. Now the effects on individual and small-group behavior of confinement, isolation, boredom, weightlessness, and sustained maintenance of alertness may be expected to be more significant. Crew responsibilities will be more complex, involving astronavigation, cabin-environment monitoring and maintenance, and pilotage to a far greater degree than before.

STAGE 3: SPACE TRAVEL UNLIMITED. As one regards the present situation in comparison with that of only ten years ago, it seems reasonable to predict that the only limits of future space operations are those imposed by the poverty of human imagination. Indeed, the acceleration of this field resulting from inventions such as nuclear power, inertial guidance, and closed ecological environmental systems, prodded by the insatiable urge of man to explore the unknown frontiers of space, open vistas of man's ultimate conquest of the entire universe. This later stage, of inhabited space satellites, military space operations, interplanetary travel, and even more fantastic developments, is beyond the scope of our present essay. Nevertheless, it does not now seem improbable. As man approaches it, he will be faced with the need for solving further problems, such as the space-time dilemma in relation to aging and others that are now regarded by many as virtually in the realm of science fiction.

**Required Operator Characteristics.** Beyer and Sells (1) in 1957 published a detailed set of proposals for the selection and training of space pilots. These covered (1) aptitude and skill requirements, (2) biological, medical, and physical requirements, and (3) required tolerances of anticipated psychological stresses. These have been reviewed carefully by the authors (8) in the light of new information developed in the interim. This review fully supported the original proposals with only minor amendments. The reported procedures for the selection of the seven astronauts for Project Mercury appear to follow this outline in most major respects.

The principal additions to the proposals of Beyer and Sells are two. The first is the concept of *making up the difference* in estimating human physiological requirements, in cases in which equipment available represents a compromise with total protection needed and additional demands must be levied on the man. The second is the estimation of priorities among problems to be faced in relation to the crude timetable of successive stages of development discussed above.

The personal requirements outlined in the following paragraphs are stated in terms of the trained and qualified space pilot. Practical and economical procurement of required numbers of such personnel must be accomplished through effective selection and training. Selection of candidates with appropriate background and experience may substantially reduce the training and indoctrination necessary. At the same time the initial selection must be regarded as a general screening measure and the subsequent training procedures as a continuing program of supplementary selection. Attrition due to inability to qualify on the psychological or physiological indoctrination phases and on flight checks and voluntary withdrawal during training may be high. This combination of initial screening and selection in depth is the most rigorous approach that can presently be visualized. It reflects a policy of attempting to achieve as nearly error-less selection as possible, even at the cost of a high false-positive rate. The responsibility for assuring success is so great that no precaution can be considered too expensive. It is expected that less drastic procedures may be tolerated as equipment is improved and operations later become more routine.

**Aptitude and Skill Requirements.** The space pilot must be able to perform at least the following types of functions with alertness, speed, and accuracy: (1) pilot a high-performance, ultrasonic aircraft through the atmosphere during boost; control the vehicle in orbit and re-entry glide; and guide it to a landing; (2) obtain and interpret information concerning vehicle operation, cabin-environment conditioning, personnel functioning, and external conditions; and make rapid and accurate computations and decisions, anticipating difficulties by advance planning and actions; and (3) check, test, observe, and report for scientific study data concerning the spacecraft, its personnel, and the environment, as directed.

These functions require personnel with special skills, knowledges, and understandings: (1) proficiency and experience as pilot of high-speed, high-performance jet and rocket aircraft; (2) competent engineering understanding of the operation and maintenance of the power plant, controls, and environmental-conditioning equipment of the spacecraft; (3) medical and psychological training in human performance and functioning, with particular emphasis on survival and efficiency in the spacecraft; the space pilot must check frequently all relevant indicators and make immediate adjustments when needed; (4) detailed understanding of the operation and maintenance of all communications and scientific observational equipment; and (5) detailed understanding of mission plan in relation to navigational and astronomical frames of reference.

It would be uneconomical to consider any personnel for such a program who are not already highly experienced in high-performance jet or rocket aircraft. Test pilots may be expected to have, in addition, engineering and scientific training and interest. Proficiency in high-performance flight and in the engineering, physiological, communications, scientific, and navigational skills required would reduce the selection problem greatly.

However, even among such highly trained and experienced applicants, there are individual differences in aptitude for the additional mathematical, physical, astronomical, and engineering training and skills required. To maximize the likelihood of success of applicants accepted, aptitude assessment of factors related to success in such technical areas is indicated.

Assessment of flying proficiency and previous flying careers can be done with confidence. Present flight-check techniques are adequate for this purpose, and new methods have recently been devised for quantitative appraisal of career experience and performance, based on information in personnel and flying records and effectiveness reports (11, 12). Adequate assessment techniques and aptitude tests are presently available for this portion of the selection of volunteer candidates, but they must be validated and cutting scores established empirically as soon as performance criteria can be obtained.

The need for thorough medical indoctrination and for continuing close monitoring of environmental-conditioning equipment was implied but not explicitly stated in the paper of Beyer and Sells. Continuous evaluation of such equipment and the experience of Simons (9) in his "manhigh II" balloon flight have emphasized the importance of these functions as a realistic requirement, at least until effective automatic control systems are produced.

**Biological, Medical, and Physical Requirements.** If and when a sealed cabin equipped with a reliable recycling, closed ecological system, to provide a complete simulated ground environment, is available on spacecraft, there should be little reason to prescribe physical standards more stringent than those presently required of rated personnel. The only exceptions might be for body dimensions, which would have to conform to cabin size, for operations of long duration involving unusual strain or fatigue, or for missions requiring personnel to leave the spacecraft in protective garments for exploratory or other purposes. Otherwise, "shirt-sleeves missions" would be possible, since such ideal cabin conditions would require no adjustments to unusual environmental stresses.

On the other hand, should the ecological system be considered unreliable or require compromises with full cabin protection, for example, as to temperature or cabin gas and pressure levels, then such differences between needed and available protection must be made up. Even if control should be increased by monitoring and adjustment of the system by the pilot, safety would require supplementary measures, such as protective garments and pressure suits, selection of personnel with superior adaptive capacities, and conditioning of personnel to the expected stresses.

At present neither selection nor physical conditioning per se offers promise of solving these problems. It must be remembered that Mother Nature has been slow to change the structure of man, and the 1960 model is very much the same as the 1560 model man. Variations in physical characteristics are slight and evolutionary adaptive change is slow. If man were exposed to a new planetary environment, eons of time would have to pass before any physiologically adaptive change might appear.

Protective garments are more realistic but require both supplementary selection and conditioning training for practical use. For example, partial or full pressure suits impose a requirement for a more thorough evaluation of *cardiovascular* status in order that personnel may successfully overcome the physiological stresses occasioned by their use. Since some failures in the use of such equipment have been due to decompression sickness, additional requirements would favor youth and reject obesity. The effects of such suits on comfort, mobility, and feelings of confinement must be evaluated in relation to time. There is as yet inadequate experience with the effects of using such equipment for periods in excess of from twelve to fourteen hours.

Personnel must be adapted to any special conditions they will experience on the spacecraft. They must be given time and guidance in training sessions to adapt their behavior to them. This applies not only to pressure suits and their component anti-g, thermal protective, and helmet sections but to warning-signal devices and any special devices that may be developed for use in conditions of weightlessness. Motivation and prior experience in the use of such devices are significant additional determiners of successful adjustment and offer powerful protection against psychological stresses.

Since early space missions could hardly be undertaken without some arrangements for "making up the difference" for environmental protection, the use of protective garments, as mentioned in the preceding paragraph, appears inevitable. Under these conditions physiological selection for tolerance of a number of stresses related to the use of protective personal equipment must be considered. These include tolerance of transverse acceleration up to 9 g for from 30 seconds to a minute, high cardiovascular efficiency, resistance to *dysbarism*, and tolerance of uncomfortable variations of temperature, humidity, gas partial pressure, and cabin pressure. Such selection must be supplemented by a well-planned conditioning program for optimal adaptation to these conditions while performing vital tasks.

There are several important psychophysiological factors for which conditioning is critical even for short missions. Notable among them are adaptation to the in-cabin rations and conditions of eating and drinking, including weightlessness; withdrawal of customary supports, such as smoking, Cokes, coffee, and snacks; and normal sleep-waking cycle, when a different schedule is to be required in flight. Additional problems of a related nature may be expected later, when mission duration is extended beyond two days and crews of two or more members are used. These may include deprivation of other needs, such as alcohol, sex, recreation, and rest, and reactions to sustained isolation, confinement, group coordination, and accumulated strain.

**Psychological Adaptability Requirements.** By the time a pilot has logged over 1,000 hours in high-performance jet aircraft, most of which are flown at altitudes requiring physiological training and cabin protection, he may be assumed to have passed a rigorous stress test of adaptability to a major portion of the rigors of the most demanding flying. Such individuals have already been cited as the most appropriate source of professional airmen of the jet age from whom the pioneers of the space age must be recruited. As a group they may be considered to have proved not only the aptitude and physiological fitness for high-speed, high-altitude flying but also psychological fitness in regard to stability, judgment under pressure, and competency to deal effectively with hazardous emergencies. From the standpoint of motivation, as well, they have the most appropriate experience and background to appraise the challenge of space realistically. Volunteers from their ranks are therefore most likely to have an enduring interest and likely satisfaction in this job. Since tolerance of stress is a direct function of strength of motivation, the requirement that qualified candidates be volunteers is obviously basic.

STRESS TOLERANCE AND MOTIVATION. The assessment of applicants with respect to stress tolerance and motivation for space operation is much simplified but not obviated by this proposed pre-selection. There remains, first, the weeding out of marginal and questionable members of the jet-qualified volunteer group by careful examination of individual life and work histories. This must be followed by further evaluation of the surviving candidates in relation to their expected ability to cope with additional stresses of spaceship operation which are over and above those characteristic of present high-altitude jet flying.

In the early stage of space operation, by far the greatest stress problems are expected to be those associated with the reliability of equipment. Beyer and Sells, when they examined this problem, assumed that it would have been minimized over a longer period of engineering development than has actually been permitted. As a result they did not even mention the probability of disaster due to equipment failure as a major stress factor. However, the race to space has waxed hot as the realization of the goal has rapidly approached, and space missions are being discussed with greater risk factors than previous thinking had entertained.

Fortunately, this problem may be considered temporary and of relatively minor concern in the broad perspective of staffing a developing space program, once the first major flight-test hurdles are past. During this period stress associated with the reliability of the craft will probably be at its most acute point; but at the same time the flight-test personnel employed are likely to be the most able. The men who have been selected for the X-15 and Project Mercury space trials, for example, are extremely dedicated and capable engineering test pilots, whose intimate knowledge of the craft and of their idiosyncrasies, ego involvement in the projects, and whose extensive training and preparatory experience must assure the ultimate in human effort and performance in carrying out the tests. Since the most effective counter to fear of unreliability of equipment is successful operation, this source of stress must abate as successful progress in engineering development and flight tests proceeds. After acceptable reliability of space vehicles has been demonstrated, from launch, through flight, to safe return, an increase in the attractiveness of the challenge of space may be predicted.

RADIATION AS STRESS FACTOR. The hazard of cosmic radiation has been mentioned above, and not much can be said about it until further research on absorption in relation to exposure is completed. This is as yet one of the major stress problems that test pilots will investigate, although valuable data have been obtained from the Explorer satellites and other experimental sources. Should radiation exposure be judged too dangerous, it is unlikely that personnel will be exposed further until efforts to conquer the protection problem produce a tolerable solution.

OTHER STRESSES. Apart from the stresses associated with the reliability of the spacecraft and its protective cocoon, the major remaining unusual stresses inferable in the situation involve adjustments to weightlessness, to sleep deprivation and fatigue on extended missions, and to the complex of factors covered by the term "isolation." These may vary in severity as functions of time of exposure, crew composition, cabin habitability, task requirements, work layout, and work schedules, and their effects may be expected to be cumulative.

WEIGHTLESSNESS. Until more is learned about weightlessness from actual experience under sustained exposure, one can only make "educated guesses" about this problem. It is not presently expected to be a serious selection problem. If a program of indoctrination and training in the use of special devices, such as squeeze bottles for drinking, belts, harnesses, and techniques of controlled movement, under a routine of progressively increased exposure, is either inadequate or unfeasible, an engineering solution will have to be provided.

PHYSIOLOGICAL CYCLES. Sleep deprivation will probably not be a serious problem for trained personnel on missions of less than two days. Although research has shown that a man in reasonable physical and mental condition may be able to miss sleep for five days without damage, the important issue is maintenance of efficiency. This involves training and conditioning to take maximum advantage of opportunities for rest and relaxation. An important aspect of conditioning is habituation to a day-night cycle of waking-work and sleep-rest consistent with the demands of the mission. Since the restorative effects of sleep can be felt even after cat naps of brief duration, learning to catch up on sleep when possible is an important thing. Even more important is the ability to stay awake and react with alertness and vigilance when one is sleepy. Activity, movement, conversation, eating and drinking, and other techniques of self-stimulation, including the controlled use of analeptic drugs, may be indicated.

Boredom and Fatigue. The subjective aspects of boredom and fatigue are similar and frequently confused. Boredom results from repetitive, monotonous activity and can be relieved by a change, whereas fatigue involves a desire and need for rest. Since the effects of boredom are carelessness and inefficiency, planning is necessary on all missions of more than a few hours to provide a schedule of continuous, diverse activity. This would also have the advantage of helping the individual resist the deleterious effects of fear and anxiety. These tend to arise most insidiously during idleness and can often be suppressed by purposeful activity. In considering extended voyages such as a round trip to Mars, the need for variety of food, reading material, recreation, and other living arrangements will need careful study.

Isolation. Isolation is psychologically complex since it involves a number of different conditions which have the common denominator of separating the individual from significant parts of his environment. One of these is *confinement* which involves restraint or restriction of freedom of movement or action. Such restraint could occur by command, by threat, by physical enclosure, or by encapsulation. Confinement produced by the dimensions of the cabin, harnesses, garments, and personal equipment, as well as the possible sharing of cabin space with other crew members, may have harmful effects on individual and group efficiency. Reactions of discomfort, fatigue, annoyance, fear, and even acute claustrophobia must be anticipated and prevented. Anthropometric limitations in selection standards may therefore be important when cabin space is tight.

For the same reason engineering for comfort and work efficiency offers additional advantages. Although experienced jet pilots are generally habituated to cabin confinement as extreme as that expected in early spacecraft, exposure has not yet been for long periods. Before exposure time is substantially extended, research is needed on the effects of prolonged exposure on thresholds both of emotional reactions and impairment of efficiency. Habituation tests under simulated conditions must also be considered part of the selection program, as well as necessary pilot conditioning.

Another dimension of isolation of probable concern in space travel is that of *aloneness* and separation from familiar supports. This has been recognized even on extremely short jet flights as the "break-off phenomenon" (1, 2), when pilots have become painfully aware of leaving and being separated from the earth's friendly environment and being alone in the hostile and limitless beyond. Some pilots have reacted to this detachment with exhilaration and feelings of omnipotence; others have felt lonely, afraid, and depressed. However, this experience has yet to be studied over greater distances and longer time. Much research is needed to understand the role of personality type, previous experience, and various component factors in the situation on individual and group reactions at different levels of exposure and in association with other stresses. Preselection should screen out the most predisposed, highly dependent individuals who are characteristically unable to adjust to new locales, routines, and associates. Conditioning of prior experience at increasing levels of exposure, effective use of supportive communication, strategic matching of personalities in composition of crews, and effective application of group dynamics in crew coordination may prove to be important means of insuring effective adaptation and performance. Until these ideas are investigated, however, they can only be regarded as speculative.

A third dimension of isolation that merits consideration in this discussion involves *sensory deprivation* or narrowing of the variability of sensory stimulation of the individual. This might occur should the monotony of the space environment and of the cabin interior become a repetitive, undifferentiated, unchanging expanse of sameness. Recent research (7) has indicated that mental alertness depends on having a variety of sensory stimulation, e.g., of sight, sound, smell, movement, and so forth, and that when the variation is drastically reduced, there are measurable effects in loss of efficiency in mental performance. Such effects are seen at a moderate level in monotonous tasks, such as repetitive, simple work, monitoring a radarscope in a quiet, dark, confined workspace, and studying uninteresting, dull material. It is believed that these effects can be overcome in a variety of ways, particularly by care in engineering the cabin interior and by appropriate arrangement of work schedules. Avoidance of monotony, as mentioned above, should adequately prevent the more serious effects discussed here. However, this problem, too, is one deserving of further intensive study toward the goal not merely of preventing onset of loss of efficiency but rather of understanding the means of maximizing efficiency.

Finally, the problems of adaptability and stress tolerance must be viewed in terms of the cumulative effects, over time, of all the stresses of the situation on the individual. The accumulation of a number of minor annoyances, strains, and fears—none of an intensity to evoke a maladaptive reaction by itself—may result after some time in a combined stress of significant proportions. Separate consideration of the problem areas discussed above is important both for planning an optimal living and work environment aboard ship and in diagnosing and reducing individual susceptibilities. But the final test of both, as a space-worthy man-machine complex, requires suitability tests in adequate simulators. The complete program makes it necessary to test trained personnel and machine systems under ground-level and space-equivalent flight conditions and then to conduct actual flight tests.

**Personnel Selection.** Popular interest in space travel has given rise to all manner of suggestions, from ridiculous to reasonable, as to the selection of spacemen. These suggestions have included such divergent and extreme proposals as one that they should be schizophrenics who would not be bothered by isolation, another that they must be supermen, and still another that they must be midgets in order to meet the size-weight allowance. One writer (10) believes that the men selected for the Mars expedition:

. . . must be in excellent health and must have great stability. They will be persons of the scientific type who combine the love of adventure with the craving for scientific knowledge—men who can set aside their personal desires in favor of the ideal of a great technical and scientific achievement. A man of this nature will not mind spending two quiet years aboard a space ship. In his normal life such a man always carries with him a backlog of unfinished scientific work which he cannot find time to complete. The prospect of being given the opportunity of two full years of undisturbed time in which to study and work on his pet projects will be for him one more dream come true when his space ship takes off for its long voyage to Mars.

In contrast to this rather idyllic view, which seems to apply more to a dedicated scientist who would go along as a passenger, is the following statement (3) by the X-15 test pilot, A. Scott Crossfield, who may well have been speaking for all pilots, when he said that:

. . . the pilot's problems are not those of capability, environment, or physiological stress, but as usual are assessed to be in the area of system and subsystem reliability and control.

The analysis of human requirements in the preceding sections must be the basis for personnel selection. It is apparent that the operator of a space vehicle must be a motivated, controlled, professional pilot whose interests are directed, as Crossfield has emphasized, toward his primary task of controlling the vehicle. The physiological and psychological stresses that concern the doctors who advise engineers and select personnel do not enter into the pilot's concept of his total job except in relation to the understanding and operation of various equipment systems and procedures. However, it is the doctors' job to screen the applicants and to identify the men most likely to measure up to all the demands of this most exacting assignment.

As indicated above, the pioneer space pilots will be men like Mr. Crossfield and his small but select band of colleagues. These men are engineering test pilots, mostly identified with the project virtually from blueprint stage. Each has been recognized and selected for proved accomplishments in the most advanced projects yet undertaken. A handful of such men will probably carry the project past its most hazardous stage of reliability testing on relatively short but highly important missions.

After their basic work is accomplished, requirements should increase numerically as more spacecraft are built and further developmental and exploratory missions are scheduled. Volunteer applicants will be required to have experience as pilots of high-performance jet and rocket aircraft, preferably in engineering flight test. Volunteers who meet experience requirements, which must be defined, may be screened initially by procedures such as the following:

1.  Weight-size restrictions, based on payload and cabin requirements.

2.  Review of career experience, based on evaluation of personnel and flying records, effectiveness reports, letters of recommendation, and ratings by fellow pilots and superior officers.

3.  Physical examination, including review of medical records, detailed medical history, comprehensive flight physical examination, and a number of special procedures related to tolerance of acceleration and heat stress and the use of pressure suits. According to present thinking, visual standards may be relaxed somewhat, but weight standards in relation to height should be more stringent to eliminate obese persons who are unduly susceptible to decompression difficulties, such as *dysbarism*. In this connection maximum-

age standards may also be prescribed. Examination for *inguinal hernias,* chest x-ray to discover *pleural blebs,* and an electrocardiogram with the patient at rest and during certain procedures may still be indicated. Such physical examinations were of greater importance in partial pressure suits, but new full pressure garments create less physiological stress. Additional clinical tests for cardiovascular reactivity may be included, such as the cold pressor, tilt-table, and Harvard-type tests.

4. Psychiatric examination, supplemented by neurological examination and routine clinical psychological examination, to assess general personality resources, areas of conflict, dependency needs, reality orientation, and motivation toward the project. Electroencephalographic examination would be included for clinical neurology, baseline studies, and follow-up research.

5. Psychological examination for general intelligence, mathematical ability, mechanical principles, dial and table reading, and technical reading and vocabulary, supplemented by a comprehensive experimental selection battery of personality questionnaires and psychophysiological and performance tests. These would be included for research purposes, to be validated later against operational criteria.

Preliminary standards for screening of candidates will of necessity be based largely on "clinical judgment," supported by available scientific research. Standards will probably be too high at first but may be relaxed as experience in the indoctrination and training program proceeds, since substantial attrition is expected as the candidates go through the schooling and conditioning experience necessary to prepare for actual space work. The initial screening will thus accept for the second stage of selection-in-training a select group of professional airmen. Each one will be qualified as an experienced jet and probably rocket pilot, highly and realistically motivated for the program, physically and mentally superior, emotionally calm and controlled, and possessed of certain technical aptitudes necessary for performance of the task ahead.

**Indoctrination and Training.** The principal areas of training may be divided into (1) survival indoctrination and habituation, (2) operation and maintenance of all equipment systems and subsystems, and (3) navigation and communication. Each of these involves didactic classroom training or ground school and practical applica-

tion in ground simulators, balloon trainers, rocket ships, and spaceships.

SURVIVAL INDOCTRINATION. Training and indoctrination for survival are basically an extension of the physiological training presently
given for high-altitude flying. For the spaceman the curriculum
must be extended to cover all components of the synthetic cabin
environment essential to life, including the physiological processes,
possible dysfunctions, and corrective action. In addition he must be
taught practical survival principles and facts concerning the physiological and psychological aspects of nutrition, fluid balance and
dehydration, temperature regulation, fatigue, sleep, boredom, isolation, anxiety, fear, and loneliness. To use this knowledge most effectively, each man's training should enable him to learn to apply it
meaningfully to himself and, when applicable, to his comrades, with
insightful knowledge of his and their physical and mental characteristics.

To complete the survival training, indoctrination must be followed up by realistic individual and later group habituation to the
actual conditions of work and living space, tasks, and equipment to
be encountered on space missions. This phase should consist of a
progressive series of practice sessions, first in the laboratory, later
in ground simulator mock-ups and balloon-gondola simulators at
altitude, and finally in rocket and spaceships. These sessions must
provide exposure to the various stresses of the type described earlier
while the pilots perform simulated required tasks. Pilots must learn
to function effectively while using flight rations, drinking from
squeeze bottles, recognizing signs and signals indicative of their
own functioning, recognizing and coping with emergencies, and
tolerating unusual bodily attitudes and motion, fatigue, discomfort,
and deprivation of smoking and other habits of long standing. In
short, they must be adapted to live comfortably and efficiently in
the spaceship.

Flight training and training in navigation and communication
must be laid out on the basis of the functioning abilities and backgrounds of the personnel selected and of the particular equipment
and operations involved. The traditional training sequence of
ground school, simulator trainer, and transition to operational craft
must be adapted to this situation.

Every aspect of the training program must also provide for further selection and attrition. As a result each graduate will actually have passed a comprehensive series of stress and performance test hurdles while going through his preparation. It is not too much to expect that they will measure up to the standard mentioned by Major General Dan C. Ogle (6), former Surgeon General of the United States Air Force, who said:

Such a person must be all that the best aviator is today as well as being constitutionally and emotionally suited for the physical and emotional traumatic influences of sealed cabins speeding, heaven knows where, through the awful silence of a timeless and a darkened sky.

## References

1. BEYER, D. H., and SELLS, S. B. 1957. Selection and training of personnel for space flight. *J. Aviation Med.* 28: 1–6.
2. CLARK, BRANT, and GRAYBIEL, ASHTON. 1957. The break-off phenomenon: A feeling of separation from the earth experienced by pilots at high altitude. *J. Aviation Med.* 28: 121–126.
3. CROSSFIELD, A. S. 1957. Space travel symposium: A test pilot's viewpoint. *J. Aviation Med.* 28: 492–495.
4. HENRY J. P., ECKSTRAND, G. A., HESSBERG, R. R., SIMONS, D. G., and WEBB, P. P. 1957. *Human Factors Research and Development Program for a Manned Satellite.* Aeromedical Division, Human Factors Directorate, Headquarters ARDC, Baltimore, Md.
5. MAYO, A. M. 1957. Space travel symposium: Some survival aspects of space travel. *J. Aviation Med.* 28: 498–503.
6. OGLE, D. C. 1957. Man in a space vehicle. *U.S. Armed Forces Med. J.* 8: 1561–1570.
7. SCOTT, T. H. 1954. Intellectual Effects of Perceptual Isolation. Unpublished Ph.D. dissertation. McGill University, Ottawa, Canada.
8. SELLS, S. B., and BERRY, C. A. 1958. Human requirements for space travel. *Air Univ. Quart. Rev.* 10: 108–120.
9. SIMONS, D. G. 1958. Pilot reactions during "manhigh II" balloon flight. *J. Aviation Med.* 29: 1–14.
10. STUHLINGER, ERNST. 1957. Outlook to space travel. *Sci. Monthly* 85: 281–287.
11. TRITES, D. K., and KUBALA, A. L. 1957. Characteristics of successful pilots. *J. Aviation Med.* 28: 34–40.
12. TUPES, E. C. 1957. *Psychometric Characteristics of Officer Effectiveness Reports of OCS Graduates.* (AFPTRC–TN–57–20 [ASTIA Document No. 098923].) Air Force Personnel and Training Research Center, USAF, Lackland Air Force Base, Tex.

# 9

# Preventive Medicine in Jet and Space Flight

## John A. Norton, M.D.*

A simple approach to the meaning of *preventive medicine* is that of thinking ahead so as to be prepared for any combination of contingencies related to maintaining good health. Any preparatory action in the field of medicine or good health may be considered a part of preventive medicine.

Preventive medicine is presented here with particular reference to high-performance jet aircraft, although some of its problems concerning the space vehicle are discussed. The topics covered include crew selection, crew conditioning, arthropod vectors, drinking water, nutritional requirements, food-service sanitation, noise, waste disposal, effective temperature index, and industrial health.

## Crew-Selection Problems

With the development of progressively higher performance aircraft and space vehicles, crew-performance reliability becomes increasingly critical. At the same time, in military aircraft the number of essential crew members has been steadily reduced in relation to the number of major functions that must be accomplished during flight. Space and weight relationships for military jet aircraft and spaceships are so critical that there can be essentially no provision for spare crew members. Single-place craft are obviously limited. Multiplace craft can provide only minor relief from duties

---

* Colonel, USAF, MC, Director of Medical Operations, Aerospace Medical Center, Brooks Air Force Base, Texas.

when crew members substitute for each other during periods of rest, eating, and sleeping. The extremely high demands upon crew members require consideration of every possible and foreseeable measure to insure reliable operator performance. An important consideration, related to crew selection, arises from the analysis of preventive medicine problems. This is the factor of immunity.

One foreseeable and generally avoidable hazard to crew effectiveness, which has not always received sufficient weight, is that of illness due to infectious disease. While quarantine prior to take-off is usually adequate to minimize such a hazard, it is appropriate to consider, as an additional factor in crew selection, immunity to the largest practicable number of heterogeneous etiological agents. Such selection, if practicable, would contribute materially to the prevention of disability due to infection.

Immunity is never absolute. The relative degree of protection is exceedingly variable. For example, there is a relatively high degree of long-lasting immunity against measles but a relatively low degree of evanescent immunity against the common cold, gonorrhea, dengue fever, and the various herpes.

In general, immunity to disease increases with age and also with the amount of prior exposure to infection. Maximum immunity from natural and artificial antigens would be realized by most personnel past the age of fifty. This age would be reduced in the case of individuals who have been exposed to a wide range of pathogens through extensive foreign travel or overseas service. The importance of extensive exposure for the development of immunity is emphasized by the fact that many field studies of the epidemiology of diseases, such as viral hepatitis (7, 30) and others (6), have indicated that there are probably far more undiagnosed, unapparent infections than there are clinical cases of the disease. In *poliomyelitis,* prior to widespread vaccination, the majority of humans experienced at least one infection prior to age thirty-five. Infectious mononucleosis probably is similar in being diagnosed less often than not.

The advantage to older crew members of increased immunity to disease must, of course, be balanced against other requirements, many of which put a premium on youth. In this case, as in many others, a compromise is necessary. It is desirable that as much advantage as possible be taken of the contribution to immunity of age and exposure. At least some protection would be gained by setting a minimum age limit of twenty-five, while at thirty-five the increased immunity would be considerably greater.

## Crew Conditioning

**Infectious Disease Prevention.** Isolation or quarantine of crew members to the maximum degree practicable is essential to prevention of infectious disease if the flight is to be of many hours' or of days' duration. Crew members should work and associate together over as long a period as possible so as not only to develop close interpersonal relations for good crew performance but also to enable some interchange of antigens, as is normally experienced in family living. This sort of communal living has been practiced in both naval aircraft carriers and with crews of the Strategic Air Command. The relatively small area of ready rooms on a carrier lends itself admirably to cross-infections with resultant wider range of antibodies developed. Similarly, Strategic Air Command crews have often been on 144 continuous hours of alert.

In considering the protection of passengers and crew for space trips of a few days' to a few weeks' duration, a quarantine for the final week prior to take-off may be a practicable measure. Its inconvenience would certainly have to be weighed judiciously. Unfortunately, many communicable diseases, such as the common cold, the various herpes, dengue fever, and gonorrhea, have no immunity of sufficient degree to be considered practicable. Some prophylaxis might be achieved against serum hepatitis by the use of immune globulin. The effectiveness of this procedure would depend primarily upon the cooperation and memory of the potential travelers. To insure that no serum hepatitis would develop on space flights of months' duration, the simplest procedure would be to *avoid any injections during the six months prior to take-off*. In accordance with current immunization criteria for aircrews, this would require very little modification. The use of immune globulin for prophylaxis against infectious hepatitis has been clearly demonstrated (6).

**Preflight Conditioning.** The flight surgeon should be an integral part of the team concerned with the planning of the flight from its inception until after actual departure. Crews should be observed scrupulously to be certain that they have met all established psychological and physical requirements. A positive effort is necessary to avoid perfunctory compliance. Examination reports should be final, complete, and also recent. Physiological training, ejection-seat training, and training for all emergency procedures should be a matter of personal knowledge to the flight surgeon as well as the crew member. Crew members selected for specialized missions should be men with exemplary personal hygiene habits, who are at most very moderate consumers of alcoholic beverages. Operations personnel should, of course, be certain that all possible personal conveniences are accorded the crews.

Continuous and effective liaison is essential between crew members, operations personnel, flight surgeons, psychologists, and physiologists who should all be active participants in preparation for flight. For a period of at least sixteen hours prior to take-off, crews should be under the detailed, personal guidance of an experienced flight surgeon.

**Immunization.** Crews for flights terminating on earth (and certainly on space stations) should be required to be prepared for world-wide immunizations in accordance with international sanitary regulations (16, 17). A program including the following immunizations should meet, within the limits of practicability, the following requirements, adjusted to be consistent with the earlier recommendation of *avoiding any injections during the six months prior to take-off:*

*Smallpox immunity.* Re-established by vaccination between twelve and six months prior to anticipated take-off.

*Typhoid-paratyphoid vaccination.* A basic series with a booster inoculation between twelve and six months prior to anticipated take-off.

*Tetanus immunization.* The basic series of tetanus toxoid or tetanus-diphtheria toxoid for adults followed by a booster inoculation sometime between four years and six months prior to take-off. This is probably best accomplished by the type of toxoid currently used by the United States Armed Forces. It contains a small amount of diphtheria toxoid for those persons who have not demonstrated a high level of diphtheria immunity by means of the Schick test.

*Yellow fever vaccine.* Given not less than six months prior to take-off but within six years. This requirement would, of course, be inapplicable to jet flights of short duration and to certain flight plans that could not conceivably terminate in any yellow fever endemic areas.

*Typhus fever immunity.* Established with a basic series of injections with a booster inoculation between twelve and six months preceding departure.

*Cholera immunization.* The basic series plus annual booster immunizations. Necessary as a prophylaxis against international complications rather than as a really potential hazard for a crewman.

*Poliomyelitis vaccination.* The basic series of inoculations. As experience with the results of this vaccine develops, it is possible that a more definite policy on booster immunizations would apply to crew members.

*Influenza immunization.* Use of a vaccine that includes the currently prevalent strains at yearly intervals.

**Immunization Records.** Meticulous attention should be given to the preparation of correct immunization records of all passengers and crew members. The form specified in the International Sanitary Regulations should be adhered to without the slightest variation in order to avoid inconvenience, aggravation, and actual detention of international travelers. Particular attention should be given to the official stamp of the vaccinating center or *Cachet d'authentification.*

For travelers or passengers, as distinguished from crew members, only the minimum number of injections possible should be given compared with those recommended earlier for pilots and crew members. For example, travelers need not be immunized against yellow fever if there is no likelihood of passing through an endemic yellow fever area.

**Sedation and Stimulation.** Under ideal conditions aircrews should receive their evening meal approximately fourteen hours prior to anticipated morning take-off in company with the flight surgeon. This meal should be as large as the aircrew can comfortably assimilate and should feature high-protein low-residue foods, such as meat and potatoes. Alcoholic appetizers should be limited to no more than 2 ounces of spirits per crew member. If it has been determined feasible to use sedation, this should be given approximately twelve hours prior to anticipated take-off. Approximately eleven hours prior to anticipated take-off, aircrew members should be in bed in as quiet an environment as possible. The flight surgeon should continue his rapport with the crew by being available in quarters shared with them, checking each one during the first few hours after retiring to be certain that the crew members are sleeping soundly.

One of the controversial aspects of crew conditioning for long-range jet crews has been the extent to which sedation before the flight and chemical stimulation during the flight should be tolerated or prescribed. As yet there is inadequate scientific information on this problem. In one series of well-controlled studies of several analeptics under laboratory and experimental conditions, all the analeptics postponed deterioration of proficiency in the performance of the experimental tasks (13). *Dextro-amphetamine* appeared to produce no marked depression in thirty-hour tests. In spite of such optimistic implications, objections properly center around the fact that it is not possible to design a long-range experiment to rule out satisfactorily the possibility of delayed adverse effects. In military operations the decision to use analeptics is based upon the premise that it is better to risk a potential slight damage for all the troops than to let physical and mental fatigue lead to mass casualties.

For special flights there is some justification for considering intelligent, supervised use of sedation prior to the flight and the *amphetamine*-derivative stimulants during flight. The absolute invariable requirement for the use of sedatives and stimulants must be actual experience with the drugs, used in flight, competently interpreted by an experienced flight surgeon. Using rigorous psychometric evaluation, the hand-picked, elite crew members must be individually and thoroughly tested with the particular sedatives and stimulants that might be used. This author prefers to start with *sodium pentobarbital*, using a dosage of 200 mg for an average crew member of some 150 to 175 lbs. body weight. There must be no doubt that each crew member so sedated will fully metabolize this dosage in twelve hours or less. This dosage worked well with jet fighter pilots in an operational wing, which participated in many long-range missions including single-place jet flights of as much as fourteen hours' duration.

In a period of eighteen months, there were no known near-accidents, incidents, or operational difficulties in which prior use of sedatives was indicated as a contributing factor. Two forms of *dextro-amphetamine sulfate* (usually in 5 mg dosage) have been used with sufficient frequency with jet pilots to confirm their usefulness in practice. The majority of pilots expressed a preference for a capsule of dextro-amphetamine sulfate in granular form, which spreads the action of the stimulant over a period of from six to eight hours. Other pilots preferred a tablet form taken for quicker action and lasting for about four hours. The use of such stimulants for flights of less than ten hours should not be considered. Critical times with jet fighter aircraft and light bombers are during air-to-air refueling and, of course, in all aircraft during let-down and landing procedures.

In at least one aircraft accident, the misuse of stimulants was believed to have been a contributing factor. The pilot mistakenly took a 10 mg capsule of the stimulant shortly after take-off so that by the end of the mission of approximately ten hours' duration, he was fatigued, and a certain element of depression possibly contributed to even slower cerebration than would have been natural after ten hours of fatiguing flight. Other incidents are reported less reliably, involving mistaken ingestion on the night before take-off of stimulants thought to be sedatives.

**Prophylactic Drugs.** In general, the use of prophylactic drugs is considered inadvisable in flight. Malaria suppressants were a military necessity during World War II and the Korean conflict, but newer curative antimalaria drugs are now available, making it unnecessary to suppress an attack of malaria. Prevention of malaria depends upon proper engineering control of the insect vector. Antibiotic prophylactics against venereal diseases can mask diagnoses. For example, a person may have had sufficient penicillin prophylaxis to prevent gonorrhea but not have had enough to prevent a spirochetal infection.

Prophylaxis against diarrheal diseases, which is frequently sought by passengers and crew members (18), is generally inadvisable. To remain free from diarrheal disease, dietary restrictions are believed to be more reliable than dependence upon any of the mycin antibiotics or other suppressants.

## Arthropod Vectors

Animate vectors might be of little consequence for crew members of most higher jet flights because of the total enclosure of flight gear worn in such flights. The necessity of sealing the crew capsule in space vehicles would likewise minimize the hazards of arthropod-borne infections. This section is concerned primarily with vector-control measures desirable and necessary for commercial jet airliners.

At the first meeting of the World Health Organization Expert Committee on Sanitation of International Airports, there was agreement that vector-borne diseases were especially in need of regulation (14). These were ranked with food and water sanitation as important areas of preventive medicine for airports.*

Cockroaches have never been too seriously considered as potential transmittors of disease. However, Roth and Willis (34), who reviewed over four hundred references, concluded that these vermin may be important as vectors, for they may acquire, maintain, and excrete viruses. Cockroaches starve to death in a galley or kitchen that is constantly immaculate. If immaculate operation is not possible, residual sprays and other forms of toxic control can be employed for control (8).

The International Sanitary Regulations and other quarantine procedures prescribing legal minimum requirements have been responsible for much common practice. The most commonly used method of control of arthropod vectors in aircraft is, of course, the use of sprays of various sorts. Built-in spray units, as seen in certain of the military transport aircraft, have been found useful, especially in spraying inaccessible areas such as wheel wells. Passenger and crew compartments are more often sprayed with a hand atomizer or a pressurized dispenser, using relatively inert, highly volatile liquids such as Freon for the propulsion and atomizing vehicle. Pyrethrum and related compounds are still commonly used for the quick kill of adult forms of mosquitoes. Lindane, dieldrin, DDT, and newer lethal agents are usually incorporated in order to provide some degree of residual control (8).

The toxicity of killing agents for arthropod vectors has been under constant study (23). The gamma isomer of benzene hexachloride, more commonly referred to as lindane, is not considered too hazardous in ordinary usage. Lindane boilers, which are used in commercial eating establishments, would be condemned as being too toxic if they were used continuously. Some of the newer agents, such as diazinon, are considerably less toxic to humans yet have a higher kill rate for arthropod vectors.

Entomological inspectors of some of the more recently independent countries have been, on occasion, unusually meticulous in demanding a detailed search of foreign aircraft for specific evidence

---

* A good set of standards is provided in *Handbook on Sanitation of Airlines*, U.S. Public Health Service (10).

of effective spraying. In some cases their standards have appeared to require the presence of at least one dead mosquito within the aircraft. Commercial jet airliner pilots landing in these countries should be prepared to demonstrate to even an unreasonable inspector that all vectors have been indubitably destroyed.

## Drinking Water

**Quantitative Requirements.** Fluid requirements for both crew and passengers on jet airliner flights should not be significantly different from previously established standards of comfort. According to Megonnell and Chapman (25), the operating experience of BOAC on flights of from five to twelve hours' duration averaged about 10 lbs. (4.7 l) per passenger for drinking and washing water. This compares with subsistence water requirements of 12 lbs. (5.68 l) per capita per day for stabilized civilian populations (8).

Fluid intake requirements for military jet crews and for space cabins need to be computed more precisely. Harrow and Mazur (12) give a fluid intake average of 1.2 l per day for fluid beverages, 1.0 l as fluid in other foods, and 0.3 l produced by normal body oxidation processes. Kleiner and Orten (19) show water intake and/or production as: drinking water, 0.4 l; water in other beverages, 5.8 l; water in solid foods, 7.2 l; and metabolic water, 0.32 l. With such a range of values, it is readily apparent that one must be exceedingly cautious in calculating just what is meant by normal fluid intake. For spacecraft this will be a very critical item to be calculated (4, 20).

Experience with single-place jet fighters indicates that meeting pilots' water requirements on flights of less than fourteen hours is not a difficult problem. A pint of water has been found to be completely adequate. Crews of light bombers and single-place jet fighter aircraft tend deliberately to limit the amount of fluid intake because of the complexity of accomplishing the relatively simple act of urination.

**Sanitary Requirements.** Sanitary standards for drinking water should meet those presently known in the United States as the Public Health Service Drinking Water Standards (5, 8, 38).

In normal locations within the United States proper, compliance with the complete drinking-water standards is most extensive.

These standards include many detailed requirements concerning the basic source of the water, for example, whether it is ground water or surface water, the size of the catchment areas, the topography, geology, potential sources of pollution, existing sewage treatment above water sites, physical characteristics of raw water, methods used in the filter plant, the coagulant system, the mixing and flocculation basins, sedimentation basins, filtered water storage, aeration, disinfection, plant operation, and control.

In establishing permanent overseas airline operations it will rarely be economically feasible to develop basic water supplies that would meet the Public Health Service standards. A probable compromise between long-term ideal sources of water and emergency sources of potable water would be akin to that provided by United States military forces during somewhat stabilized operations in overseas communications zones. Here, the Corps of Engineers of the United States Army develops water points utilizing portable water filters with a slurry method of developing a reasonably efficient filtration using diatomaceous earth for the slurry (24, 43). The diatomite filter lessens the necessity for pretreatment or chemicals. This will remove physical particles, such as cyclops, that might otherwise be a vector of protozoan diseases and in all probability removes the cysts of *Endamoeba histolytica*. There is also a good probability of removing or inactivating some of the virus pathogens (2, 6). The product of such rapid filtration might leave much to be desired as far as taste and turbidity are concerned.

It is essential that chlorinating equipment be of the automatic type, which would require the least possible intellect and motivation on the part of the operator. However, chlorination or any other chemical disinfection of water can never be a complete water treatment. "Sterilizing" water and leafy vegetables is not possible with the use of such agents as potassium permanganate or chlorine solutions. In waters of high organic content or containing other interfering agents, chlorination to the point of safe degree will often render the water markedly unpalatable. Storage for several days, both before and after treatment, is one of the most certain of the age-old methods of reducing the likelihood of transmitting water-borne disease. Microorganisms capable of causing disease in humans do not usually multiply or thrive in water without significant nutrients.

For commercial jet passenger liners or for other craft departing from sites not convenient to established potable water supplies, it is possible that the most practical method might be that in use at Tainan Air Base on Taiwan. The ingenious Chinese airmen built from salvage wing-tip tanks a "Rube Goldberg" water sanitizer. Using low-grade coal, they were able to deliver a product that was consistently above 190° F and that had been held at that temperature for several minutes. This method of water sanitizing is most reliable for inactivating all types of parasites (viral, fungous, protozoan, rickettsial, and bacterial). The vexing difficulties of inactivating the cysts of *Endamoeba histolytica* are well known.

In establishing independent sources of water in overseas operations, proper plumbing should be emphasized to provide absolute assurance that there are no cross-connections, open connections, or back-flow connections that could in any way result in non-potable water contaminating an otherwise potable product.

**Ice.** The use of ice for beverages and drinking water for airliners is fraught with many problems, particularly overseas. Crushed ice in the United States is one of the least sanitary products permitted for public consumption. In overseas operations, possibly the only practicable safe source of ice would be automatic ice-making machines connected to a fully reliable source of potable water. Even then the handling of a potable product from such a machine would be hazardous in the hands of indigenous employees. Mechanical refrigeration should be relied upon to the greatest extent practicable for cooling beverages and drinking water while they are still in sanitary dispensing containers similar to those currently in use for homogenized milk.

## Nutritional Requirements

For flights of twelve hours' duration or less, nutritional requirements are not extensive from the standpoint of nutritional adequacy per se. In jet airliners, as in existing passenger aircraft, the serving of food in the most palatable and pleasing manner possible is related almost exclusively to competitive considerations and to the relief of passenger boredom rather than to any need to furnish a correctly computed diet of fats, carbohydrates, proteins, vitamins, and minerals.

In military jet aircraft, in spite of the many years of conscientious and fruitful research on palatable meals, it has been found that crew acceptability of many of these highly specialized foods has been rather low. Military pilots rarely eat as much during flights lasting up to twelve hours as they would in an equal amount of time on the ground. Much effort has been expended to provide attractive flight lunches (41). Yet, it is a very common thing to see a large proportion of the in-flight rations left uneaten at the conclusion of the flight. For military flights or for space travel of one week's duration or less, there is no serious requirement for a balanced diet. A high-calorie, high-protein, low-residue diet is a desirable objective. The development of quite palatable commercial instant beverages makes long trips less onerous. Instant tea, coffee, cocoa, as well as bouillons, can be prepared aloft with relatively little difficulty.

During periods of weightlessness, there arises a problem of getting food to the posterior portion of the oral cavity in order to start the normal deglutition reflex. It is possible that there will be more *aerophagia* than normally expected under conventional gravity conditions. In a normal gravitational field and with the body in an upright position, this is easily accomplished by voluntary or reflex eructation. In a state of weightlessness, there would be no reason for the air trapped in the stomach to gravitate toward the cardiac sphincter. At the other end of the alimentary canal, other problems would be potentially disturbing, since the entrapped air bubbles might not coalesce in the terminal portion of the large bowel. It would therefore be difficult, if not impossible, for the reflexes that normally actuate the anal sphincter to determine when to pass flatus and when to pass gas-impregnated fecal matter. Food concentrates prepared in collapsible metal tubes, like toothpaste, offer some promise for better feeding with less last-minute preparation.

For prolonged space flights it is a logistical necessity to provide for the recycling of organic matter to furnish a miniature of the terrestrial biological balance. *Chlorella* and other lower forms of plant life have been demonstrated in laboratory and analytical studies to be a potentially acceptable food source for space vehicles. Several species contain a reasonably proper balance of proteins, carbohydrates, fats, and vitamins. If a large enough quantity could be harvested, it is entirely possible for a person to survive with no other food than algae for many weeks. To date there has been no enthusiastic acceptance of the palatability of various forms of these plant cells for use as foods. Even when this food is produced from relatively esthetic chemicals to which there is attached no relatively lifelong abhorrence of the source of some of the organic matter, the algae food is not truly palatable. In prolonged space flights, assuming that a practicable recycling system may be developed, it would be essential for crew members to take a detached, objective view toward urine, perspiration, and feces as the sole sources of organic matter that would be converted into their only source of food and water. In the consideration of crew selection, it might not be completely impracticable to select for crew members those who, in addition to all other attributes, have developed anosmia since much of the sensation of taste is actually associated with the sense of smell.

The packaging, storage, and refrigeration of food on aircraft is, of course, exceedingly important. In recent years commercial airliners have developed packaged food with minimum weight and bulk required for the food containers. Refrigeration of milk and other perishables, which cannot be completely resanitized through thorough heating, is a serious space, weight, and energy problem. In commercial jet airliners this will simply have to be the best possible compromise with payload efficiency.

## Food-Service Sanitation

**Sanitary Principles.** It is not too essential to be concerned about attempting to break a link in the chain of infection for the various people in a closed group. For example, any infectious disease that is easily communicable will be rapidly communicated to all other members of the family group during the first stage of the illness of the members first infected. But public eating facilities must be constructed and operated in a much more sanitary fashion than a home kitchen, since there is a constant intermingling of new strains of new pathogens. This is a most important consideration for jet airliners which hasten, to the greatest extent yet experienced, the transportation of persons during the incubation phases of communicable diseases of all sorts.

**Model Restaurant Code.** The United States Public Health Service has developed a model ordinance and code related to eating and drinking establishments (8). International airliners should consider nothing less than invariable, strict compliance with those portions of this code for a grade "A" restaurant. It is imperative that menus avoid foods which have been shown by epidemiological experts to be frequent vehicles of food poisoning, such as potato salad, salad-type sandwiches, and cream-filled and custard-filled pastries (26).

One of the most misunderstood features of clean food-service operations in overseas areas has been the value of food-handler's examinations. Experience in the United States has demonstrated that the time, money, and effort that go into food-handler's examinations are more likely to produce less benefit than the same energies devoted toward better health education and proper supervision of food-handling employees. Emphasis on the physical examination of food-handlers usually leads to a false sense of security. It is not possible even for the most thorough examination to assure freedom from communicable disease in a person the day after his examination. It is far better to train all food-handlers on the assumption that each one is a carrier of typhoid fever, amebiasis, and ascariasis.

One deficiency that has not yet been overcome in the education and management of indigenous food-handlers in the many overseas areas in which American interests are involved, is the provision for effective health-education material. American motion pictures and animated cartoons are popular in every country of the world. In order to reach people of many ethnic backgrounds with heterogeneous mores, there is need for a small film library of motion-picture cartoons illustrating the do's and don't's of good sanitary procedures. Such films could avoid offending racial and ethnic groups by featuring non-identifying human figures or animal caricatures. Although scores of health-education films produced in the United States and other western nations are available in many overseas film libraries, these depict conditions of sanitation and American mores that are often totally incomprehensible to the native audience.

The model code of the Public Health Service requires restaurant inspections at least once each six months. Airline medical directors almost invariably inspect food-service facilities far more frequently. These facilities for both in-flight and terminal-restaurant food are well planned, properly supervised medically, and permit no reduction in the high standards of sanitation. Hand-washing facilities for food-handlers in accordance with the code include separate toilet rooms, hot and cold running water, adequate clean towels, plenty of soap, and, of course, hand-washing signs. The use of the common towel is prohibited by the code.

In dishware sanitation the model code permits a choice of heat or chemical sterilization of utensils. Considering the diversified facilities available on overseas airline operations, it is highly desirable that only heat-sanitizing methods be employed. The complete dependence upon the understanding cooperation of indigenous employees in using bacteriocidal compounds is such that they simply require too much time and effort for supervision. The only type of dish sanitizer providing adequate protection is one that uses rinse water of not less than 180° F for at least 10 seconds with a volume of at least 3.8 gal. of fresh water per 100 sq. in. of dish area. Automatic devices are available which cut off and display a warning light whenever the rinse temperature drops below 180° F. Manually operated devices for emergency operation are a valuable safeguard. If such heat-sanitizing methods are used, many of the bacteriological examinations of utensils and foods can probably be eliminated.

The common travelers' belief that "a change of water" is responsible for watery bowel movements is, of course, almost always wrong. The vast majority of diarrheal diseases are caused by serving unsanitary food. *Staphylococcus* and *Salmonella* food poisonings are world-wide and not restricted to travelers.[*]

**Food Preservation.** It seems simple enough to prescribe food sanitation based upon keeping perishable foods below 40°F and reheating all foods prior to serving to a point far beyond pasteurization. Nevertheless, breaks in technique occur with disturbing repetition (18, 25). Newer proposals for the safe preservation of food must be considered. *Chlortetracycline* as a preservative of food (3) has been studied with considerable optimism (36). The basic position of the United States Food and Drug Administration is that about 10 per cent of the public have a proneness to allergies. Use of effective amounts of antibiotics for food preservation would lead to large numbers of allergic reactions. The use of a residual of not more than seven parts per million chlortetracycline remaining in any portion of poultry is approved since cooking will destroy such a small concentration. This amount merely augments refrigeration as the choice basic method of food preservation.

Gamma rays or x-rays for irradiation preservation have been studied (21, 29). The dosage of radiation sufficient to preserve food adequately is one which will sterilize it. The relatively high radiation resistance of *Clostridium botulinum* requires dosages much higher than those which will kill animals. At such higher dosage

[*] A most practical small manual for use in investigating such outbreaks is entitled *Procedures for the Investigation of Food-borne Disease Outbreaks* (33).

there is considerable change in colors, odors, and palatability. Milk and dairy products are most likely to deteriorate. Eggs, vegetables, and fruit also suffer. Until further studies bring new knowledge to light, it is probable that antibiotics and radiation will have very little application for food preservation for jet or space travel.

## Noise

Technical and scientific literature on the subject of noise is voluminous (1, 11). Much interest in this problem has resulted from recent decisions involving Workmen's Compensation claims. Not long ago there was a cumulative total of over two billion dollars in claims against employers for alleged hearing loss from excessive noise in industry. There are many presumably deleterious effects of noise beyond that of sheer hearing loss brought on by high noise levels over a period of many years. Operators of jet airliners must deal with the alleged nuisance noise when these planes use existing commercial airports. Noise is also a factor in the comfort level of the paying passengers in the airliner's cabin. Fatigue, mental distraction, inattention, or failure to understand warning sounds all contribute to the total problem of noise in jet travel.

Noise of a fairly constant intensity and pitch is called "white" or "steady-state" noise. The intermittent or impact noise produced by such things as a drop forge is much more annoying to most humans than the equivalent noise from a steady-state source. The noise from jet aircraft falls into the steady-state noise category. The crew members of military jet aircraft should experience little or no noise problem from the standpoint of comfort or from that of hearing loss so long as the present requirement for a helmet of some sort remains. If jet aircraft are developed in which the pilot is in a small sealed capsule, it is conceivable that noise levels might be sufficiently high to be of some clinical or compensational importance. This is highly improbable so long as there is a requirement for a relatively low threshold of noise where conversation by voice radio is a necessity.

The noise factor for the passengers of jet airliners is of much more concern. The concern is not so much for the potential hearing loss that could reasonably be attributed to noise levels within the aircraft but simply a matter of passenger annoyance and loss of revenue from people who would not travel by jet aircraft. The impression that many people have concerning the quiet of the jet airliner is, in part, due to the difference in the character of the noise. The noise from propellers and piston-driven engines combined with the more noticeable vibration levels gives the subjective impression of there being a greater noise level in the case of piston-driven aircraft. Lederer (22) compared noise and vibration characteristics of piston-driven and turboprop aircraft. Neither is as low as the comfort level curve (S.A.E.-Janeway curve) which is the maximum level tolerated by the automobile industry of the United States. The turboprop vibration curve is well below that which Getline (9) found to cause complaints in military passengers. Pure jet transports should have a vibration characteristic that more closely resembles the S.A.E.-Janeway curve. The problem of noise and the public's reaction against it were already well known during the design phases of the engineering development of American jet aircraft. Thus, it is anticipated that there will not be any major problem from the standpoint of the noise level in American jet transports as far as passengers are concerned.

There will be a need to watch carefully and periodically to evaluate the crews of jet airliners. The high noise level of the steady-state noise, with its deceptive impression of being less severe, coupled with the many man-hours of exposure of the crew, might create some actual acoustic trauma of sufficient degree to cause perceptive deafness.

In industrial medicine it was long ago recognized that management in industry needed very specific guides in order to determine safe tolerances of various industrial hazards. The most widely accepted standards called "threshold limit values" are published each spring at the annual meeting of the American Conference of Governmental Industrial Hygienists (42).

The threshold limit values for noise for an entire vocational career have not yet been completely established. The tremendous complexity of designing worthwhile experiments to determine what the values might be is such that it may be another decade or more before such a standard can be agreed upon. The aggregate of considerations along these lines can be referred to as "damage risk criteria." *It is highly improbable that sound levels of 90 decibels or less for eight hours per day or less would be likely to cause any permanent hearing loss or premature presbycusis in a person whose hearing organs were otherwise normal* (32). Very few people in jet operations are exposed to noise levels of more than 90 decibels

for significant periods approaching forty hours per week. When the
F-100 series of aircraft were introduced into the United States Air
Force operational inventory, considerable apprehension was expressed by many persons regarding the hazards to hearing. Operating experience over the past several years has indicated that most of
these fears have been groundless. Certain ground operations require
prolonged exposure. Most of these can be carried out on properly
designed engine-test stands where the principal operators are in a
sound-protective booth. The operator needed outside the booth
can be protected by a helmet similar to that worn by pilots. The
helmet has the advantage over the ear defenders which are inserted
into the external auditory canals, because much of the noise energy
is deflected away from the skull and therefore cannot reach the
acoustic branch of the eighth cranial nerve in damaging levels even
through the skull.

## Waste Disposal

**Gaseous Wastes.** The only significant gaseous waste product
from human metabolism is carbon dioxide. In jet transports the
problem of carbon dioxide must be solved in conjunction with that
of the recirculation of cabin air and the introduction of pressurized
ambient atmosphere coupled with occasional use of oxygen during
in-flight emergencies. It would be virtually impossible for the carbon dioxide level in the cabin to build up to a toxic level of 5,000
ppm unless there were concurrent difficulties in the over-all supply
of air in the ventilating system. Similarly, in military jet aircraft
utilizing present-day oxygen equipment, there is no foreseeable
problem since it is merely a matter of exhausting the carbon dioxide
into the cabin air with replacement by oxygen and ambient air mixtures. For the most part the higher altitude jets with which this
book is concerned will be using pure liquid oxygen systems.

Carbon dioxide will be a major problem in any aircraft with a
crew capsule or in any space vehicle. This was well demonstrated
during one high-altitude balloon flight when a malfunction of the
carbon dioxide resorption mechanism occurred. This resulted in a
toxic level of carbon dioxide within the gondola. Subsequent deleterious effects on the crew member were noted (37).

**Perspiration.** Moisture and odor products are the two principal
problems resultant from perspiration of humans in jet and space

flights. The normal airline passenger, with average amounts of insensible perspiration and relatively minor production of body odors, constitutes no major additional problem. As with carbon dioxide content, the concomitant problems of ventilation and oxygen supply are such that humidity and odor control are not thought to be sources of great difficulty for design engineers. The relative humidity of the compressed ambient air at high altitudes is rather low, so that the water from perspiration is in reality a welcome by-product of human metabolism. In a high-altitude military jet aircraft the flying gear is relatively impervious to any interchange of air and water vapor. The perspiration generated by the aircrews during ground operation is of relatively short duration and is minor in importance. The removal of body odors from the flight clothes of military pilots is something that has not uniformly received all desirable attention. Ready rooms in military aircraft operations often have the odor of a second-rate gymnasium.

In space cabins and capsule cockpits, the problem of the disposal of perspiration may be something much more significant (37). This may develop into a difficult engineering problem but is not insurmountable. Certain oxidizing agents for odor control cannot be considered because of their toxicity. A specific example is ozone which would effectively remove many odors, but its irritant qualities, which became best publicized during smog studies of metropolitan areas, are such that resulting conjunctival and nasal irritation render it completely unsuitable. Absorption agents, such as activated carbon, while effective and harmless, may be of little practicability due to the weight and bulk involved. One partial solution to this problem might be the selection of anosmic crew members. Activated charcoal functioned satisfactorily during the one-week confinement of a subject in a simulated space cabin in 1959. Although the protection was satisfactory to the occupant, the stench was considered nauseating to other humans when the chamber was opened at the end of the week. The space and weight required for the charcoal was entirely compatible with the physical limitations of this experimental cabin (39). Nader (28) has developed an odor-evaluation apparatus that may prove useful in future simulated space cabin design.

**Urine.** The disposition of urine from aircraft in flight is a problem that has, in many respects, been side-stepped rather than solved.

The International Sanitary Regulations (17), adopted in 1951, state in Article 31: "no matter capable of causing any epidemic diseases shall be thrown or allowed to fall from any aircraft when it is in flight." This has been generally interpreted to mean that urine may not be discharged from an aircraft in flight. Many thousands of private and military aircraft today rather casually disregard this article with no apparent public furor resulting. In the United States the public has passively accepted the strewing of human feces across the railroad roadbeds of the country and has not developed any keen awareness of, or concern about, a theoretical urine mist from any aircraft flying over an international boundary.

While it is theoretically possible to transmit leptospirosis and typhoid fever by urine from an infected patient, it is completely beyond the realm of possibility that discharges at altitudes of 40,000 ft. or higher could endanger the health of any other persons in the aircraft or on the ground. The vaporization and dispersion of fluids coming from such a high altitude would make this solely a theoretical situation. A further practical consideration is that persons who are passing viable pathogenic microorganisms through the urinary tract are, in general, in the invasive and early states of an infection, which would most likely render them too ill to consider travel.

For jet transports the problem of urine disposal will not be significantly different from that of piston-driven aircraft with the use of so-called chemical toilets. With proper sanitary precautions at terminals, these should take care of the sanitation and esthetic problems involved. Any method by which urine is allowed to accumulate at a temperature above 40° F will create the problem of putrefaction. Various chemical preparations are, to varying degrees, satisfactory for the control of these odors, and the resulting odors are somewhat less annoying than those of protein destruction (25). Progress in colloid chemistry is such that it is hoped that eventually there may be developed a practical colloid resin ion exchanger in a simple, small, light-weight device to alter some of the chemicals of urine to lessen the noxious odors from this putrefaction.

In the space cabin on extended flights, the problem of urine will be tremendous in comparison to that of other modes of transportation. The necessity for conservation of each molecule of water is so great that reuse of the water components of urine will be a necessity. Clark (4) suggested that the best ultimate method may be a chemical or physical chemistry process. This would eliminate objections to a biological exchange system with mutations from radiation, diseases of algae, and other problems. The possibility of using ion-exchange resins, such as Amberlite MB-5, urease from jack beans, and an electroosmotic system utilizing selective permeable membranes has also been considered. Any of these systems would require a large input of energy. At present this is a challenge to physicists and engineers to provide efficient utilization of solar or nuclear energy so that biochemists can develop a practical solution to the problem.

Feces. For tactical jet aircraft when the duration of flight is twenty-four hours or less, it has been the practice of aircrews to abstain from defecation as the primary means of solving the problem of feces disposal in flight. In B-66 crews, which participate in long-range over-water missions, it has been the practice to plan every tactical or operational situation sufficiently far in advance to enable the crews to subsist on a very low residue diet for seventy-two hours prior to take-off. This deliberate, induced constipation has not proved too great a problem to the crews at the completion of the flight. One of the many reasons why crews have resorted to this rather undesirable procedure is that the survival suits worn on a long, over-water flight make it nearly impossible in a cramped aircraft to have a bowel movement.

It is generally conceded by aircrew members that should a bowel movement be inescapable, the survival suit itself would be the receptacle for the feces. Injudicious intake of unsanitary foods with copious diarrhea resulting leads to a completely unacceptable situation. At best, flyers accept the survival suits with great reluctance because of the excessive weight, the physical discomfort, and the total lack of evaporative cooling of the body usually resulting from normal perspiration.

Feces disposal in jet transports will not be significantly different from that now accomplished in pressurized, piston-driven aircraft using the so-called chemical toilet (25). The existing requirements for thorough cleaning of all components of these systems will remain a definite requirement for an indefinite time. Live steam will coagulate the protein of viral, fungous, rickettsial, protozoan, and bacterial pathogens. No other method of sanitizing can be so reliable in the hands of slightly skilled airport maintenance employees.

In space cabins, if the duration of the flight is only a few days, the most probable method of feces disposal will be with impermeable plastic bags. The bulk of a few days will not be too great, and the completely unesthetic putrefactive decomposition will be kept from the olfactory organs of the crew members by the physical barrier of the plastic bag. For medium-length voyages incineration may ultimately prove to be the best method of disposal of feces. Although no such apparatus has yet been designed to meet all major criteria, some models accomplish the primary objective. For trips involving many months, the use of the incinerator might be incorporated in an atomic conservation system utilizing a synthetic diet with physicochemical syntheses to convert carbon and nitrogen atoms into molecules suitable for food and energy. A biological system for reuse of feces may prove to be the unavoidable and best compromise.

## Effective Temperature Index

One of the most important factors in cabin habitability is the effective temperature index (15). This index is a mathematical means of expressing body comfort, correlating three interdependent variables, namely, temperature, humidity, and air velocity. The public has been somewhat educated to the fact that humidity is important in relation to tolerances to high temperatures, but is not fully cognizant of the complete interdependence of these three factors. A fourth factor of varying importance is radiation. A person may be in an environment that has an essentially ideal effective temperature index and yet be close to a very cold or very hot surface. His body may radiate heat toward a cold surface in quantities sufficient to develop a subjective sense of chill. Conversely, a radiant electric heater close to him may produce discomfort in the presence of an ideal combination of ambient air temperature, relative humidity, and air velocity.

Through studies, which were as objective as could be made, on hundreds of subjects in various parts of the country, heating and ventilating engineers have developed nomograms by which the effective temperature index can be computed. When the dry-bulb temperature and air velocity are known, an effective temperature index of 85° F can be found on the nomogram. One combination would be a reading of 85° F on the dry thermometer, 85° F on the wet-bulb thermometer, and air movement of zero linear feet per minute. Expressed another way, this is ambient air in which there is 85° of heat with 100 per cent relative humidity and no breeze. If we increase the velocity and decrease the wet-bulb reading, the dry-bulb reading can move much higher without increasing discomfort, as indicated by the effective temperature index. A dry-bulb reading into the nineties can still have an effective temperature index as low as 85°, if there is a low enough humidity and high enough velocity of air movement.

The advantages of air conditioning can be had simply by other means at low cost. For example, a house can be partially air-conditioned so that the dry-bulb reading is 85° and the relative humidity is down to 20 per cent. If the ventilation in this house is increased by the use of an ordinary, quiet, oscillating fan so that the air velocity approaches 100 linear feet per minute, then the effective temperature index moves down into the low seventies, and the occupants are much more comfortable.

In adapting the information of the above example to a consideration of passenger and crew comfort, it is apparent that the weight and energy involved in the air conditioning of the plane can be most effectively utilized if the highest tolerable comfort level of air movement is provided. This, of course, is applicable only when excessive heat is a problem. Conversely, in heating a cool cabin, which is the problem at altitude, the air velocity should be dropped to the minimum consistent with odor and humidity control, otherwise it will be necessary to maintain a high dry-bulb temperature.

Ground operations of any of the types of jet aircraft or spacecraft will involve serious air-conditioning problems if they take off at latitudes and seasons when the ambient effective temperature index is 75° or higher. Newer transport planes are being designed to handle adequately the problem of air conditioning required on the ground. In addition to the physical discomfort which might indirectly result in the loss of revenue passengers, there is the problem of an increased tendency toward motion sickness in persons who are uncomfortable and unhappy due to the excess heat and humidity experienced during ground operations. The vast majority of commercial and military aircraft presently flying have air-conditioning equipment incapable of providing a tolerable effective temperature index in less than fifteen minutes after take-off, if the effective temperature index was as high as 85° while the aircraft was on the ground.

In consideration of the effective temperature index and air-conditioning requirements, it should be remembered that these vary tremendously with the type and phase of flight. In jet aircraft flight there will be no heat dissipation problem at altitudes from 5,000 ft. upward and at speeds below Mach 1. As the speed approaches the "thermal thicket," problems in dissipation of heat multiply with exceeding rapidity. In vehicles that have been in outer space and are returning, there will be a tremendous thermal dispersion problem in which the principles of the effective temperature index will have to be carefully considered if the human components of the vehicle are to return relatively intact. This phase of the problem is such a tremendous engineering challenge that no simple statement in this section could adequately convey the total requirements that must be met.

Under prolonged use of 100 per cent oxygen, toxicity frequently results (27). One fact concerning breathing oxygen, which is often overlooked, is the fact that this is an almost totally anhydrous gas. It is necessary to keep oxygen dry to prevent blocking of the oxygen supply at high altitudes by freezing of moisture in the oxygen lines. Breathing of completely dry oxygen results in considerable drying of the mucous membranes of the respiratory tract. This in turn involves the desire for a higher water intake of crew members who are on 100 per cent oxygen. The water-vapor control in cabin space vehicles must be planned, bearing in mind that the liquid oxygen supply contributes nothing to the humidity comfort of the crew. Some desirable level of humidity will have to be found.

Excessive heat, humidity, and odors are frequently a great problem during ground operations. Hence, it is highly desirable to have the maximum tolerable velocity of air.

## Industrial Health

Several aspects of industrial health have already been mentioned. This section presents a brief summary of other problems in this field particularly related to modern jet and space travel.

Air pollution per se should be of no great concern in view of the unavoidable need for proper ventilation and air conditioning. It is desirable that overseas air terminals be located where smog and smaze are known to be infrequent problems.

Nuttall (31) has reviewed major aircraft accidents and incidents in the United States Air Force and analyzed them in regard to toxic hazards. *Carbon monoxide,* JP-4 fuel, trichloroethylene, and other agents have contributed to accidents and near-accidents.

Schreuder (35) has outlined the broad requirements for the establishment of an industrial health program for an international airline using jet transports. His views merit careful consideration in all stages of planning for expansion of routes, especially for airlines that have not previously engaged in overseas operations. Newer fuels and propellants of aircraft and rockets are variable in their toxicity. Some are more lethal than the hydrogen cyanide used in the execution chambers of state penitentiaries. Stumpe (40) has considered the health hazards of the borones (boron hydrides), ethyl alcohol, methyl alcohol, asymmetric dimethylhydrazine, ammonia, JP-4, red fuming nitric acid, fluorine, 90 per cent hydrogen peroxide, ozone, and liquid oxygen. Some of these agents are so new and so different in application that they have not yet been included in the latest threshold limit values (42).

## References

1. *An Annotated Bibliography on Noise, Its Measurements, Effects, and Control.* Industrial Hygiene Foundation of America, Inc., Mellon Institute, Pittsburgh, Pa., 1955. P. 364.
2. CHANG, S. L., STEVENSON, R. E., BRYANT, A. R., WOODWARD, R. L., and KABLER, P. S. 1958. Removal of Coxsackie and bacterial viruses in water by flocculation. *Am. J. Public Health* 48: 159–169.
3. Chlortetracycline as a preservative. *Public Health Repts.* (*U.S.*) 71: 66, 1956.
4. CLARK, C. C. 1958. A closed food cycle atomic conservation for space flight. *J. Aviation Med.* 29: 535–540.
5. *Drinking Water Standards.* U.S. Department of Health, Education, and Welfare, Public Health Report (Reprint No. 2679). 1946.
6. EICHENWALD, H. F. 1955. *Viral Hepatitis.* (Public Health Service Pub. No. 435.) U.S. Department of Health, Education, and Welfare, Washington, D.C.
7. *First Report, Expert Committee on Hepatitis.* (World Health Organization Tech. Rep. Ser., No. 62.) Columbia University Press, New York, 1953.
8. FREEDMAN, B. 1957. *Sanitarians Handbook.* Peerless Publishing Co., New Orleans.
9. GETLINE, G. L. 1955. *Vibration Tolerance Levels in Military Aircraft, Supplement to the 22d Shock and Vibration Bulletin.* (U.S. Navy Research Laboratory Bull. No. 22.)
10. *Handbook on Sanitation of Airlines.* (Public Health Service Pub. No. 308.) Washington, D.C., 1953.
11. HARRIS, C. M. 1957. *Handbook of Noise Control.* McGraw-Hill Book Co., Inc., New York.

12. HARROW, B., and MAZUR, A. 1954. *Textbook of Biochemistry.* 6th ed. W. B. Saunders Co., Philadelphia.

13. HAUTY, G. T., and PAYNE, R. B. 1958. Effects of analeptic and depressant drugs upon psychological behavior. *Am. J. Pub. Health* 48: 571–577.

14. *Health Protection for Air Travelers Planned by W.H.O. J. Aviation Med.* 29: 628–629, 1958.

15. *Heating Ventilating Air Conditioning Guide.* 36th ed. American Society of Heating, Refrigerating and Air-Conditioning Engineers, Inc., New York. 1958.

16. *Immunization Information for International Travel.* (Supplement to Public Health Service Publ. No. 384.) U.S. Department of Health, Education, and Welfare. 1957.

17. *International Sanitary Regulations.* (World Health Organization Tech. Rep. Ser., No. 41.) Columbia University Press, New York. 1951.

18. KEAN, B. H., and WATERS, S. 1958. The diarrhea of travelers. *A.M.A. Arch. Ind. Health* 18: 148–150.

19. KLEINER, I. S., and ORTEN, J. M. 1958. *Human Biochemistry.* C. V. Mosby Company, St. Louis.

20. KONECCI, E. B. 1958. Human factors in space flight. *Aero/Space Eng.* 17: 34–40.

21. KRAYBIEL, H. F. 1957. Radiation preservation of food. *Public Health Repts.* (U.S.) 72: 675–680.

22. LEDERER, L. G. 1956. The aeromedical aspects of turbo-prop commercial aircraft. *J. Aviation Med.* 27: 293.

23. LINDQUIST, D. A., and FAY, P. W. 1956. Laboratory comparison of eight organic phosphorus insecticides as larvacides against non-resistant house flies. *J. Econ. Entomol.* 49: 463–465.

24. MAXCY, K. F. 1956. *Preventive Medicine and Public Health.* 8th ed. Appleton-Century-Crofts, Inc., New York.

25. MEGONNELL, W. H., and CHAPMAN, H. W. 1956. Sanitation of domestic airlines. *Public Health Repts.* (U.S.) 71: 360–368.

26. MEGONNELL, W. H., and GARTHE, E. C. 1955. Dining car sanitation. *Public Health Repts.* (U.S.) 70: 25–34.

27. MULLINAX, P. F., and BEISCHER, D. E. 1958. Oxygen toxicity in aviation medicine. *J. Aviation Med.* 29: 660–667.

28. NADER, J. S. 1958. An odor evaluation apparatus for field and laboratory use. *Am. Ind. Hyg. Assoc. Quart.* 19: 1–7.

29. NICKERSON, J. T. R., PROCTOR, B. E., and GOLDBLITH, S. A. 1958. Freezing and irradiation. *Am. J. Public Health* 48: 1041–1048.

30. NORTON, J. A. 1939. Acute infectious jaundice. *J. Am. Med. Assoc.* 113: 916–917.

31. NUTTALL, J. B. 1958. Toxic hazards in the aviation environment. *J. Aviation Med.* 29: 641–649.

32. PARRACK, H. O. 1956. Noise, vibration, and people. *Noise Control* 2: 10–24.

33. *Procedures for the Investigation of Food-borne Disease Outbreaks.* International Association of Milk and Food Sanitarians, Shelbyville, Ind. 1957.

34. ROTH, M. R., and WILLIS, E. R. 1957. *The Medical and Veterinary Importance of Cockroaches.* (Smithsonian Inst. Misc. Coll. 134, No. 10, Pub. No. 4299.) Government Printing Office, Washington, D.C.

35. SCHREUDER, O. B. 1958. Occupational health in international airline operation. *J. Aviation Med.* 29: 37–39.

36. Sees future for antibiotics as food preservatives. *Public Health Repts.* (U.S.) 72: 231–232, 1957.

37. SIMONS, D. G. 1958. Pilot reactions during "manhigh II" balloon flight. *J. Aviation Med.* 29: 1–14.

38. *Standard Methods for the Examination of Water, Sewage, and Industrial Wastes.* 10th ed. American Public Health Association, New York. 1955.

39. STEINKAMP, G. R. Personal communication. October 3, 1958.

40. STUMPE, A. R. 1958. Health hazards of new aircraft and rocket propellants. *J. Aviation Med.* 29: 650–659.

41. TAYLOR, A. A., and FINKELSTEIN, B. 1958. Preventive medicine aspects of flight feeding. *Am. J. Public Health* 48: 604–609.

42. Threshold Limit Values for 1958. *A.M.A. Arch. Ind. Health* 18: 178–182, 1958.

43. *Water Quality and Treatment.* 2nd ed. The American Water Works Association, Inc., New York. 1951.

# 10

# Aircraft Accidents and Flight Safety

HARRY G. MOSELEY, M.D.[*]

It is probable that one of the most significant deterrents to future progress in jet and space flight will be losses through accidents. Such accidents will be costly from a material viewpoint and disastrous as far as loss of life is concerned, because increasing velocities will provoke increasing destruction when mishaps occur. Inasmuch as human factors have been the primary cause of accidents in the past and will probably be the primary cause of most accidents in the future, the problem of preventing these losses will remain a highly important challenge.

## Magnitude

**Loss of Life.** Among accidents involving mankind those concerned with aircraft and their occupants are characterized by a high incidence of loss of life. Although accidents occurring when velocities are relatively low, such as in landing or take-off stages, may have little traumatic potential, those occurring when high velocities are suddenly interrupted are accompanied by severe to extreme traumatic forces in the form of deceleration, explosion, and fire. In military flying where the risk is relatively high, aircraft accidents are the foremost cause of death among personnel on flying status (Table 10–1). These percentages, incidentally, have not varied significantly during the history of military aviation, and sudden or marked

[*] Colonel, USAF, MC, (Late) Chief, Aeromedical Safety Division, Directorate of Flight Safety Research, Office of The Inspector General, USAF, Norton Air Force Base, California.

TABLE 10–1

Causes of Death, USAF Personnel on Flying Status, 1954–1955 *

| Cause of Death | Number | Percentage |
|---|---|---|
| Neoplasms | 16 | 1 |
| Circulatory disease | 26 | 2 |
| Other disease | 15 | 1 |
| Firearms and violence | 61 | 4 |
| Traffic (land vehicles) | 95 | 7 |
| Aircraft accidents | 1,176 | 85 |
| TOTAL | 1,389 | 100 |

* Department of the Air Force: Fourth Annual Report of the USAF Medical Service.

change is not therefore anticipated unless there are radical changes in the safety of future aircraft or flight-operating procedures. However, even in non-military aircraft, loss of life is significant (Table 10–2). Scheduled domestic flying where aircraft reliability is well established and where the crews are highly experienced has a relatively small risk factor. Nevertheless as a result of the large numbers of miles flown, the cumulative loss of life is serious. This indicates that, up to the present at least, even with aircraft of great mechanical and structural reliability and with well-trained aircrews, significant loss of life occurs. With any relaxation of safety standards, such losses could increase.

TABLE 10–2

Accidents and Fatalities, United States Civil Flying *

| Year | Revenue Operations | | Non-Air Carrier | |
|---|---|---|---|---|
| | Number Accidents | Number Fatalities | Number Accidents | Number Fatalities |
| 1946 | 33 | 75 | 7,618 | 1,009 |
| 1947 | 44 | 222 | 9,253 | 1,352 |
| 1948 | 56 | 98 | 7,850 | 1,384 |
| 1949 | 35 | 113 | 5,459 | 896 |
| 1950 | 39 | 109 | 4,505 | 871 |
| 1951 | 45 | 170 | 3,824 | 750 |
| 1952 | 44 | 54 | 3,657 | 691 |
| 1953 | 37 | 103 | 3,232 | 635 |
| 1954 | 49 | 23 | 3,381 | 684 |
| 1955 | 45 | 179 | 3,308 | 613 † |

* Bureau of Safety, CAB.
† There has been a steady fall in accident rates from 1 accident per 114,825 miles flown in 1946 to 1 per 367,594 in 1955.

**Other Losses.** Jet aircraft are extraordinarily expensive. Large aircraft, such as jet bombers and transports, are in the multimillion-dollar class. As advancements are made in vehicles capable of carrying personnel at higher speeds and to greater altitudes, the costs are expected to continue to increase. Thus, future accidents resulting in the destruction of jet or space vehicles will also represent a serious economic loss (11). The significance of such losses will be great, although difficult to interpret if only the financial aspect is considered. However, if human effort is considered, it is probable that each accident will represent the loss of hundreds of man-years of skilled, productive effort. Therefore, large numbers of such accidents could constitute an intolerable economic wastage.

In addition, aircraft catastrophes cause a setback in aeronautical progress which is defiant of accurate measurement. The adversities of public opinion, withdrawal of financial support, and even diversion of human ingenuity into other enterprises are some of the results. The avoidance of aircraft accidents, therefore, is of great significance to all who are engaged in the support of aviation.

## Types of Major Aircraft Accidents

Major aircraft accidents are usually categorized by the event or circumstance affecting the aircraft at the time of the accident. In this respect the terms used to describe the type of accident are ordinarily synonymous with the phase of flight at the time of the accident, i.e., undershoot, wheels-up landing, etc. Accident types give a valuable indication as to areas of concern and where preventive effort should be directed (4). Table 10–3 is a review of the frequency of various types of accidents in both civilian and Air Force flying which occurred in the United States during the calendar year 1956. There are at least two significant observations to be made in relation to this table. The first is that most accidents are associated with the landing process. This includes the first seven categories listed in the table and some of the accidents listed for "Other collision, aircraft." All accidents in this latter category are ground collisions during landing or take-off roll or during taxiing. In the past, accidents in the landing phase have usually been associated with moderate velocities, and the fatality rate has been relatively low. However, in jet aircraft accidents when there are high approach and landing speeds, such mishaps are much more serious, and therefore the prevention of accidents in this category is becoming of increasing concern.

A category of even greater concern is in-flight collisions. These are grouped in the two categories "Mid-air collision" and "Other collision, object." The latter are usually collisions with the terrain or objects incident thereto such as trees and poles. Accidents in this

TABLE 10–3

Types of Aircraft Accidents, USAF and United States Civilian Aircraft,
Calendar Year 1956 *

| Type of Aircraft Accident | U.S. Civil Non-Air Carrier | U.S. Civil Air Carrier | USAF |
|---|---|---|---|
| Ground loop | 570 | 8 | 79 |
| Wheels-up landing | 142 | 6 | 197 |
| Hard landing | 198 | 8 | 95 |
| Collapse-retract landing gear | 99 | 10 | 71 |
| Undershoot | 215 | 4 | 66 |
| Overshoot | 176 | 5 | 55 |
| Nose up or over | 183 | 1 | 10 |
| Mid-air collision | 14 | 2 | 61 |
| Other collision, aircraft | 50 | 1 | 157 |
| Other collision, object (ground or water) | 760 | 26 | 205 |
| Spin and stall | 606 | 3 | 70 |
| Fire in air | 9 | 2 | 119 |
| Air-frame failure, ground or air | 25 | 7 | 39 |
| Other | 100 | 22 | 216 † |
| TOTAL | 3,147 | 105 | 1,440 |

* U.S. Civil: CAB Bureau of Safety; USAF: Directorate of Flight Safety Research, USAF.
† Of these, 120 were abandoned in air.

category are characterized by relatively high fatality rates, as high velocities and abrupt deceleration are frequent. As supersonic speeds are attained, survival from an in-flight collision cannot be expected except under the most unusual circumstances. Prevention of in-flight collisions is, therefore, a major issue in flight safety.

## Causes of Aircraft Accidents

Aircraft accidents, like other vehicular accidents, do not just happen; they are caused (3, 9, 12, 13). They are caused by unsafe acts or omissions on the part of the pilot or his crew members or by unsafe conditions beyond their control. For example, if a pilot forgets to put the wheels down and tears up his aircraft in the subsequent bellylanding, he has committed an unsafe act. On the other hand, if the engine fails in flight and the aircraft is destroyed in the crashlanding, the accident is due to an unsafe condition. Table 10–3 includes all causes, both primary and secondary, for Air Force and United States civilian aircraft for the year 1956.

Most accidents are considered to have a primary cause that is the act or condition that made the accident most inevitable and one or more secondary causes that also contributed to the accident. An example is a mishap when the pilot ground-looped while landing in a strong cross-wind. The primary cause is attributed to the pilot's mishandling of the aircraft (most pilots would not have ground-looped), and the secondary cause is the weather. Often contributing causes are not identified. When a pilot flies into the ground under instrument conditions, as a result of misreading his altimeter, the cause is usually attributed to an unsafe act on the part of the aircraft operator. The fact that misreading the altimeter is unsafe cannot be contested. However, the additional fact that the altimeter is difficult to interpret is often overlooked in accident investigations. Careful identification of all causes is essential if adequate corrective action is to be taken.

**Unsafe Acts.** Pilot-factor accidents are discussed in detail below. In addition, errors and omissions on the part of supervisory and maintenance personnel can be direct causes of aircraft accidents. The most obvious of these involves maintenance personnel when inadequate attention to essential maintenance procedures, such as preflight lubrication, may result in materiel failure and cause an accident. When the aircraft subsequently is totally destroyed, it is frequently difficult or impossible to isolate maintenance oversight as the definitive factor. Thus, the role of inadequate maintenance is deserving of more consideration than afforded by its identification with accidents. Supervisory personnel may likewise lead to an aircraft accident by inadequate supervision or insufficient direction of essential aircraft upkeep.

The most frequent type of supervisory error leading to an aircraft accident lies in the establishment of unsafe flight procedures or failure to monitor the flight properly. This may occur when instructor pilots or aircraft commanders allow an inexperienced pilot or crew member to commit an unsafe act or to omit an essential procedure while they are aboard in a supervisory capacity. More seriously, supervisors may commit an inexperienced pilot to a flight beyond his capability. If an accident results, it is ordinarily charged to the pilot for failing to meet the demands of the occasion. The supervisor who directed him to undertake the flight may or may not be implicated. Under such circumstances failure to recognize supervisory error is not in the best interest of accident prevention. Such accidents can only be avoided when supervisors realize the accident potential of inexperience and similar factors and avoid commitments that exceed the capabilities of their flight crews.

**Unsafe Conditions.** Accidents attributable to failure of the aircraft are primarily of design or engineering concern. Detailed reviews of air-frame and power-plant problems and their relation to aircraft accidents are presented in various aeronautical engineering publications. In addition both civilian and governmental agencies maintain up-to-date information on facilities, navigational aids, air-traffic control, and other matters related to support of flight. The human-factors interest with regard to unsafe conditions is primarily in the field of industrial hygiene and is beyond the scope of this publication. However, materiel-failure accidents are seldom the result of catastrophic in-flight conditions. Such accidents usually result subsequent to problems such as engine failure, malfunction of an aircraft system, e.g., the fuel or hydraulic system, or from mechanical or electrical irregularities which are of concern but not of a critical nature. Under such circumstances it is usually possible to continue controlled flight temporarily, and remedial measures often can be taken. However, the handling of in-flight mechanical adversities is a serious challenge, even to highly trained aircraft pilots. When such emergencies confront an inexperienced pilot or when they occur during critical stages of flight, they often cannot be effectively countered and an accident occurs. Therefore, human capability to handle mechanical malfunctions becomes a matter of concern.

## Pilot-Factor Accidents

Because of its importance this topic is extracted from other cause factors and considered separately. There are four different ways in which an aircraft operator may commit or become responsible for an act or omission leading to an aircraft accident: (1) He may be physically unable to meet the demands of operating the vehicle in a particular situation. (2) He may be the victim of physiological compromise. (3) He may be unable to make an appropriate adaptive response requiring intellectual application. (4) The demands of the flight may exceed the fundamental limitations of his capacity to respond to stimuli encountered. These are considered separately.

**Physical Ability.** From the viewpoint of accident prevention, the physical requirements of an aircraft operator are relatively simple to define. Flying requires certain medians of size and strength, acuity of the physical senses, reasonable stamina and resistance to stress, and immunity insofar as possible from sudden physical incapacitation. The criteria for selecting such individuals are well defined with the result that when adequate screening methods are used and when proper medical surveillance is practiced, aircraft operators are able to meet the physical requirements of aircraft operation (1). As a result accidents due to physical incapacity are a rarity.

Almost the only defiant problem in this category is that of sudden and unexpected incapacitation. This may not appear to be a problem in younger age groups. Accidents, however, have been caused by such conditions as *epilepsy, syncope,* and *cardiovascular* phenomena (i.e., *paroxysmal tachycardia*). Inasmuch as the potentiality of sudden incapacitation from deteriorative disease increases with advancing age, there is a concomitant increase of accident potentials in this area in the older pilot population. However, such conditions are well understood and health factors are well monitored, and accidents attributable to such conditions have been a rarity to the present time.

**Physiological Compromise.** Physiological compromise is of much greater concern (2). In any flight in which high velocities are involved and areas of low barometric pressure are traversed, the effectiveness of the aircraft occupant is directly dependent upon the proper functioning of the artificial environment. It is obvious that whenever there is inadequacy or failure of environment control, rapid incapacitation may result. In this regard the potential harm of radiation is still to be determined. Even though the dangers of incapacitation from such physiological compromise are well known, the problem has not been solved insofar as flight is concerned. The military services experience repeated instances of in-flight *hypoxia* and *dysbarism*. In single-place aircraft these can lead to accidents. Usually such accidents are so destructive that the cause can only be surmised. Thus, the role of physiological compromise often escapes detection.

Two important conditions of physiological compromise are frequently overlooked. These are fatigue and disorientation.

*Fatigue* is not amenable to accurate measurement. Therefore, its role in detracting from an aircraft operator's efficiency of performance is seldom defined. However, it is obvious that the accomplishment of any complex and highly critical task will suffer some comparative delay or imperfection if the individual concerned has applied himself for such a prolonged period that physical and mental efficiency is impaired. Landing an aircraft, especially under adverse weather conditions or when the operation is complicated by mechanical irregularities, is a complex task. Under such circumstances fatigue may be a significant factor of accident potential.

*Disorientation* is of exceptional importance in high-performance flight (8). In some respects it may be inappropriate to include this phenomenon in the category of physiological compromise. Except in instances of severe *vertigo,* disorientation does not lead to profound incapacitation as in the case of oxygen deprivation. However, insofar as flight safety is concerned, a disoriented aircraft operator is in great jeopardy. High-velocity aircraft cover enormous distances in a brief space of time, and the structure of these vehicles is such that sudden changes in flight path can lead to structural disintegration. If the pilot becomes confused as to the direction he is traveling or is subjected to *vertiginous* stimuli, he could establish a flight path that might commit the aircraft to striking the ground or to structural disintegration before recovery could be effected.

There are several factors that contribute to disorientation. One is the simple condition of mistaken direction which might arise from poor flight planning, faulty compasses, misinterpreted radio signals, and the like. This is the least dangerous of the various disorientations, as often there is ample opportunity to gather new information and correct the error before an accident results. This might well be called "misorientation."

Much more serious is the disorientation that arises from the false sensations of flight. In instrument flight the altimeter, the air-speed indicator, and the attitude indicators replace or augment the physical senses. Whenever anything detracts from surveillance of these instruments, such as diversions to maps or radio, the operator is deprived of accurate information concerning external events and is vulnerable to misinformation. Under such circumstances the only information he may receive concerning the flight is from the proprioceptive senses and the inner ear, both of which orient him to the aircraft and not to his true position or direction in space. Reactions to these stimuli often lead the pilot to place the aircraft in a dive or abnormal attitude from which recovery cannot be effected.

**Judgment and Decision.** Errors of judgment and erroneous decisions have always been the foremost reasons why aircraft operators become responsible for aircraft accidents. In spite of the potential physiological adversities in future jet and space flight, such deficiencies will probably remain the greatest deterrent to successful flight. Reviews have suggested that there are several fundamental psychological requirements for the aircraft operator if flight is to be successful. Failure to meet any of them virtually constitutes an accident potential of a magnitude in direct ratio to the degree of deficiency.

CAPACITY. The operation of aircraft requires a certain minimum of competency and emotional stability. When an individual fails to meet these minimums, an aircraft accident can result. In the past careful screening requirements have made accidents due to mental or emotional deficiencies rare. However, increased complexity of aircraft operation is placing an increased demand upon basic ability and personality factors.

KNOWLEDGE AND EXPERIENCE. The operation of modern, high-performance aircraft requires a high degree of skill, specialized knowledge concerning the operation of the aircraft power plants, and familiarity with multitudinous instruments which give information concerning mechanical and physical factors encountered in flight. In addition it requires an acquaintance with high velocity, extreme closing speeds, and unnatural attitudes in space. The required degree of skill and level of knowledge must be attained through careful indoctrination and practice. There is probably no other occupation in which mistakes made in the learning process can be so tragic or costly. And this does not apply solely to initial indoctrination in the art of flying. Due to the rapid progress of aeronautics, new and more complex aircraft succeed each other with great rapidity. Newer models may incorporate radical changes in systems and require special handling techniques. Therefore, even experienced pilots must continually broaden their knowledge of aircraft operation. Failure to respect the need for careful indoctrination in each new aircraft has led to the loss of many skilled pilots during transition flying.

A major requirement in the area of knowledge and experience is that of maintaining proficiency. Inasmuch as the operation of modern aircraft is a complex technical skill, proficiency, once attained, must not be allowed to deteriorate. Although the amount of flying that must be peformed in a given period to prevent such deterioration varies with different aircraft, experience in the Air Force has indicated that when a jet pilot flies less than 50 hours in a six-month period, his accident potential significantly increases.

APPLICATION. The operation of modern aircraft requires a high degree of concentration and mental alertness. This applies particularly to critical stages of flight such as landing or take-off and during aerial maneuvers. The pilot's performance must be sufficiently reliable to assure correct interpretation of all things observed and to encompass multiple sources of vital information. Failure to meet these requirements can manifestly result in oversights leading to an accident. The most obvious are such accidents as wheels-up landings, because the pilot fails to notice position of the landing lever, the gear indicator, or gear-up warning lights. In the same category are many more serious accidents such as those that sometimes occur during high-angle strafing passes when the pilot, intent upon his target, fails to notice the air speed or altimeter and initiates a pull-out too low to avoid striking the ground.

Another aspect of the judgment and alertness requirement is the vital necessity for thorough preconsideration prior to flight. This includes careful development of the flight plan and detailed pre-flight inspection of the aircraft. As explained below, the rapidity of in-flight events often allows no leeway for correcting preflight errors or omissions. Thus, the planning exercised prior to flight is one of the vital measures in accident prevention.

ATTITUDE. The aircraft operator's attitude toward flying conditions his performance. It also strongly influences his reaction to many critical factors in flight. The successful pilot must have a positive orientation and a willing attitude toward his occupation, as any adversity of attitude may result in rejection or overreaction to the feared or disliked subject matter. Pronounced cases of maladaptive attitude can arise from disturbances of mood or general adjustment. In such cases pilots may not only fail to accept but may flatly rebel at rules and regulations. Conversely, excessive motivation can also interfere with the pilot's proper acceptance of guidance and information. These are the cases in which enthusiasm for flying or desire to obtain an objective can cause a pilot to minimize hazardous conditions or take unwarranted chances. In addition, situational apprehension, though usually transitory, can condition the pilot against ready and unprejudiced acceptance of facts or instructions. In typical cases excessive concern over such a condition as a short runway has caused pilots to deviate from recommended approach procedures. Such deviations illustrate what is meant by pilot error, and too frequently they result in aircraft accidents.

**Stimulus-Response Relations.** Survival in flight is basically dependent on the pilot's ability to respond quickly and accurately to a wide range of stimuli. Specifically, the pilot's proficiency can be defined in terms of the following functions: (1) how he perceives his world and cockpit about him and interprets the meaning and significance of what he perceives, (2) how he decides from such observations the course of action that will best assure unhampered continuance of his flight, and (3) how he reacts to on-going events not only to make the aircraft respond to his decisions but also to maintain it in flight and bring it to a safe landing in spite of his preoccupations and distractions.

These complex behaviors can be analyzed in terms of stimulus-response sequences measurable in time varying from the few seconds required to make simple reactions to signals to minutes or hours involved in meeting and solving more complex problems. During high-speed flight, a pilot traverses space at 1,000 ft. or more per second. Thus, unlike most terrestrial occupations, flying often requires instant perception, split-second decision, and immediate response. Every observation, decision, and act must be correct because even minor deficiencies may lead to an irrevocable course of action and end in a destructive accident.

OPPORTUNITY. In view of these requirements, there are several different although somewhat overlapping aspects of human ability to be considered in evaluating the successful operation of aircraft. The first of these is opportunity. Obviously, an essential condition for an adequate response to a stimulus must be the provision of sufficient time to complete the response. It is not uncommon for events incident to high-velocity flight to occur with such rapidity that there is no time for the simplest sequence of reaction. Such would be the case of an aircraft operator flying at night or on instruments who suddenly perceives a mountain 100 ft. or less ahead of him. In the same category are mid-air collisions between converging high-speed aircraft. Closing speeds are such that even though an aircraft operator may perceive another aircraft on a collision course as much as one mile away, the collision would take place before the remaining processes of interpretation, decision, and response could be completed. In this respect many aspects of flight control involving high-velocity jet and space flight are moving beyond the ability of the unaided human aircraft operator. Successful flight, therefore, will depend upon how well the time requirements of human reaction are understood and to what extent appropriate remedial action can be taken.

COMPROMISES. A related problem involves the limitations of attention span and task load on the human operator. The normal individual is able to sustain a high degree of concentration and attention on a task or situation for only a limited time; his attention span is also limited to a small number of tasks at any given time. Both the accuracy of sustained performance and the number of problems to which the individual can simultaneously attend are subject to compromise. Accurate performance can be compromised by distractions that demand attention or by fatigue that lowers efficiency. Distractions during flight planning, for example, may lead to the establishment of a flight course that scatters the aircraft on a mountainside. The requirement for a prolonged flight without relief may lead to a reduction of efficiency of performance that in an emergency situation might cause a landing accident.

An individual may be able to divide his attention between several problems and attend to them in sequence almost simultaneously. But when any one task becomes too demanding, the other problems tend to be neglected. These factors have considerable significance when related to the problem of pilot error, because flying demands a degree of concentration and a range of attention that allows very little compromise. The pilot must be able to perceive, decide, and react rapidly and correctly to any emergency during all stages of flight from the planning of the mission to its successful completion. An illustration of compromise of span of attention is the case in which a pilot, in his desire for exact marksmanship on a high-angle strafing mission, concentrates on the target and overlooks essential observations of speed and altitude, thus failing to pull up in time to avert striking the earth. However, most pertinent of all is the situation in which the requirements of the occasion overwhelm human ability to respond adequately. The following example is typical of this problem:

A multijet aircraft with relatively high gross weight was engaged in a night take-off mission. Water-alcohol engine augmentation was started just prior to the take-off roll. As the aircraft became airborne, the No. 4 engine began to overspeed. Meanwhile, the landing gear which had been activated for retraction failed to retract completely. In order to reduce the drag of the unretracted gear, the mechanism had to be recycled to the "up" position. To control the overspeeding, the No. 4 engine was retarded. Flaps were started up; however, this action took place before the aircraft had attained the minimum speed for flap retraction considering the gross weight of the aircraft. The aircraft began to buffet; the nose was dropped to increase speed; however, the descending path thus established was too steep, and the aircraft struck the ground before it could be leveled. It slid for approximately one-half mile and was destroyed by impact and fire. The four crew members escaped with major injuries.

The pilot was considered responsible for this accident because he attempted flap retraction too soon for the gross weight of the aircraft. However, it is apparent that he was confronted almost simultaneously with an engine malfunction that demanded attention, with gear malfunction that required manipulation, with water-alcohol engine augmentation that required attention, with other essential procedures such as flap retraction, and with *monitorship of attitude, air-speed, and other instruments* during the night take-off. It is entirely understandable that the pilot was unable to analyze clearly and react correctly to all these demands in the brief period of time consumed by this series of events. Although the accident was the direct result of erroneous handling, the events and conditions that influenced the pilot made these erroneous actions almost inevitable.

COMPLICATIONS. Although there are many factors that may divert or confuse an aircraft operator and give him faulty or inadequate stimuli, those most frequently encountered in flight and most often distracting him are complications within the cockpit itself. The cockpit is an artificial, man-made environment, designed to assist the pilot in performing his mission. To do this it should facilitate his requirement for perceiving, deciding, and reacting. Review of aircraft accidents, however, reveals that design sometimes not only fails to facilitate the pilot's task but may on occasion intensify and complicate the fundamental requirements of flying to a point at which aircraft accidents result. The numerous accidents due to such cockpit complications may be grouped in the following general categories:

1. *Instruments and Their Interpretation.* Many accidents have resulted from misreading essential flight instruments. In some cases the difficulty could be attributed to malpositioning or inadequate lighting of critical instruments. But usually the problem has reflected a faulty basic design which resulted in presentation of several different types of information in a confusing or misleading manner. A common example of a confusing instrument is the standard altimeter. This instrument is subject to many misreading errors. On occasion it has become evident that pilots have misread their altitude by 10,000 ft. during critical stages of flight, such as in let-downs. Any instrument that cannot be rapidly and clearly interpreted is obviously detrimental to safe flight.

2. *Instrument Malfunction.* Although it is obvious that instrument malfunction cannot always be prevented, some instruments are so essential to flight that their malfunction can make an accident almost inevitable. An example is a malfunction of attitude indicators during take-off on instrument conditions. A number of accidents that have proved fatal have resulted from this cause. It is apparent that either exceptional reliability or stand-by instruments must be provided if problems in this area are to be solved.

3. *Cockpit Arrangement.* This is perhaps the source of the greatest number of complications. It is also the most resistant to change, partly because correction may require complete redesign but also because of opposition on the part of pilots. Instruments and controls may be so arranged in the cockpit that they seriously divert the pilot during critical stages of flight. Location of the radio channel selector on the rear of the right console is an example. Attending this selector during instrument let-downs has precipitated

many fatal disorientation accidents. The following typical pilot report emphasizes this problem:

It may be well to review what this requires of a pilot. The pilot executes a penetration dive with his left hand on the throttle where the microphone button and the dive brake controls are located. His right hand is on the control stick feeling for the proper pressure and trim tab control. He continually scans the instruments to arrive at the right aircraft altitude and airspeed. He also attempts to keep on (or get to) the correct penetration track by comparing ADF pointer indications and gyro compass headings. Steering corrections for wind-drift are made while the altimeter unwinds, four to six thousand feet per minute down. About this time the controller may break in with several requests for a radio channel change. To comply, the pilot's right hand must leave the stick, and the left hand must leave the throttle to go over to the stick. The left hand may not know what the right was doing; and it takes a few seconds for it to adjust to the feel of its new job. Now the right hand has to feel along a ledge to the right and somewhat to the rear for the radio channel selector. If the pilot is real proficient, he may remember, by feel, the desired positions for the wafer and toggle switch controls. However, he may have to turn his head and body around to get an awkward look at the control switch. The oxygen mask protrudes over his nose in such a way that he has to hold the head and body askew to even see the control box. When he turns back to his instruments, he may find that his penetration dive, which he had intended as a thing of beauty, has degenerated into uncontrolled gyrations.

However, the accident potential may lie in the basic concept of cockpit design. An anachronistic example is found in tandem-seat jet training aircraft in which the instructor pilot, who is far removed from the student pilot, cannot observe the erroneous acts or omissions the student may make. This not only interferes with adequate training but has frequently caused accidents when the instructor could not detect the student pilot's error in time to take over and avert the accident. The tandem-seat arrangement in multiengine, high-performance aircraft is another example. Here a single operator is required to attend to duties normally shared by two or more crew members. This inevitably leads to accidents such as the case of the night take-off crash cited earlier.

## Aeromedical Investigation of Aircraft Accidents

Inasmuch as human factors are involved in the majority of aircraft accidents, specialists in aviation medicine, psychology, and related fields have an important responsibility in aircraft accident investigation. Their participation should contribute both to the isolation of the adverse influences or conditions that may have been present and to the formulation and promotion of recommendations for remedial action (5).

**Conduct of Investigation.** Normally, flight surgeons and other human-factors specialists serve as assistants on the board appointed to conduct an accident investigation. Such boards are composed of experts who understand the complexity of aircraft accident investigation in addition to having specialized training and experience in engineering, operational procedures, communications, or other critical components. The role of human-factors specialists is primarily to ascertain, in those accidents presumed to be due to some human act or omission, whether or not there was physiological adversity, compromise of the aircraft operator's ability, or similar factors. In addition, flight surgeons should have a responsibility to review injuries sustained and their causes in order to provide information on which remedial action may be considered.

**Lines of Inquiry.** Specialized inquiry into accident causes can be conducted along the following lines:

ENVIRONMENTAL ADVERSITIES. In the majority of instances in which the environment becomes extremely adverse, the pilot is overwhelmed so that he cannot mentally or physically respond to the demands of flight (6). On occasions such as in cases of severe hypoxia, he may become unconscious. As a result the aircraft usually plunges to earth with little or no effective human guidance. Investigation of the wreckage reveals no evidence of mechanical malfunction, and inasmuch as these accidents are highly destructive, postmortem clues are usually non-existent. As a result such accidents are often "cause undetermined." However, the probability of environmental compromise often can be implicated. This is done by review of preceding circumstances, especially the altitude and attitude of the aircraft at the onset of the emergency, and then by postulating the operational irregularities or conditions to which the pilot might have been subjected. Supporting clues may sometimes be found in historical data such as inadequate or faulty cabin pressurization or faulty personal equipment such as worn-out or ill-fitting oxygen masks. Particularly pertinent is a review of the probable actions of the pilot at the onset of the accident sequence. For example, a strong basis for influence may exist if it should become evident that the pilot's last act was of a diversionary nature such as attending a poorly positioned control. When the condition of the body permits, analysis of blood and tissues and evidence of exposure to toxic substances or of conditions such as hypoxia may be investigated.

BEHAVIORAL FACTORS. In contrast to accidents resulting from environmental adversities, those resulting from behavioral variables are almost always characterized by evidence of purposeful control of the aircraft prior to the crash. In these cases the pilot may be flying straight and level or attempting a landing or take-off when, as a result of some inadequacy, the accident occurs. Whenever mechanical malfunction can be positively ruled out, all accidents of this type should be reviewed in order to learn as accurately as possible what human acts or omissions in design, mission planning, and pilotage may have been involved and what were the circumstances in which they occurred. To conclude that the pilot mishandled the aircraft and label the accident poor pilot technique may be both entirely inadequate and misleading. Such crucial factors as pilot-task overloads and inadequacy of design, mission planning, training, or supervision will not be recognized unless all the factors contributing to operator error are carefully analyzed.

OTHER FACTORS. Factors such as physical disability, physical deterioration, and temporary performance impairment due to strain or fatigue merit special aeromedical attention. In fatal accidents such conditions may be very difficult to establish, except when postmortem examination (10) may reveal evidence of conditions such as coronary occlusion. A review of the pilot's medical history, including recent temporary illness and use of medication, may also offer clues. As in any other diagnostic problem, the validity of conclusions will be directly proportional to the thoroughness of observation in all areas permitting inquiry.

## Accident Prevention

The successful prevention of operator-factor accidents in future jet and space travel will depend directly upon how well accident cause factors are understood and engaged. To consider that human-factor accidents are inevitable will make them inevitable. On the contrary, firm conviction that they are remediable will do much to lower their incidence. Every cause factor can be minimized. Some can be virtually eliminated. The following are the principal areas in which preventive action is indicated.

**Physical Screening of Aircrew Candidates.** This requirement is frequently oversimplified. It is obvious that pilots and other aircrew members need to have an acuity of the physical senses and mental and emotional equanimity and should be free from disease or significant physical defects. This reflects a definition of physical and psychological standards based on the requirements of particular types of flight duty and selection of applicants who meet these standards. The traditional approach in this area has been the establishment of standards that are too rigid rather than too liberal. It is relatively easy to require very high physical standards with the intention of assuring that accidents could not possibly be attributable to physical defects. This, however, results in screening many highly motivated and talented individuals from the aircrew population. Furthermore, the physically superior specimens selected are not uniformly superior in motivation and talent.

Aviation medicine could make a distinct contribution to the safety of flight by careful appraisal of the validity of current physical standards for various flight duties and by maintaining future review of the practicality of such standards in relation to changing operational concepts. It is probable that in the future flying will depend increasingly upon the monitoring of cockpit displays in the forms of illuminated scopes, dials, and instruments and on the utilization of engineering and mathematical concepts for aircraft control and guidance. Under these circumstances the requirements for mental capacity and specific abilities would far exceed such physical requirements as perfection of distance vision or faultless color discrimination.

**Maintenance of Aircrew Health and Well-being.** There are two requirements in this area. One is monitorship of the aircrew physical condition in order that illness and defects may be recognized early. This permits prompt remedial action or removal of the individual from flying duties during the period that his physical incapacity constitutes an accident potential. The second requirement is that of monitoring aircrew mental equanimity. Inasmuch as most accidents happen as a result of human error in relation to the requirements of flying, it is obvious that emotional conflicts and mental disturbances are incompatible with optimum aircrew performance.

These requirements are met by periodic physical examinations and by having readily available medical consultation. To the extent that the medical consultant is sympathetic to the problems of the crew members, effective rapport may be achieved and effective aeromedical surveillance practiced. The importance of the doctor-patient relationship in this situation cannot be overemphasized.

**Prevention of Physiological Compromise.** Accident-prevention activities in this area are of necessity largely educational. They consist of education and indoctrination directed both at supervisors and aircrews. The primary requirement with reference to supervisors is to familiarize them with the adverse effects of all physiological compromises. Understanding of such human limitations is essential to the establishment of intelligent mission profiles. Concerning aircrews, it is not only necessary to inform them of the physiological adversities that may be encountered in flight, but also it is advisable to give them physiological training so that symptoms may be recognized. Many pilots have recognized incipient hypoxia because of previous experience with this phenomenon in pressure chambers. As a result they have been able to take corrective action in time and avoid incapacitation.

However, the only satisfactory method of eliminating the danger of physiological compromise is to prevent failure of environmental protective equipment. Although the installation and functioning of the equipment is an engineering problem, the safety standards regarded as acceptable may depend on the position taken by aeromedical authorities (7). For example, if it is determined that pressurization systems are not 100 per cent reliable and, therefore, occasions of severe physiological compromise will arise, it is the responsibility of aeromedical advisors to insist upon either greater basic reliability or stand-by systems in order that life and materiel may be preserved.

**Effectiveness of Operator Performance.** As aircraft increase in performance and complexity, their successful operation will involve commensurately higher levels of operator competency. The aircraft operator will be unable to get along only on general familiarity with the machines and their systems. He will require knowledge of electronics and communications, of the physics of the space being traversed, and of the chemistry of the fuels being utilized. He will also require relevant knowledge of human tolerances and human physiology. And knowledge of emergency procedures will need to be as nearly infallible as human ability permits. In this respect the operation of jet and space vehicles is becoming primarily an applied-science profession although still a technical skill. To meet these requirements of flying, therefore, it is reasonable that this profession should be controlled by the same disciplines that apply to other highly technical professions. This implies definite and appropriately high standards of scholarship and motivation, with provision for intense and prolonged training in simulators and in training aircraft so arranged that mistakes may be made in the learning process without resulting catastrophic accidents taking hundreds of lives. To a certain extent aviation is already evolving toward this goal. As higher standards of selection and training are achieved, we may expect reduction of the enormous number of accidents now resulting from avoidable errors on the part of pilot or aircrew.

**Providing Opportunity.** To eliminate or reduce accidents caused by the types of factors discussed under Stimulus-Response Relations, above, it is necessary to provide the aircrew with reasonable opportunity to meet the demands of flight. To do this the following approaches are urgently indicated:

DEFINITION OF THE MAN. Although precise measurements have been made of numerous stimulus-response reaction times, little practical knowledge exists concerning the time required for perception, interpretation, decision, and reaction in connection with specific problems associated with flight. Yet, there have been many accidents in which pilots have unknowingly placed themselves or found themselves placed in an in-flight situation from which they could not recover. For example, if a particular maneuver requires a median of 20 seconds and an extreme of 30 seconds for proper perception, analysis, and response, flight paths that require alteration prior to the expiration of this period are impossible to execute. As long as time requirements such as these remain unknown, unreasonable demands can be placed upon aircraft operators.

There is also a need for careful definition of the variables affecting human dependability under varying conditions of stress and emergency task load. If definitive research data could predict the transition from the confused reaction patterns of inexperienced pilots to the prompt and correct responses of experienced pilots in emergency situations, it is probable that more effective training curriculums would be established and many accidents avoided. The need for research in this area is almost inexhaustible. Never before has the human element been confronted with time and velocity factors that have such a direct bearing upon both aeromedical progress and human survival. To date, the majority of questions concerning human ability to meet the demands of flight have been answered either on the basis of past experience, which is completely inapplicable to future flight, or by conjecture.

DEFINITION OF THE TASK. Although the time required to perform essential tasks may be established by research such as mentioned above, there is an additional responsibility to determine whether or not the task has aspects that may be detrimental to flight. For example, the time required for a pilot to change radio channel selectors could be easily established. However, the answer would be most incomplete if inquiry did not reveal that the process, in addition to taking a given number of seconds, was also diverting the pilot and leading to disorientation. In this respect in-flight tasks need to be carefully evaluated to determine whether or not their accomplishment, in addition to taking time, in any way compromises proper handling of the aircraft.

COCKPIT IMPROVEMENT. This is a meaningless term unless it is applied to the parameters of normal human ability. In other words the cockpit must be adapted to the operator's basic capabilities. However, even pending more exact definition of human parameters, there are basic principles that, if observed, will prevent many accidents. It is essential that the aircraft operator have opportunity to perceive critical stimuli with time to react effectively, that his interpretation of such stimuli be facilitated, that the requirement for decision be minimized, and that performance be facilitated by controls designed for smooth, easy, and prompt manipulation. There are two problem areas currently in great need of remedial action. The first is that of preventing massive work overloads, and the second involves improvement of information displays.

*Work overload* is an increasing problem. Whenever aircraft are so complex or situations so confusing that a single operator can be subjected to a sudden multiplicity of demands, an acute accident potential is created. Although problems in this area may be partially solved by mechanical simplifications, the most obvious remedial action is cockpit construction that provides for two or more operators where tasks can be jointly engaged. In the case of pilots, they should be so seated as to provide the optimum of remedial understanding and cooperation, such as side-by-side seating where observation of each other's acts is often essential.

The development of *information displays* facilitating interpretation needs prompt engagement if accidents due to time pressure in critical stimulus-response relations are to be prevented. This applies particularly to instruments that take considerable time to interpret and are subject to misinterpretation as well as to the arrangement of information displays and presentation systems generally. A great many accidents are currently being occasioned by the time consumed and the errors made in such interpretation. In the future, due to the greater velocities, misinterpretations and delayed interpretations will constitute a great hazard.

**Assuring Essential Assistance.** When events encountered in flight are obviously beyond the ability of the aircraft operator to engage, he must be given assistance. This assistance may include air traffic-control warning devices to avoid mid-air collisions, radar guidance during let-down, and aids such as runway lights, distance markers, and many others. As speeds of flight increase, success in flight will rely more and more upon human guidance and mechanical assistance to avoid situations or conditions beyond the capability of the aircraft operator.

**Anticipation.** Perhaps this is the most vital aspect of accident prevention in current and future flight. Success will depend to a great extent upon the degree to which in-flight events are anticipated. During the flight itself the aircraft will traverse great distances while the operator is making even relatively simple decisions concerning routine matters such as changes of route. Enormous distances will be traversed while the operator is making more complex decisions such as the method of handling mechanical malfunctions or emergencies. Insofar as every potential event or adversity is anticipated in advance and corrective or remedial measures are thoroughly understood and immediately available for action, the time-consuming factors of in-flight decision will be minimized. The sequence for in-flight survival may then be reduced almost to the immediacy of a response to a simple stimulus. In this respect the familiar behavior sequence of perception, interpretation, decision, and response will be replaced by preflight decision and in-flight response to expected stimulus.  It appears as if this may become the law of survival in future flight.

## References

1. ARMSTRONG, H. G.  1952.  *Principles and Practices of Aviation Medicine.* 3rd ed.  Williams & Wilkins Co., Baltimore.
2. KONECCI, E. B.  1957.  Physiologic factors in aircraft accidents in the U.S. Air Force.  *J. Aviation Med.* 28: 553–559.
3. McFARLAND, R. A.  1953.  *Human Factors in Air Transportation.*  McGraw-Hill Book Co., Inc., New York.
4. MOSELEY, H. G.  1957.  *An Analysis of 2400 Pilot Error Accidents.*  (Publication No. M–40–56.)  Office of The Inspector General, USAF.
5. MOSELEY, H. G.  1957.  Aeromedical investigation of aircraft accidents.  *Aeronaut. Eng. Rev.* 16: 74–76.
6. MOSELEY, H. G., and STEMBRIDGE, V. A.  1957.  The hostile environment as a cause of aircraft accidents.  *J. Aviation Med.* 28: 535–540.
7. NUTTALL, J. B.  1958.  Toxic hazards in the aviation environment.  *J. Aviation Med.* 29: 641–650.
8. TALBOT, J. M.  1958.  Unexplained accidents in the U.S. Air Force in Europe.  *J. Aviation Med.* 29: 111–117.
9. THORNDIKE, R. L.  1950.  *Human Factors in Accidents.*  USAF, Air University, School of Aviation Medicine, Randolph Air Force Base, Tex.
10. TOWNSEND, F. M.  1957.  The pathologic investigation of aircraft accident fatalities.  *J. Aviation Med.* 28: 461–469.
11. WHITE, H. S.  1958.  The aeromedical realities of space travel.  *J. Aviation Med.* 29: 707–715.
12. ZELLER, A. F.  1957.  The search for the human cause of aircraft accidents.  *Skyways,* August, 1957.  P. 18.
13. ZELLER, A. F., and MOSELEY, H. G.  1957.  Aircraft accidents as related to pilot age and experience.  *J. Aviation Med.* 28: 171–180.

# 11

# Human Factors Related to Jet Aircraft

THRIFT G. HANKS, M.D.*

The manner in which an aircraft or weapons system is developed affects significantly the application of human-factors concepts to the system. The manufacture of aircraft is a highly competitive business in which the customer is in a position to dictate the choice of subsidiary systems so that, far from being a homogeneous effort, the ultimate design and installation may be subject to many wills and opinions, operational and administrative demands and philosophies, and, in the opinion of some, just pure cussedness. Thus, cost or weight factors may overshadow important human operational considerations, especially if competency in human-factors analysis is lacking on the part of the customer, the subsidiary, or the prime contractor.

This particular difficulty in the application of human-factors concepts predates jet aircraft. With the advent of the jet, however, some urgency in their use was added because of two important differences between piston-engined and jet airplanes, namely, the advanced speed and the very high altitudes attained by the latter. For example, the problem of escape from conventional aircraft during World War II was primarily that of clearance of aircraft structures. However, the jet introduced the possibility of severe trauma from windblast and high decelerative stresses. Piston-engine aircraft employ oxygen and pressurized cabins, but jet aircraft now reach altitudes at which the simpler protective measures against lack of oxygen and depressurization are ineffectual.

---

* Director of Health and Safety, Boeing Airplane Company, Seattle, Washington.

This chapter discusses some of the human factors arising out of jet speeds and altitudes. In relation to that purpose, the limiting altitude of turbojet aircraft is considered to be 100,000 ft. and the limiting speed, Mach 3.5. That these are not excessive is supported by the present speed record of 1,404 mph and the altitude record of 91,249 ft., held by a jet fighter, as well as the reported drawing-board status of a supersonic jet airliner of Mach 3 speed and 80,000-ft. altitude capability. Military and civil jet aircraft are not differentiated except as their peculiarities affect the specific topic. The intent is to suggest methods of approach to human factors rather than solutions. Calculations are representative and not necessarily definitive.

## Air Conditioning

With present air-conditioning techniques it is possible to be comfortably cooled or heated in jet aircraft. How successfully comfort is assured depends on many factors, among them the frequently overriding one of cost, not of the equipment but in carrying the weight of equipment through the air month after month. An oft-quoted approximation relative to this cost is that for every pound of load added to a plane as much as 9 lbs. of material may be required in the form of airplane structure, fuel, etc., to transport that pound. For example, if an engineer can supply 15 cu. ft. per minute of air flow per passenger with one design and it takes 200 lbs. more weight of equipment to supply 20 cu. ft. per minute, the total weight to be added might be 2,000 lbs. The airline would have to haul the equivalent of 12 passengers on every flight in extra weight just to provide the extra 5 cu. ft. of ventilation. Obviously, the necessity of the higher ventilation rate to comfort or health must be weighed carefully.

Air conditioning, in its usual sense, has the goal of providing a fairly uniform, pleasant temperature balance, a feeling of "freshness," and freedom from disagreeable odors and contaminants in the environmental air.

In another sense air conditioning becomes a necessary protective device, shielding the occupants of an enclosure from dangerous temperatures and atmospheric contaminants. In either situation it becomes concerned with entangling physical, physiological, and psychological factors.

**Physical Factors.** Among physical factors the thermal influences involved are those of convection, conduction, and radiation (12). The first two involve molecular and the last involves radiant mechanisms of heat exchange.

In *convection* heat exchange is accomplished between the body and the atmosphere mainly by movement of the air mass which disturbs the air layer immediately adjacent to the body. This layer, undisturbed, tends to come to equilibrium with the skin temperature, thus slowing down heat transfer to or from the body. In the presence of ambient air temperatures either well below or well above skin temperature, the air layer next to the skin may set up a movement of its own because of the difference between its density and that of the surrounding air; but this convective action is small compared to that caused by movement of the major air mass surrounding the body. Thus, the body has a small insulating layer of air which can be blown away, bringing other air molecules in contact with the skin surface and making possible a more rapid exchange of heat. Arctic research has shown that the Eskimo uses the air-insulation principle by trapping the air warmed by his body within his specialized garments (16).

In general the cooling or heating action of a moving air mass is a function of its velocity. This action is exploited in the use of convection in air conditioning. It is clear that convective heat exchange can be modified by interposing material such as clothing between the body and the air mass. The material used is important, however, and a simple illustration can be given by recalling an experience common to almost everyone. On a chilly, windy day neither a thin raincoat lying close to the skin nor a heavy, loosely knit sweater provides much comfort in itself, but if the raincoat is applied as a wind-breaker over the sweater, the air cells in the sweater can trap warmed air, and this combination of clothing provides protection and comfort.

In *conduction* there is a direct transfer of heat between materials in contact, as any farm boy will testify on a cold winter morning. The heat exchange here is proportional to the difference in temperature, but the conductivity of the materials also affects the rate of exchange. Conduction is important to comfort under ordinary circumstances and to safety in the emergency situation.

*Radiant* heat is typified by the sun's warmth. As a form of electromagnetic energy, it can be reflected and refracted. The net heat exchange in the form of radiation between two bodies is from the body of higher to the body of lower temperature. The rate of exchange further depends on the nature of the bodies, that is, their reflective, absorptive, and conductive properties.

Between two radiating surfaces that have the quality of "perfect" absorption of heat and reradiation of the absorbed heat, the so-called black-body state, a special relation exists with respect to the exchange of radiant energy. This relation, first proposed by Stefan (1879), is that the transfer of radiant energy is proportional to the difference between the fourth powers of the absolute temperatures of the two surfaces. This means that with increasing temperature differences between two such surfaces, the transfer of heat rises very rapidly with the temperature rise of the hotter surface. Such a situation can exist between the surrounding cockpit heated by air friction at increasing speeds and the body of the pilot.

Conversely, the occupant of a plane flying at speeds below which significant frictional heating occurs but at altitudes of extreme cold will suffer a reversal of heat transfer, in this case from the body of the occupant to the cold walls of the cabin.

Another physical factor of importance to air conditioning is the vapor pressure of water. Temperature governs the kinetic energy of the molecules in a gas or liquid. It therefore determines the rate of entry of water molecules from a water surface into a space adjoining the surface and also the pressure exerted by these molecules once they are within the space. Temperature is the sole determinant of the total *amount* of vapor that can be held within the space.

If one encloses a space above a pure-water surface, water molecules will enter the space until a state of equilibrium is reached between the molecules entering the space and those returning to the liquid, provided there is thermal equilibrium of this arrangement as well. At the point of vapor-pressure equilibrium, the space is said to be saturated with water vapor. If at this time the pressure in the space above the fluid is reduced by pumping away some of the water vapor, a state of imbalance is created between the pressures of the molecules in the liquid and those within the space. Water molecules will now leave the fluid surface in greater numbers, entering the space at a rate that depends both on the temperature of the water and the total pressure within the space. (A higher temperature of the liquid would increase the rate as does the lower pressure above the liquid (27).) On reaching equilibrium again, however, the total water-vapor pressure will be the same as before, provided the same temperature is maintained, since the pressure reached is dependent only on the temperature of the enclosed system.

This vapor pressure will be the same whether or not the original space was filled with air or consisted of a vacuum; hence, the water-vapor content is unaffected by the total gas pressure, should other gases be present. So long as a source of water molecules is present, they will tend to enter the space until the saturation pressure is reached. As indicated, this *rate* of entry, though not their final number, will depend in part on the total pressure of the gas above the liquid. This will have consequences to be discussed later.

In going from a liquid to a gaseous state or vice versa, water molecules gain or lose energy, respectively, in the form of motion (heat). The amount of work performed in this transfer between states is 540 times that required to raise the temperature of the same number of molecules in the form of water just one degree centigrade. In escaping from the fluid state, then, a water molecule in the form of vapor has 540 times the energy it had in the form of liquid and takes with it, that is, subtracts from the fluid, an equivalent amount of heat. Conversely, on returning to a fluid state, it releases this heat. The energy so represented is termed the latent heat of the vapor and varies according to the substance. Thus, a water molecule escaping from the body surface or the surface of the respiratory tract takes with it a relatively large amount of heat.

In meteorological and air-conditioning parlance, the amount of moisture that actually is contained in the air, expressed as a percentage of the amount that could be held at the saturated state of the air at a particular temperature, is called the "relative humidity" (RH). Completely dry air would thus have an RH of 0 per cent and saturated air 100 per cent. Other things being equal, a maximum evaporative heat loss from the body surface will occur at 0 per cent RH. No net heat exchange as a function of vapor pressure can occur between the body and the atmosphere at 100 per cent RH.

Recalling the warmed air layer that tends to accumulate around the body, it is possible to visualize a similar stabilizing moisture layer. In the former instance the equilibrium that tends to be established is that of heat. In the latter it is that of vapor pressure. The movement of unsaturated air across the body surface has similar consequences for effecting the escape of water vapor to those of movement of cool air for the escape of the heat of convection. Air movement can thus affect body temperature in two ways: through increasing the convective and evaporative heat exchange.

**Physiological Factors.** Physiological factors affecting heat exchange are still a subject of investigation. The unprotected body is unable to cope with the full range of environmental factors influencing heat exchange but still is capable of withstanding limited fluctuations among these factors while maintaining a stable thermal state. Heat production within the body is the result of chemical processes whose chief stimulus beyond the vegetative state is muscular activity (3). Differences between the vegetative (resting or basal) state and that of activity can vary more than tenfold (25). Because of the effects of age, state of nutrition, and other factors, the bodily heat production for the twenty- to forty-year-old male will range from about 0.6 to 0.7 Cal. per square meter of body surface per minute at the basal level, that is, with the body at rest and in the absence of digestive stimuli or the residual effects of activity (3).

The large calorie (abbreviated Cal.) is that amount of heat necessary to raise the temperature of 1,000 gm of water from 15° to 16° C and is 1,000 times the value of the small calorie (abbreviated cal.), the amount of heat used to raise the temperature of 1 gm of water from 15° to 16° C. (The large calorie is sometimes called the "kilocalorie," abbreviated kcal.) The large calorie is also that quantity used to express the unit of metabolic and food-energy value. The evaporation of 2 gm of sweat, removing 1,080 cal. of heat from the body, is approximately balanced by the combustion of a twentieth of a teaspoon of sugar, representing one large calorie, in the body. Expressed in another way, the evaporation of 1 gm of sweat (heat loss equals 540 cal.) just about matches the basal heat-production rate of 0.6 Cal/m²/min (600 cal/m²/min). Under normal conditions of comfort and sedentary circumstances, however, perhaps only 25 per cent of bodily heat loss is due to evaporation.

A passenger, sitting quietly, may produce heat at a rate of 0.7 Cal/m²/min (26). A pilot may expend up to about 1.0 Cal/m²/min under cruise conditions or in combat 1.3 Cal/m²/min (32). Using an autopilot, a pilot may produce little more heat than his passenger.

The organism can react in several ways to those physical factors in the environment affecting bodily heat exchange. It can conserve heat by reducing the flow of blood in the skin, thereby decreasing the surface temperature and thus the heat loss by convection and radiation. To a certain extent it can reduce evaporative heat loss. To counteract increasing loss, the body resorts to muscular activity, either voluntary or involuntary (shivering), thus producing more heat. Some conservation can be obtained by curling the body into a ball, thus reducing the amount of exposed surface. Having exhausted such measures and still faced with increasing heat loss, man must use artificial methods of protection.

To meet increasing heat in the environment, the organism resorts to the reverse of these mechanisms. Especially effective is the use of evaporative heat loss, effective, that is, in the absence of high relative humidity. In the hot air of a desert resort, one can be tolerant of the environment, while on the banks of the Potomac in July at much lower air temperatures, *comfort* is not even a polite word.

As the body reaches its own limitations in effecting heat loss, body temperature rises unless artificial cooling is available and may reach injurious or fatal heights.

**Psychological Factors.** There are some purely psychological factors in man's adjustment to the thermal environment. For example, heat producing sweating may not be obnoxious at the seashore, but in a working environment it may be poorly tolerated. At a football game sleet and ice are not so unbearable if the "right" team is winning. Subjective feeling and motivation are therefore important factors in tolerance. Some so-called psychological factors are probably physiological, the result of acclimatization or lack of it, racial and individual characteristics, diet, etc. (16). Nevertheless, most psychophysiological factors in this adjustment are associated with a gradient of localized or generalized thermal or other stresses and the time of their action. The organism seems to be more receptive to surroundings that do not call into play, to an unusual degree, use of those physiological adjustmental factors mentioned above. Yet the body is not comfortable in a completely static environment. Some change, especially in air movement, seems necessary to comfort even in the complete absence of thermal stress (2).

**Factorial Interactions and Their Artificial Modifications.** The number and nature of the variables just discussed give some idea of the complexity of their possible interactions. These interactions can be made much more complicated by artificial manipulation of the environment and of the human, by imposing physical parameters more extreme than those found in the usual natural environment, or by modifying the human through the use of special clothing and artificial heat-exchange mechanisms within the clothing complex.

Extremes of heat and cold can be expected as a result of the high altitudes and great speeds made possible by jet aircraft operation. Varying according to seasons and latitudes, air temperatures decrease with altitude, tending to become fixed at about −67° F at the operating altitudes of jet airplanes, although lower temperatures than this can be experienced. Moisture content of the air is reduced to almost nothing at these altitudes (12). As air speed increases, so does frictional heating of aircraft surfaces, whose temperatures may reach as much as 1,000° F within the speed-range capabilities of jet-propelled planes (11, 12, 21). What cannot be accomplished by the general engineering control of these environmental extremes must be done by measures directed at the human occupant, a matter complicated by factors of escape, by those of survival following escape, and by possible failure of the engineering controls systems (29, 30). The purpose for which the type of aircraft is designed will determine the type of these measures and the human tolerances the extent.

Customarily three parameters of tolerance are referred to, namely, those of comfort, of functional deficiency, and of survival. The first is the predominant goal in civil transport design except in the event of emergency. It is a desired quality in military plane design. In combat aircraft, however, performance requirements may demand departure from standards of comfort and the imposition of limits within which a crew will retain normal functional capacity in spite of possible discomfort. In all craft the emergency situation may call for meeting tolerances just short of causing injury to the occupants. In some situations the element of risk must be accepted.

Tolerances depend ordinarily on two variables, namely, the degree of the imposed stress and the time over which the stress operates. Juggling a hot potato is illustrative. At first, it must be flipped in and out of the hand rapidly to allow only a brief period of heat transfer to the hand, and a high toss must be given it to allow a long period for the heat added to the hand to be dissipated. As the potato cools, longer periods of contact with the hand are possible as are shorter periods away from the hand. Finally, the potato can be held indefinitely because the rate of heating of the hand does not exceed its ability to get rid of the added heat. At one stage, if the potato is held too long, a burn results; at another no burn but discomfort is evident; and at last the potato may feel pleasantly warm.

Some of the first scientific attempts to relate comfort to the atmospheric environment were made by Sheppard and E. V. Hill in 1913. These were expanded by the American Society of Heating and Ventilating Engineers through research programs beginning a few years later (12). Research on tolerances related to functional efficiency was directed chiefly at the industrial worker prior to World War II (2). Research on survival tolerances was chiefly an outgrowth of World War II and the continuing race for air supremacy (4, 6, 8, 33). Numerous investigations directed at the environment of the industrial worker or the effect of the medical use of heat have aided in the understanding of human heat-exchange problems (1, 5, 7, 10, 13, 15, 18-20, 23, 31). Most of these efforts have attempted to describe the parameters in a specific environment, but others have attempted to provide the formulas or indices by which calculations or extrapolations could be carried to other circumstances.

An effective temperature scale was developed in the United States (14, 15). This index, applicable to sensations of comfort, takes into account air temperatures of limited ranges (those found in the temperate zone), humidity, and limited air-flow rates. It neglects the effect of radiation, of high ventilation rates, and of wearing other than ordinary indoor clothing.

An equivalent temperature index was developed in Great Britain. Of the three factors just mentioned, it neglects humidity (2).

Other efforts attempted correction of the radiant factor in the effective temperatures scale, giving a "corrected effective temperature" factor and a "mean radiant temperature" factor (1, 15).

These formulations have been especially helpful in planning for air conditioning in the ordinary circumstances of living, working, and flying but have fallen short in predicting the requirements of extraordinary circumstances possible in jet flight. For this reason increasing attention has been given to the relation between very high environmental temperatures and human tolerance (17).

Increasing temperatures call for increasing protection of the body against heat gain. The rapid transfer of heat to the body from radiant sources of high temperature has been mentioned. Radiant heat gain cannot be prevented short of using reflective garments or shielding, but it can be counteracted by increasing convective loss (increased air-flow velocities and lower air temperatures) and evaporative loss. The latter is aided by the increased air-flow rates and also by the very dry air and the reduced atmospheric pressure in an airplane cabin at high altitude. If an aircrewman is wearing clothing impervious to moisture, however, evaporative heat loss is impossible, and heat tolerances become those of the worker exposed to high heats and high humidities in industrial work.

Too rapid air-flow rates may cause discomfort because of excessive cooling or, if the available air is at a higher temperature, may actually add to the total bodily heat gain. It is these combined factors of varying radiant temperatures, air temperatures, and air-flow rates that must be determined, as well as the different tolerance states related to them, with respect to the time of exposure. They must be examined further in connection with the effect of protective garments. The work of Blockley, McCutchan, and Taylor is representative of the theoretical and practical difficulties met in attempting formulation of these relations but also of the progress in this field (4).

Localized heat-exchange factors are important to comfort. For example, air- and floor-temperatures at foot level are important (2, 9, 22). The relationships among air temperatures, conductivity of the floor material, and radiant heating in terms of effects on foot comfort have not been firmly established. It would appear that the lower part of the air-temperature range (from 55° to 65° F), noted by Munro and Chrenko (22) in relation to nullifying the effect of floor conductivity, is too low in many circumstances of air-flow rate and floor temperatures possible in aircraft, especially for lightly shod women.

Air temperatures of from 55° to 58° F at floor level associated with from 64° to 68° air temperature at head level, combined with cold walls and moderate air movement, were observed by the writer to result in shivering in men well shod and clothed (tweed suits) working on asphalt tile over concrete. In this instance it was necessary to use electric heaters with circulating fans located within from 3 to 4 ft. of the worker at floor level to alleviate the heat loss and restore some sense of comfort. The authors cited were undoubtedly correct, however, in attributing the decisive thermal effect in preventing cold feet to the air temperature over the feet, provided it is high enough. Floor temperatures that are too high can cause discomfort. Chrenko has identified the threshold for discomfort as being between 75° and 77° F (9).

It should be remembered that skin temperature is closely associated with thermal comfort and that the blood vessels in the extremities respond quickly to low temperatures, cutting down blood flow and lowering the local skin temperature markedly. Chilling of the hands and feet can cause generalized constriction of the skin blood vessels and produce general sensations of chilling. Of course, on commercial airliners passengers commonly introduce modifications to thermal factors through the various types of clothing worn (24).

**Humidity Control.** The basic role of humidity control remains unsolved for high-altitude flight and becomes important because of penalties imposed by weight and condensation hazards when humidification of jet aircraft is attempted. Water vapor permeates linings and insulation; it condenses on the aircraft's structures and material exposed to the cold of high altitudes. Air-frame manufacturers tend to let the customer make the decision on installation of humidifiers of which several types exist (29, 30).

In that coffee-bar otherwise known as the crew compartment, a good deal of armchair research has gone into this matter of humidity. One subject not yet exhausted concerns the effects on the eyes, nose, and throat of the dry cabin air present at high altitudes, but two arch contributors to the symptoms complained of are seldom given the attention they deserve. These are excessively high cabin-air temperatures and tobacco smoke.

In air free of irritants, the nose is capable of rapidly humidifying inspired air without significant symptoms, provided the air temperature is not excessive. In civil air transports the air is relatively free of dust, but, especially following meals, it becomes concentrated with tobacco smoke which provides an irritating, inflammatory stimulus to the mucous membranes of the respiratory tract. At the same time cabin temperatures often are maintained at 80° F or above; at these temperatures dry air takes up moisture from the nasal turbinates and other mucous membranes at rates well above those existing for dry-bulb temperatures of from 68° to 70° F (28). The combined result is a dry, raw, or burning sensation appearing on prolonged flight and usually blamed upon dry air alone.

Examination of non-smoking pilots fails to reveal evidence of nasal or conjunctival inflammation following high-altitude flight. Smoking pilots constantly reveal nasal, pharyngeal, and frequently conjunctival inflammation. Non-smokers complain of ocular and nasal symptoms in the presence of smoke in dry air but find relief in uncontaminated dry air if temperatures are within the lower ranges of from 65° to 75° F, dry bulb. Smokers' responses to questioning on subjective reactions to cabin air are not dependable in that smoking may provide temporary relief by causing increased mucous flow. Ultimately, the symptoms experienced by smokers are probably more marked, however, than if there had been no smoking.

High temperatures as well as decreased atmospheric pressure increase total fluid loss from the body through increased evaporation, but the effect of this loss on local nasal and ocular symptoms has not been studied. At air temperatures from 84° F and above (dry bulb), evaporative losses are increasingly relied upon for thermal equilibrium, and such generalized fluid losses may aggravate local symptoms (2). In-flight cabin temperatures of 85° F are not uncommonly encountered. These are not the fault of the air-conditioning systems but of their regulation by the crew who are given manual control over a wide range of temperatures, for example, from 65° to 85° F in a representative passenger aircraft. With "hot wall" heating, lower air temperatures are possible than are predicted by the effective temperature.

It is certain that lower cabin temperatures and control of tobacco smoke would reduce significantly ocular and nasal symptoms in flight. Filters are generally used on recirculating air-conditioning systems and are fairly effective in the removal of tobacco smoke, but airline operators may remove or fail to service these filters and so render them ineffectual. Whether or not non-recirculating systems in jet aircraft that use only fresh air for cabin ventilation are effective in providing relief from air contamination remains to be seen. Supersonic commercial jets operating at very high altitudes may have to conserve air and resort to recirculation. Effective filtration again will be a problem.

**Ground-Level Comfort.** Another problem of air conditioning common to conventional aircraft will continue into the jet age. This concerns ground-level comfort. A jet plane can develop ovenlike temperatures in hot desert airports such as are found in the southwestern states or take on a load of water vapor in the southern and southeastern states. Climbing rapidly to high altitude following such an exposure, the plane would subject the wringing-wet passenger to a refrigerating heat loss through evaporation. The solution, of course, is ground-level air conditioning, an increasingly effective service rendered by the aviation industry. The available equipment takes advantage of another dividend of the jet era, the gas-turbine engine used in ground-servicing carts.

## Toxicology

Aside from the ever-changing technology in air-frame manufacture and its attendant chemical hazards, the jet introduces some special problems of its own. These are chiefly associated with fuels, sealants, solvents, lubricants, hydraulic fluids, special plastics, fire extinguishants, and the possibility of atmospheric contamination at high altitudes (34, 35).

**Jet Fuels.** Present jet-fuel formulations require the same general precautions in handling and storage as aviation gasoline. Military formulas, such as JP-4, are more flammable than civil jet formulas, represented by JP-6 fuel. The former carry varying concentrations of aromatic hydrocarbons; otherwise, they are similar to aviation gasoline in regard to toxicity. The latter involve essentially the same hazard as kerosene.

The fact that "integral" fuel tanks, that is, tanks that are structurally a part of the airplane, are increasingly used carries with it the need for particular precautions in maintenance. To prevent fire or explosion during maintenance, it is necessary to render such tanks inert by means of a gas such as nitrogen in order to reduce the oxygen content of the tank vapor-gas mixture. The oxygen tension then becomes too low to sustain life, and entry into an "inerted" tank may result in asphyxiation unless air is provided through a respirator under positive pressure.

Entry into open fuel tanks must be preceded by forced air ventilation until tests of the vapor content show it to be below hazardous concentrations. Ventilation must be continuous because of the vapor given off by pools of fuel still present in the tanks and because of the restricted air space once the fuel is mopped up.

The continued development of jet airplanes proposes additional problems for environmental health. The search for high-energy fuels has led to the investigation of such compounds as the boron hydrides (37). They are toxic both in their precombustive and post-combustive states. At present boron fuel exposures are limited to employees manufacturing or carrying out research on relatively small quantities. Should use of the compounds become practical, the aviation industry will have greater cause for concern than with present fuels in the protection of employees and the public.

Jet aircraft with nuclear-power sources would seem to be assured if only for the range to be gained, but airborne reactors cannot be shielded in the same manner as submarine reactors because of the weight factor. The safety requirements for nuclear-propelled air-craft would seem to impose a whole new mechanism of operation for protection of aircrew, passengers, maintenance crew, and the general public.

**Sealants.** Sealing of the tanks requires its own precautions in that the sealants used contain solvents that may produce toxic concentrations within the small air space present; in addition, solvent cleaners are used to prepare the surfaces for sealing, and sealing is followed by the application of a coating material which adds to the potential hazard (36). Inspection and maintenance of integral fuel tanks, therefore, demand the strictest adherence to standards of safety in regard to toxic hazard and possible asphyxiation.

The size of the enclosures and their relative inaccessibility raise another problem, that of physical fitness on the part of the employee. The employment for this purpose of persons suffering from cardiac disease, diabetes, epilepsy, and the like, whose incapacitation within a tank can cause serious consequences to victim and plane alike, is unwise.

**Solvents.** The widespread use of solvents in maintenance and manufacture imposes the threat of dermatoses and minor ocular injury. The defatting action of many solvents is well known and predisposes the skin to further injury and possible sensitization from other materials. The use of solvent cleaners without eye protection results in chemical eye injury which, though not serious in itself for the most part, causes significant time loss and may lead to complications. The commonest accident is from splashing or dripping of the solvent from the cloth with which it is applied.

**Lubricants.** The special lubricants used in deference to the range of temperatures existing in the operation of jet engines pose a possible hazard if seals should leak. If the air conditioning-pressurizing system "bleeds" air from the first-stage compressors, a leak can cause the introduction (into the aircraft cabin) of thermal breakdown products of synthetic oils. Air so contaminated causes irritation of the eyes and can produce haze in the cockpit which could possibly be confused with smoke from fire. Filter systems can effectively reduce the threat of contamination.

American commercial jets avoid this possibility by using separate compressors. The British, claiming superiority of their compressor-bearing seals, bleed air from the engine (38).

**Hydraulic Fluids.** Non-flammable hydraulic fluid that resists the freezing cold of high altitude is a requirement for jet operations. At the present time the most widely used fluid is not a toxic hazard but contains a corrosion inhibitor which is a sensitizer and a source of dermatosis for those in intimate contact with it. The manufacturer is searching for a non-sensitizing substitute. Behind this search is an example of effective cooperation between vendor and user in the interests of occupational health.

**Resins.** The use of "epoxy" resins in paint formulas and other applications in air-frame manufacture and maintenance provides another potential source of employee exposure to toxic irritant or sensitizing substances. Exhaust ventilation, respirators, protective clothing, and skin-coating creams have been found necessary to protect adequately employees engaged in spray painting with resin-based paints of this type. Scrupulous personal hygiene is as important here as in the presence of any materials capable of causing dermatosis.

**Extinguishants.** There are no new fire extinguishants associated with jet aircraft in flight, and there are no ideal extinguishants. In-flight fire safety is an engineering problem which must also deal with the side effects of fire-fighting chemicals. One approach is to isolate as well as possible the potential sources of fire and so permit the use of extinguishants without danger of cabin-air contamination by the combustion products, extinguishants, or their thermal breakdown products if these exist. A second is to choose materials in the component systems that will not support combustion, such as non-flammable insulating materials, ducts, lubricants, flame-resistant fabrics, and the like.

The choice of extinguishants is not clear-cut. Smothering agents used in large quantities are potential asphyxiants. Some excellent agents are in themselves toxic and may have even more toxic break-down products. Some concern is to be had for the combined effects of a toxic or asphyxiant agent and lowered oxygen tension should reduction of cabin pressure be associated with fire. The crew and passenger oxygen equipment can provide a considerable measure of protection in this event.

In the final analysis the actual ability of an agent to cope with fire, combined with structural isolation of fire sources, use of non-flammable electric and electronic materials, and the use of oxygen equipment for crew and passengers, will provide the best over-all safety.

Compounds combining fluorine and carbon fluorine, carbon, and chlorine have been found to be of great value in the wide environmental range of jet operations. Examples are *polytetrafluoroethylene* and *polytrifluorochloroethylene*. Some of these compounds, innocuous in themselves, can produce toxic breakdown products on excessive heating. Such heating is unlikely to occur outside laboratory experimentation and testing or actual fire aboard an aircraft.

**Ozone.** The presence of ozone at high altitudes has led to speculation as to its possible effects on occupants of jet aircraft. There is little that can be said on the practical implications of the ozone layer, since the concentration of ozone in the atmosphere cannot be directly related to its concentration within the cabin of jet aircraft and no reliable data have been obtained on the latter.

Wilkins briefly summarizes the present physical and biological data on atmospheric ozone (39). There appears to be a lack of agreement between these data and flight experience. It is possible that ozone is rapidly reconverted to molecular oxygen during compression and heating in pressurization systems. Reliable cabin-ozone measurements are needed in the 50,000- to 90,000-ft. range of altitude at different latitudes and seasons. There seems to be little cause for concern at altitudes of 40,000 ft. and below. Some flights between 40,000 and 50,000 ft. have raised a suspicion of cabin-ozone levels at the olfactory threshold, but measurements indicating cabin concentrations of up to 0.075 ppm by volume of air do not appear to be entirely reliable.

It is difficult to say what additional environmental hazards will be introduced in successive generations of air-breathing aircraft, but the almost exponential developments in chemistry and the slower but significant advances in metallurgy, ceramics, and nuclear physics will increasingly burden the organizations in industry responsible for the control of environmental hazards.

It has become apparent that air-frame manufacture and airline operation require continuous surveillance in the field of environmental health. Such coverage is not and cannot be supplied by insurance carriers or governmental agencies but must be an integral part of the industry itself.

## Decompression

The possible effects of loss of cabin pressure at altitudes above 30,000 ft. are: (1) physical injury, (2) dysbarism, (3) ebullism, and (4) hypoxia. In each the hazard is a function of time and is considered in the light of circumstances that could initiate decompression and of the type and operational status of the affected aircraft.

Decompression accidents have occurred principally through the loss of hatches and canopies, less often through the loss of doors, astrodomes, and windows or by pressure-system failure. Infrequently, though at times catastrophically, they have resulted from structural failure or from damage caused by propellers or other aircraft. Thus, while the intent of the designer is to avoid completely the risk of decompression, its possibility introduces the need for special measures in the jet era.

Major structural failure can be combated effectively by "tear-stop" design, which tends to prevent small structural failures from spreading. Multiple compression units and pressure valves with fail-safe features limit the possibility of complete pressurization failure. Inward-opening doors act as plugs to prevent accidental opening. Warning devices sound and oxygen masks are presented automatically to passengers if cabin altitudes exceed certain limits. The aircraft itself is a safeguard in view of its ability to descend rapidly to safe altitudes.

The degree and rate of decompression are essentially (though not entirely) dependent on the initial differential between the cabin pressure and the air pressure outside the cabin, on the size of the cabin and on the size of the opening responsible for the loss of pressure. With an opening of similar size, a small cabin will be evacuated much more rapidly than a large cabin at the same altitude.

For example, since cabin size may vary from less than 50 cu. ft. in fighter aircraft to more than 10,000 cu. ft. in airliners, the loss of a window in the former could result in decompression in less than one second, but from 15 to 30 seconds would be required for decompression in the latter cabin with an opening of similar size.

**Hazard from Physical Injury.** A limiting factor in decompression rates is the speed of sound. In other words there is a critical value in the ratio between cabin and ambient pressures above which the rate of decompression will not increase through a given orifice. Interpreted in respect to the modes of decompression that might occur in craft with large cabins (except those resulting in destruction of the aircraft through collision or similar catastrophe), this means that decompression rates would not approach those capable of causing injury to bodily tissues.

On the other hand, in small cabins with relatively large potential openings, very rapid decompression can occur as indicated above. To the writer's knowledge numerous decompressions in aircraft, including canopy loss, have not resulted in decompression injury provided respiratory passages were kept open. However, combat aircraft operate at cabin pressures considerably below those practical for commercial aircraft because of decompression and escape hazards associated with combat and since the crews can use oxygen or pressure equipment. In rapid decompression the rate and total change in pressure are less for combat aircraft than they would be were the initial pressure equal to those of commercial jets. Thus, the possibility of physical injury is limited in civil aircraft by large cabin size and limited orifices and in combat planes by low-pressure differentials.

**Hazard from Dysbarism.** Following decompression, unless altitude is maintained for a time beyond safe limits for hypoxia in commercial aircraft,* bends and their equivalents will not occur. Expansion of gases in bodily cavities can cause pain and in the presence of lesions, such as pneumothorax, more serious consequences. The relative expansion of a gas is dependent on its pressure, on the pressure of the ambient atmosphere, and on the water-vapor content of the gas. Since bodily gases are saturated, inability to vent them becomes increasingly serious with gain in

---

* See Oxygen Requirements below.

altitude, because their expansion is not dependent on simple inverse pressure laws that hold for dry gases.

The difference between the relative expansions of a saturated gas and a dry gas at the usual operating levels of the first generation of jet airliners (about 35,000 ft.) is not significant. At altitudes reached by present military craft and future civil craft, however, the difference and hence hazard is increasingly great. To illustrate, the expression for the relative expansion of a saturated gas at 37° C is

$$\frac{V_2}{V_1} = \frac{P_1 - 47}{P_2 - 47},$$

where $\frac{V_2}{V_1}$ = ratio between the final volume of the gas ($V_2$) and the initial volume ($V_1$), $P_1$ and $P_2$ are the pressures before and after decompression, and 47 is the vapor pressure of water at body temperature expressed in millimeters of Hg.

Thus, if the initial pressure is that of a cabin altitude of 8,000 ft. (564.4 mm Hg) and the final pressure that at a cruising altitude of 35,000 ft. (178.7 mm Hg), the ratio $\frac{V_2}{V_1}$ equals $\frac{564.4 - 47}{178.7 - 47}$ or about 4:1 for saturated bodily gas as compared to $\frac{564.4}{178.7}$ or a little more than 3:1 for a dry gas.

If the expansion were to occur between the pressures equivalent to the altitudes of 8,000 and 50,000 ft., however, the ratio would become $\frac{564.4 - 47}{87.3 - 47}$ or 12:1 for the saturated gas as opposed to 6.5:1.0 for a dry gas. At 60,000 ft., where the ambient pressure is 54.1, the ratio would become $\frac{564.4 - 47}{54.1 - 47}$ or about 80:1 for the saturated gas. That of dry gas would be about 10:1. These ratios, of course, are for an unopposed expansion and do not mean that trapped bodily gas would so expand. The resistance of the walls of the cavity containing the gas tends to resist the expansion, so that the important factor becomes that pressure exerted by the gas which is not countered by the ambient atmospheric pressure. This gas pressure then acts against blood vessels, nerve endings, resisting muscles, and cells, causing pain and interference with function.

In estimating the physical effect of gas expansion, it should be remembered that the amount of gas initially present is as important as the ratio of expansion. Expanding a pinpoint-size bubble 10 times is less significant than the same ratio applied to a bubble containing 5 ml of gas; the greatest pressure thus produced by gas entrapped at sea level would be that of 1 atmosphere (at extra-atmospheric altitudes) were it not for the added source of water vapor within the body.

In combat aircraft the hazard of dysbarism is not entirely avoided, even though the differential pressure drop is purposely small and the crew may have been on 100 per cent oxygen (that is, have experienced some denitrogenation) for some time prior to decompression. Decompression thus becomes a threat to mission accomplishment.

**Hazard from Ebullism.** At altitudes above 63,000 ft., the vapor pressure of water at bodily temperatures exceeds that of the atmospheric pressure. Under these conditions the phenomenon of *ebullism* is exhibited, namely, the boiling of fluid without the addition of heat. At these altitudes only the relative inelasticity of bodily tissues serves to contain expanding water molecules and then only for a limited time. Hence, 63,000 ft. creates a critical altitude for commercial aircraft and manufacturers, whose sales representatives are not overly enthusiastic about proposing the use of pressure suits for passengers.

Safety, in the event of decompression above this critical altitude, becomes increasingly a matter of structural and systemic reliability in commercial aircraft, but again, with decompression always a possibility, if not a probability, designers must consider various countermeasures. These may take the form of compartmentation and stand-by pressurization units or of windowless passenger cabins. The speed of the aircraft may serve to maintain partial pressurization. As usual, advance experience with military jet aircraft and present civil operational experience may point to problem areas and suggest solutions prior to the placing in service of the ultimate jet superairliner.

**Hazard from Hypoxia.** The great and immediate hazard of decompression to occupants of jet aircraft at operating altitudes is oxygen-want. In spite of the safety features built into jet airliners in the event of decompression at high altitudes, only operational procedures stand between the occupants and serious consequences. The limiting factor is that time period beyond which brain tissue may be irreversibly damaged by severe or complete lack of oxygen.

This time has been variously estimated at from 2 to 10 minutes. A reasonable limit is considered to be 4 minutes.

Within this time a pilot must recognize and react to the decompression, initiate descent, and take the aircraft to a safe altitude. If decompression is insidious, recognition might be delayed, hence the importance of an automatic warning device. To react in a reasonable fashion, however, the pilot must retain his best critical judgment. This he cannot do if he is affected by hypoxia; he may fail to recognize the situation or may make the wrong decision.

Until such time as commercial airliners carrying upward of 150 passengers are proved decompression-proof, the pilot who does not recognize the crushing responsibility that is his in the event of decompression will be the major hazard to the lives of his passengers. There are compelling reasons why this is so, why his employers must insist on operational procedures and discipline to assure the *wearing* of oxygen equipment by at least one crew member at all times, and why, above all, the pilot himself must overcome possible prejudice relative to his personal comfort and inconvenience.

First of all, the available time is extremely short. While it is true that under *controlled* circumstances the pilot can easily demonstrate a short reaction time and a capacity for early initiation of descent, aircraft accidents do not occur under controlled conditions. Any delay that might compromise so many lives is unforgivable. Pilots have been known to forget to don oxygen masks while attempting descent procedures under the stress of decompression emergencies. Others have attempted to don masks without success in decompressions of even several seconds' duration and have succumbed to hypoxia.

There is no guaranty that all passengers will successfully obtain and use the oxygen equipment provided them. The only reliable protection lies in descent, and if that protection were compromised by a crew made ineffectual by hypoxia, a minor incident could be translated into a major disaster.

The jet airliner is capable of safe descents at high rates of speed. Most cruise conditions will not call for altitudes above 35,000 ft., but descent, once it has been initiated, can be made from 42,000 to 14,000 ft. in 2 minutes (12,000–16,000 ft/min) in one type of jet airliner. Given a time for crew reaction and initiation of descent of from 45 to 60 seconds (slow for uncomplicated situations) and a time of descent to survivable altitudes of from 2 to 2½ minutes, the exposure of the passengers to serious hypoxia would be well within the 4-minute period mentioned, regardless of whether they used the individual oxygen supplies provided.

Actually, in a cabin containing some 10,000 to 11,000 cu. ft. of air space, decompression resulting from anything short of collision would not take place in much less than from 15 to 30 seconds, thus preventing the cabin from reaching ambient altitudes if the crew reaction is timely.

Other safety factors provide protection by extending the available time in which to recognize and react to the condition before very high altitude is reached within the cabin. Under most conditions in which decompression could occur, at least half a minute (and possibly several minutes) is available before the cabin reaches ambient altitude, and this should provide an alert and protected crew sufficient time to reduce altitude before pressure equalization is reached. It also provides cabin attendants time to ensure their own oxygen supplies and to assist passengers in securing theirs.

Tests of passengers' emergency oxygen equipment have shown it to be reliable at actual altitudes of 42,000 ft. in supplying oxygen flow sufficient to permit some activity. Sustained (20 minute) flight at 23,000 ft. to simulate emergent cruise altitudes faced by some airlines has been made to verify similar reliability of the oxygen equipment under these conditions. In one test decompression was initiated at 42,000 ft. ambient (8,000 ft. cabin altitude). Passenger masks were ejected automatically at 13,400 ft. and donned within a few seconds. When cabin altitude reached 42,000 ft., the flight was continued for 30 seconds before descent was initiated. The simulated passengers suffered no signs of hypoxia. One passenger experienced abdominal gas pains of moderate severity but did not fail to maintain his oxygen supply through the hand-held mask.

Descent was then begun to 23,000 ft. at emergency descent rates. Two persons experienced ear pain but no residual effects in the ear. At 23,000 ft. flight was continued for 20 minutes without incident, and the test was terminated by cabin repressurization.

**Oxygen Requirements.** In the event of decompression, oxygen requirements are dependent on the following factors:

1. Altitude at which decompression occurs
2. Type of oxygen system used
3. Time of descent to survivable altitudes

4. Terrain factors limiting descent
5. Duration of flight
6. Metabolic demands of the occupants
7. Proportion of passengers requiring an additional but limited period of oxygen inhalation
8. Proportion of passengers requiring extended or therapeutic use of oxygen
9. Transportation of known pathological cases requiring oxygen
10. Miscellaneous factors associated with the emergency.

In considering the following discussion of these factors, it should be understood that the problem is that of an emergent situation in which the primary object is prevention of harm. In such extreme circumstances the comfort of passengers must necessarily be subordinated.

1. The actual altitude reached within the cabin governs the partial pressure ($pO_2$) of the oxygen to be supplied at the time of the emergency and until descent is accomplished. It also affects the volume of oxygen available from the oxygen system.

The $pO_2$ can be varied by the use of different percentages of oxygen in the inspired gas, by supplying oxygen under pressure above the ambient, or by physiological means such as hyperventilation.

Without hyperventilation or additional pressure, a $pO_2$ equivalent to that at sea level (100 mm Hg, mean value) can be maintained in the alveoli of the lungs by the breathing of "100 per cent" oxygen at an actual altitude of about 34,000 ft. Similarly, a 10,000-ft. equivalent can be maintained at an actual altitude of about 39,000 ft. and 14,000-ft. equivalent at 41,000 ft. in the normal individual. At 14,000 ft., the altitude of Pikes Peak, unacclimatized tourists have often been observed to function without noticeable discomfort. Under these circumstances, with some pulmonary hyperventilation the alveolar $pO_2$ would amount only to about 44 mm Hg and the arterial oxygen saturation to 80 per cent.

There is little reason to believe that the average airline passenger cannot stand up to this performance *in an emergency*, even considering a prior exposure to higher altitude. Passengers now fly in unpressurized vintage aircraft at above 14,000 ft.

The effect of altitude on the original volume of stored oxygen (STPD) in the body can be calculated by using the gas laws; and the effect of body temperature and of water vapor on gas expansion can be calculated according to the formula

$$V_{BTPS} = V_{STPD} \times \frac{760}{BP - 47} \times \frac{310}{273}$$

where $V_{BTPS}$ = volume of the gas at body temperature and body pressure, saturated, and $V_{STPD}$ = volume at standard temperature and pressure, dry; $BP$ = the ambient barometric pressure; 310 = body temperature in degrees Kelvin; and 273 = 0° C in degrees Kelvin.

Thus, the volume of oxygen contained in a tank at sea level (STPD) would expand more than nine times at 40,000 ft. ($BP$ = 140.7 mm Hg) by the time it reached the alveoli (BTPS). At a 14,000-ft. altitude ($BP$ = 446.4), however, the expansion would be only about two and one-third times the volume at sea level.

Following emergency descent as a result of decompression, it may be necessary to choose an emergency cruising altitude that would protect the majority of passengers without requiring their use of oxygen and still not compromise the range capabilities of the aircraft, especially in the absence of nearby landing facilities such as in long overwater flights.

At 14,000 ft., however, the aircrew would be at levels of ambient $pO_2$ too low for safe control of the aircraft. The crew would then require continuous oxygen throughout the remainder of the flight.

At the peak operating altitudes of present jet transports, oxygen pressures supportive of consciousness and of some activity can be maintained without pressure-breathing devices, provided adequate flow rates are permitted.

2. The type of oxygen system used will affect the total amount of oxygen required. A demand system conserves oxygen by furnishing it only during inhalation, but available demand systems are too complicated and unwieldy for use by passengers. A simple continuous-flow system can also conserve oxygen through the use of a reservoir of sufficient capacity. It thus stores oxygen during exhalation and so does not depend on constantly high flow rates which otherwise would be needed to satisfy peak inspiratory flow rates which may exceed 50 l per minute.

Such a reservoir should not be confused with a rebreathing bag. Conservation of oxygen by the use of rebreathing techniques at high altitudes would lower still further the already borderline alveolar

$pO_2$. The required capacity of and the flow rate to a reservoir is determined by tidal volume and ventilatory rate. Each can increase from resting values because of physical exertion or emotional stress. In passengers the physical status is one of rest. What the emotional status will be in the event of decompression is unknown. On the basis that some increase in minute volume should be prepared for, either because of emotional or initial hypoxic hyperventilation, some factor might be chosen by which the resting minute volume can be multiplied, and on this basis the emergency flow rate could be predicted, disregarding for the moment other factors in this rate.

If a resting minute respiratory rate of 12 to 16 and a tidal volume of 500 ml are assumed (BTPS), the resting requirement would be from 6 to 8 l of oxygen per minute. If the above "emotional" factor were 2, the flow would be from 12 to 16 l per minute, but the effect of emotion on the ratio rate to depth of respiration has not been established. Consequently, one can only hazard a guess at reservoir volume. In hyperventilation due to anxiety, for example, it is often difficult to discover overt evidence of increased respiration. The condition ordinarily develops over a period of time in which the respiratory rate or depth is maintained only a little above the normal.

Maintaining the same factor of 2, if one assumes that only depth of respiration will increase, a maximum reservoir volume of 1000 ml would be predicted.

In the absence of reliable experimental or clinical data, guesses such as these are the only present solution for engineers responsible for oxygen systems.

These "calculations" assume also, of course, no effect of dead space, leakage, or improper operation of mask and reservoir valves. Should these exist to any extent, increased flow rates would be necessary. Mask efficiency tests do not provide information on the human parameters involved but only on performance under the test conditions.

3. The time of descent to safe altitudes is based on the limiting capacity of brain tissue to withstand hypoxia. This has been suggested above as 4 minutes and provides a fixed figure for calculating the total oxygen supply for the aircraft occupants during descent.

4. Terrain factors, such as high mountain ranges, may dictate cruise altitudes, following decompression, of above 22,000 ft. If normal speeds could be maintained, perhaps 20 minutes of flight would permit further descent to altitudes at which passenger oxygen

would not be necessary. Consideration for continuous oxygen consumption by all occupants during this time would be required.

5. The distance to the destination or to an emergency landing following decompression determines the amount of oxygen required by the crew and those passengers requiring oxygen during emergency-cruise conditions. The condition most demanding of oxygen would be at the point of no return in a long overwater route. This could amount to 3 or 3½ hours.

6. The passenger already has been considered as at rest. The crew, dealing with an emergency restricted to decompression alone, could be considered not much above resting level in caloric expenditures after the first few minutes (49).

The cabin attendants, as the most active physically, must be assured an oxygen supply sufficient to their needs while ministering to the safety and comfort of the passengers. Their energy expenditure may reach three times that of the resting state in the first 10 minutes or so following decompression, assuming no incapacitation and perhaps twice that of the resting rate for an extended period. Tables for caloric expenditures are available (48) for estimating oxygen requirements, for which 5 Cal. amount to about 1 l. Other tables (47) permit surface-area calculations based on weight, height, and sex.

One aspect of function apart from caloric requirements is the integrity of the cortical cells of the brain in those pilots and crewmen responsible for control of the airplane. This integrity is not universally maintained at cruising altitudes above 10,000 ft. It is important that oxygen be supplied continuously at altitudes higher than this to crewmen whose judgment and efficiency is critical to the success of the flight.

7. The proportion of passengers who might require limited amounts of oxygen following descent and extended flight at 14,000 ft. cannot be estimated readily. Assuming the worst possible circumstances (that in which no passenger succeeds in obtaining oxygen during descent), it might be assumed that all passengers would benefit from oxygen administration for a limited time following descent.

In decompression accidents healthy aircrewmen who have succumbed to a hypoxic state of unconsciousness have usually been observed to recover spontaneously (without oxygen) with rapid descent to about 18,000 to 20,000 ft. and without assistance don oxygen gear at that time. The implication for most transport passengers is that they, too, may recover sufficiently to secure their own oxygen supply, especially at the lower altitude of 14,000 ft. Assuming that oxygen is warranted following descent, the question is: How long should it be continued and what should be its concentration?

Disregarding serious and pertinent pre-existing pathology for the moment, a very few minutes on supplementary oxygen at 14,000 ft. should return tissue oxygenation to normal. The amount of oxygen required is no more than that needed to provide physiological oxyhemoglobin concentration.

Low-pressure chamber experience shows that both young, healthy men and men of middle age brought to the point of unconsciousness by oxygen-mask removal at high altitudes recover within a few seconds when provided oxygen. Decompression and oxygen-equipment accidents leading to unconsciousness in actual flight also point to rapid recovery with administration of oxygen provided neural damage has not occurred.

A 10-minute oxygen supply for the period following descent should provide reasonable safety margins for the normal and near-normal person. Any passenger who does not respond under this regimen would be a candidate for extended therapeutic use of oxygen.

Such a reserve supply probably would not be used completely in the initial period following descent and could be used in prolonged emergent cruising conditions for occasional administration to persons not entirely comfortable at ambient pressures. Such administration has been used in unpressurized aircraft but, unhappily, with no record as to the actual need for oxygen. Oxygen is often given uncritically for airsickness, hang-overs, and almost any sign of debility on the part of passengers.

8. One cannot assume the absence of *cardiopulmonary* or other disease among passengers in whom lack of oxygen might precipitate serious complications. Morbidity tables for aviation passenger populations are not available, however, and autopsy statistics dealing with diseases most suspect in decompressive emergencies are too greatly skewed by reason of their origin to assist in estimating passenger morbidity.

For long postdecompression flights the oxygen requirements in these conditions would assume significant proportions if a large number of passengers were involved. The concern for passenger safety, which could be compromised either by inadequate oxygen supplies or by the extra weight of superfluous oxygen, has caused considerable exploration of empirical means of estimation.

While it has been stated that any passenger who can climb the steps to the airplane cabin is eligible for flight, even that test will be removed by the installation of escalators and plane-level boarding devices. This approach will not provide the necessary information.

Airlines do not maintain age data on their passengers, and consequently age-related estimates are not available. Since mere ambulatory capacity has no meaning and since air travel is increasingly cosmopolitan, one is left to guess at the extent of significant oxygen-related morbidity among air travelers. Such a guess might be that from 1 to 2 per cent of passengers would suffer from serious *emphysema* and other pulmonary disease, cardiac ailments bordering on decompensation, and severe *anemia*. At least it would appear to the flight surgeon experienced in commercial air travel that the proportion would exceed 4 per cent but rarely.

While this figure is only an estimate, it is probably reasonable if one considers it in the light of all other probabilities that must be satisfied for decompression to occur and of the total safety factors assigned to them.

In consequence a basic estimate of 2 per cent and a safety factor of 2 should provide an approach to protective efforts within reasonable expectation of probabilities. In the event of decompensation in a passenger, one asks what amount of oxygen is required and how long should it be given.

In the experience of the writer, discussions on oxygen requirements often have been carried on as if the administration of oxygen were the sole desideratum in cardiopulmonary emergencies. As one who has stood perplexed at the bedside of emphysematous victims of various complications, he is unimpressed by pleas for more and more oxygen. If decompensation does ensue in decompression and if the patient does not respond to oxygen tensions simulating those of from 30 to 40 per cent concentration at sea level (alveolar $pO_2$ of from 174 to 245 mm Hg), it is improbable that higher concentrations as the sole therapeutic measure will be helpful. It is more likely that achieving these tensions by means of positive intermittent pressure will be of greater benefit than if they are administered at ambient pressure (40).

In the absence of diagnostic capability aboard an airliner, how-

ever, arguments on behalf of pressure breathing or high concentrations of oxygen in these cases are academic; either could be harmful
according to the specific pathology present. And in this regard any
regulation promulgated by a committee or regulatory agency lacking
adequate clinical representation, to be carried out by non-medical
personnel under circumstances that might confuse an astute clinician,
could be predicted to produce as many potential hazards as it pre-
tends to allay. One might as well consider standards for the use of
supportive drugs at stipulated altitudes.

9. The transportation of patients suffering known cardiopulmonary diseases, severe anemia, or other oxygen-related illness bordering on decompensation should be specially arranged by the
patient's physician with the provision of a separate, additional
oxygen supply consistent with the physician's estimate of the need
in the event of a decompression accident and at the normal operating
cabin altitudes to be reached.

10. The one miscellaneous factor that requires attention in order
to provide perspective in analyzing oxygen requirements is that of
probability.

In each of the above considerations, the worst possible situation
for decompression, short of disaster, has been assumed. A probability of one, or certainty, that decompression would occur was assigned
to the problem. It was accepted that the incident would occur at
the highest operating altitude, with the shortest time of decompression, over limiting terrain or at the farthest point from land, that all
passengers would require oxygen for 10 minutes following descent,
and that a high percentage of unrecognized and severe pathology
susceptible to lack of oxygen existed among the passengers. It was
also assumed that no passenger would successfully don an oxygen
mask and that conditions would not permit any time for flight below
14,000 ft.

It is obvious that a probability of one for decompression must be
retained for calculation of oxygen needed, for the requirement could
not otherwise be established. The only relevant probabilities are
those that affect the choice of safety factors to be used once basic
criteria are laid down. In dealing with these probabilities, one is
concerned with assuring that no passenger needing oxygen faces a
risk of being without it because of inadequate amounts aboard the
aircraft.

Individual safety factors do not stand singly against this risk, but each is applicable to some degree in support of the others. For example, if each of 100 passengers is provided enough oxygen for 10 minutes, a reserve remains sufficient to give 2 hours of continuous oxygen to 6 people. These 6 would be in addition to those for whom continuous oxygen has been provided. Thus, if 2 per cent of passengers were estimated as being candidates for continuous oxygen following a decompression and if a safety factor of two were applied to this estimate, the original supply would have been for 4 persons. Adding 6 to this figure provides coverage for 10, giving a safety factor of 5 over the original estimate.

From this and other examples, it can be demonstrated that the calculation of oxygen requirements must consider over-all probability factors if unrealistic safety factors are not to be imposed at each point of consideration.

## Ionizing Radiation

**Jet Operational Factors and Cosmic-Ray Data.** Ionizing radiation * constitutes a factor of interest in jet operations for two reasons: (1) it is increasingly evident that there is probably no threshold of radiation for causing radiation injury to living tissue (specifically to genetic material) and (2) there is essentially an increasing intensity of the cosmic radiation with altitude, with ionization effects reaching a peak within the altitude range of present military and future civil turbojet aircraft (58).

The problem is to place these factors in proper perspective, both with respect to the possible effect on the individual and on future generations. From the ethical standpoint the choice is relatively simple for the individual: the possible risk of radiation effects can be assayed against the effects of other types of exposures and against rewarding aspects of the associated activity (76, p. 1127). The choice is not so simple for a society contemplating the effects of its acts on individuals yet unborn (66, 68).

In its reaction with the particles in the earth's atmosphere, the energy of primary cosmic radiation is reduced by a number of physical effects ranging from simple excitation of atoms and molecules to

* For a general reference to the terms and concepts on ionizing radiation used here, see Reference 53 in its entirety and Reference 54, pages 554–587, for a discussion of cosmic radiation.

their complete disintegration (60). By the time the primary radiations have traversed the atmosphere to an altitude of about 60,000 to 70,000 ft., practically all their energy has been transmitted to atmospheric matter which in turn produces secondary radiation and so on, until the initial energy is dissipated by degradation into the form of heat (80). The effect of this energy is inconsequential except perhaps when it interacts with living tissue.

Below about 60,000 ft., the resulting forms of energy are such that they may be said to have a relative biological effect (RBE) of one, that is, they are equal in effect on living tissue to x-rays of 0.1 to 3.0 million electron volts (mev) (80). The first generation of civil turbojets, operating to 40,000 ft., will be exposed only to this secondary component of cosmic radiation. The radiation exposure due to cosmic radiation at altitudes up to 60,000 ft. is variously estimated as in Table 11–1.

Primary cosmic radiation increases with altitude (as a percentage of the total cosmic radiation) to the edge of the atmosphere, and the heavier nuclei begin to appear significantly above 60,000 ft. The importance of this fact for effects on tissue is related to the larger RBE of the primary particles as compared with those of the secondary radiations. The RBE, in turn, is associated with the specific ionization of the radiation, that is, its proportionate ability to produce ionization of the matter through which it passes per unit length of its path. The specific ionization is dependent on the relative energy loss (REL) experienced by the radiation in its passage (60, 80). The REL of heavy nuclei changes constantly in their passage through tissue, reaching the greatest loss-value, and therefore causing the greatest ionization, toward the end of their paths (73).

The primary radiations are said to be composed of hydrogen nuclei (protons), helium nuclei (alpha particles), and heavier nuclei in the ratio of 79:20:1 (51). Estimates range from 70 to 90 per cent protons, from 29 to 9 per cent alpha particles, and under 1 per cent heavy nuclei (59). Energies of these particles range up to 10 billion electron volts (bev) (54, 79). Some idea of their intensity at the top of the atmosphere is presented by Schaefer (73, 74). At this height particle intensity, that is, the number of particles traversing a spherical space of 1 cm$^2$ cross section per hour from all directions, is given as 4,460:633:45 ($H^+$:$He^+$:heavy nuclei) at geomagnet latitude 55°, ranging down to 1010:124:9 at latitude 30°.

## TABLE 11-1

### Radiation Exposure in Millirads per Year (Equivalent) due to Cosmic Radiation at Altitudes up to 60,000 Feet *

| Altitude (Feet) | Source | | | | | |
|---|---|---|---|---|---|---|
| | Libby (62) | Neher (67) | Clay and Burch, quoted by U.K. Med. Res. Council (78) | Laughlin and Pullman (61) | H. Jones (76, p. 1131) | After Van Allen (80) |
| Sea level | 31–34 | | 28 | 28 | 35 | Absolute maximum exposure from cosmic radiation for a shielded or unshielded body at any altitude up to 60,000 ft. 13,700 |
| 10,000 | 80–120 | | | | 40 | |
| 20,000 | 300–450 | | | | | |
| 30,000 | | 1,400 | | | | |
| 40,000 | | 2,800 | | | | |
| 50,000 | | 4,200 | | | | |
| 60,000 | | 5,200 | | | | |

* Adapted from Kinsman (58).

Due to their large cross section and charge, heavy nuclei rapidly dissipate their energy by interaction with the atmosphere. Haber (56) states that the lower limit of heavy nuclei is found at about 11.2 miles (60,000 ft.) and that only about one-half of the primary protons penetrate to 12.5 miles (66,000 ft.).

Gray (55) and others (60, 70) have dramatized the possible effects on tissue of $He^+$ and heavy nuclei by superimposing their ionization tracks (in scale) over photomicrographs of cells and cell complexes. Illustration of the localized destructive effects of this type of radiation is well borne out by such methods. Schaefer (72) has discussed the statistical probability of a destructive lesion caused by a heavy nucleus in an embryo exposed to the full intensity of the primary radiation (asymptotic above about 120,000 ft.) and has concluded that, in an embryo of 1,000,000 cells, a high-energy hit would occur on the average for each 200 hours of extra-atmospheric flight per embryo.

The rapid reduction in energy of these multicharged nuclei between 100,000 and 66,000 ft., their relatively low particle intensity, and their limitation to latitudes above 50° N decrease significantly the probability of disastrous lesions such as the above in operation of the second generation of civil jet airliners that may operate at these heights.

The total dosage in thousandths of roentgen equivalent physical (mrep) * from cosmic radiation at these latitudes rises to a peak at 75,000 ft. (15 mrep/24 hrs), showing an estimated dosage of about 13 mrep/24 hrs at 60,000 and 100,000 ft. (70, 73). Between 60,000 and 80,000 ft. alpha particles and heavy nuclei contribute no more than 2.5 mrep/24 hrs to this total dosage (70).

The difficulty in judging the effects of primary radiation lies in the lack of criteria or experimental data for establishing a satisfactory RBE of the components, especially of heavy nuclei (52, 71, 74). Dosage in rep (roentgen equivalent physical) is not a measure of dosage in tissue. Dosage in rem (roentgen equivalent man) that does provide tissue dosage can only be determined experimentally. Dosage in rem is approximately equal to the dose in rep times the RBE and is defined as the dose in rad (radiation unit) times the RBE.

---

* For a brief discussion of dosage and radiation units, see Reference 54, pages 594–596.

Possible Somatic Effects of Cosmic Radiation on Aircrew Members.
The data in Table 11–1 provide a basis for estimating the maximum
dose to a pilot or aircrewmen of a commercial airliner operating at
40,000 ft. in latitudes above 50° (geomagnetic). On the assumption that all the flight time is spent at 40,000 ft. and that there would
be an average of 80 hours of flight time per month, the individual
would sustain a whole-body exposure increment above that of the
cosmic radiation at sea level of about 300 mrem *per year*. This is
equivalent to the present maximum permissible *weekly* exposure
above the natural background dosage for workers potentially exposed to radiation in industry. (It has been recommended by scientific advisory groups that this be lowered to 100 mrem per week
because of genetic considerations.) Flight at other altitudes under
the same assumption leads to a dosage estimation of 150 mrem/yr
at 30,000 ft. (turboprop maximum operating level), 460 mrem/yr
at 50,000 ft. (subsonic bomber altitude), and upwards of 570 mrem/
yr above 60,000 (jet-fighter operating range).

At 75,000 ft., the operating altitude of future commercial and a
small number of present military jet aircraft, is found the peak ionization of 15 mrep/24 hrs. Taking into account the intensifying effects
of aircraft cabin materials installed above the crew, we might double
this dosage to 30 mrep/24 hrs or 1200 mrep/yr (80, p. 257). If
half of this dosage in rep were assigned an RBE of 1 and the other
half an RBE of 5, a dosage of about 3.6 rem/yr would be obtained.
This may be compared with the present maximum permissible yearly
exposure of 15 rem or the recently recommended maximum of 5
rem/yr. Considering that assumptions such as were made above
concerning RBE are probably not tenable (69) and the improbability
of an airman's spending all his time at high altitude and high latitude, this estimated dosage would represent too great an amount by
a factor of at least 2 and probably more.

To achieve the perspective already mentioned, one might compare these figures with other human exposure data and their estimated effects on the life span of the individual.

The total whole-body radiation exposure due to natural external
sources at sea level, assuming average background levels from terrain
and dwellings, has been placed at from 50 to over 200 mrad/yr (58,
62, 77), although large variations occur due to type of dwelling and
terrain. This latter exposure, essentially gamma radiation (from
uranium, thorium, potassium), arises from the radioactivity of rocks

and earth and from materials used in building. The activity over bodies of fresh and sea water is reduced to 0.001 and 0.5 mrad/yr, respectively.

Thus, on converting from conventional aircraft to turboprops (30,000 ft.), the pilot who now lives in a brick home (100 mrad/yr) could move into a frame house (50 mrad/yr) and spend his waking hours off the job water skiing, swimming, and fishing to balance the expected increase in cosmic-radiation exposure of 150 mrad/yr! This entirely facetious remark is made only to indicate how variable are the already existing radiation exposures resulting from natural sources. For statistical purposes, however, the average whole-body exposure at sea level from natural sources is said to be about 100 mrad/yr (England) (61, 78) or 140–160 milliroentgens per year (mr/yr) (United States) (54).

Other variables in human exposure arise from medical diagnostic and therapeutic use of radiation, the wearing of radium-dial watches, exposure to radium on instrument dials, fallout from nuclear explosions, consumption of food and water, employment in certain occupations, and the like.

Laughlin and Pullman have estimated that in the United States the average person may have received 5 r (5,000 mr) by age thirty from medical x-ray exposure. This is equivalent to about 160 mrad/yr (61). A full-mouth dental x-ray can administer as much as 1,000 mr (970 mrem) to the whole body (76, p. 1132). Chest x-rays may add about 50 mr per examination and spinal or pelvic series as much as 9,000 mr. In luminous watches the dosage is dependent on the amount of radium present on the dial. In one study (64), this amount was found to vary from 0.01 to 2.2 microcuries (μc), the latter amount capable of producing a gonadal dose of up to 1,000 mrem/yr. Other estimates are of the order of 1,000 mrem of gonadal dosage per microcurie of radium per watch (76).

Based on 3 μc of radium per dial, four radium-painted instrument dials would radiate the pilot's area (distance 3 ft.) with about 50 mr/yr (62). This would amount to about 5 mrem/yr for 80 hours flight time per month. In some jet airliners no radiation source is present in instrument dials.

What particular meaning do radiation dosages have for the possible effect of cosmic radiation on an aircrew? Hardin Jones has made an attempt to assess the effect of radiation on life span of the exposed individual (76, p. 1103) in which, statistically, 1 r (0.97 rad for gamma rays) is said to cause a loss of five days from an individual's life. (See also Reference 76, p. 1049.) Translated to turbo-jet operation at 40,000 ft. (see above), this would amount to about 45 days for cosmic-radiation exposure increment experienced by the pilot, assuming he spent all his flight time at that altitude and at high latitudes for a 30-year career. If we assign a maximum possible 30-year exposure to a pilot spending all his flight time at 75,000 ft., a dosage of 3.6 rem/yr, the total exposure would amount to 108 rem, statistically equivalent to 540 days or 1½ year's reduction in life span. This same study estimates a life-span shortening of from 7 to 10 years (3,000 to 3,650 days) from the daily smoking of one and two packs of cigarettes, respectively, and 1,300 days' shortening for a condition of 25 per cent overweight.

It should be remembered that these figures on radiation effects are statistical derivatives, often from tenuous or incomplete data, but they serve to orient one in evaluating a situation that otherwise could lead to either overemphasis or underemphasis of the problem as applied to the individual.

**Possible Genetic Effects of Cosmic Radiation on Aircrew Members.** The researches of Muller (66) have directed a world's uncomfortable attention to the effect of radiation on genetic structures. As a result many attempts have been made to correlate radiation dosage to genetic mutations with the result that there seems to be essentially unanimous agreement among geneticists and other scientists engaged in radiobiology that there is no threshold of radiation for genetic effects. In this respect every radiation exposure of a population adds to its burden of mutations, the significance of which is that the great majority of mutations are considered harmful.

While these mutations mainly are recessive when inherited from one parent, that is, more or less hidden by the effects of corresponding normal genes from the second parent, they may cause deviations from the normal which, though slight, may reduce survival to maturity (76, p. 1055). Inherited from both parents, a mutation may be experienced as a gross malfunction or as structural defects and may further reduce survival to maturity.

Applied to an entire population, the total potential of even small doses of radiation for producing harmful effects in future generations, while extremely small in proportion to the total numbers of people in these generations, is very large when considered as to the actual number of persons affected (76, p. 1057). With increasing exposures the burden of harmful genes may increase significantly. A doubling of the natural mutation rate might be induced in a population by a radiation-dosage increment of perhaps 37 r per individual in a generation (66, p. 336). Other estimates for the doubling dose range from 3.1 r as the lowest possible exposure (54, p. 1036; 57) to over 75 r (76, p. 336). This doubling of mutations would occur only over many generations.

The effect on a population, genetically speaking, of increased exposures of a small group among that population, such as aircrews, would be minute. The ethically disturbing fact is that it would be finite, thus at some point in time affecting one or more human beings.

For an excellent and absorbing compilation of data and viewpoints on the effects of radiation, see References 75 and 76 in their entirety.

**Contamination of Aircraft Due to Atmospheric Radioisotopes.** Nuclear explosions are responsible to some degree for radioactive contamination of the atmosphere (75, 76, 79). Fission products are of special interest to the public but may contribute less than 2 per cent of that atmospheric contamination due to the naturally occurring radon (63).

Radioactive particles can be trapped on aircraft surfaces made sticky by oil and fuel films, in filters, and on the surfaces of air inlets. The significance of such contamination lies in its possible hazard to maintenance and servicing personnel, not to passengers or aircrew, according to present information.

Nuclear-reaction products do not become evenly distributed geographically in the atmosphere. There appears likewise to be uneven distribution in atmospheric depth (79).

In tests on high-altitude jet bombers, tankers, and transports, early findings indicated that there was some contamination to be expected from the operational altitude of the higher flying bombers and little from that of commercial jets (65). Recent operating experience on the North Atlantic commercial air route indicates that radioactive atmospheric particles may be found at lower stratospheric heights in quantity sufficient to cause contamination of commercial aircraft. Small amounts of contamination were found on aircraft flying at heights not exceeding 36,000 ft.

In determining the degree of aircraft-surface contamination, it is customary to measure the counts per minute emanating from a specified area. Analysis of the radiation is required if any idea of the sources and the biologically effective dose rate are to be estimated. Monitoring of jet aircraft (known to the writer) as of March, 1959, has indicated the following (65): Positive identification of *cerium* 141 and 144, *zirconium* 95, *yttrium* 91, *strontium* 89, and *ruthenium* 103 has been established in wipe tests of contaminated aircraft surfaces. *Cesium* 137 was not identified (57, 75, 76). Filters have given an initially high but rapidly falling emanation ascribed to the short-lived radon (63).

Beta particles of the middle range of energies are emitted by fission products. Strontium 89, for example, gives off beta particles of 1.48 mev; cerium 141, 0.44 and 0.58 mev; cerium 144, 0.30 mev; yttrium 91, 0.55 and 1.55 mev; zirconium 95, 0.39 and 1.0 mev; and ruthenium 103, 0.20 and 0.68 mev.

Gamma rays amounted to about 2.2 per cent of the total dosage from gamma and beta radiation over the most highly contaminated areas. Wipe tests on 100 $cm^2$ areas indicated a gamma dose rate of less than 0.055 mr/hr. Gamma radiation on the most highly contaminated commercial jet airliner so far examined at the time of writing, therefore, would amount to only 2 mr/wk for an employee continuously and intimately exposed to the contaminated surface during the entire 40 hours of the usual workweek. This is 1/150 of the present Atomic Energy Commission limit for occupationally exposed workers (300 mr/wk) and 1/50 of the recommended weekly exposure (100 mr/wk).

The gloves of a workman exposed during a field-service trip gave the highest reading obtained from clothing, namely, 3000 counts per minute, an amount equivalent to a dosage rate of about 1 mr/hr or 40 mr/wk (local radiation to the hands for continuous wearing of the gloves). Gamma radiation was responsible for only about 2 per cent of the total. Prior monitoring and controlled decontamination of aircraft would largely eliminate such contamination of clothing.

The potential hazards from external beta and gamma emission can be avoided by decontamination of aircraft, reasonable personal hygiene, surveillance of employees' clothing with laundering, and disposal as indicated.

The potential hazard from accidental ingestion and inhalation is remote. Its exact definition from operational experience would have to depend on elaborate procedures based on measurements of fission products in bodily excreta and of whole-body emission from internal radiation. Such an approach does not appear warranted at this time.

The very nature of the surface contamination, that is, its entrapment by adhesive films, would tend to allay concern for accidental inhalation or ingestion. Again, reasonable personal hygiene and protection of food at mealtime should avoid ingestion of fission products.

Filters leading to the cabin showed contamination of external layers only. Cabin interiors revealed no contamination by radioisotopes.

In these continuing studies flight-line measurements for aircraft contamination are made with a Geiger-Müller counter with an open-end window probe and are taken as close as possible to the suspected surface. Wipe samples are also taken from 100 cm² area on absorbent paper and counted on a scaler used in conjunction with a windowless flow counter.

An arbitrary limit on maximal permissible contamination of any aircraft surface was set at 2,000 counts per minute (as read by a Nuclear of Chicago Geiger-Müller counter). This limit was chosen by considering such factors as the nature of the fission products, dates formed, the decay system involved, the biological hazard, possible hazard from inhalation and ingestion, and available facilities as well as the fact that flight-line personnel are considered non-occupationally exposed.

If levels above this limit are found, decontamination of metal surfaces is carried out by use of cleaning solvent, soap, and water. A single, thorough cleaning usually has sufficed to lower the radiation to below the imposed limit.

Filters, according to the level of contamination and the number of filters involved, possibly could require disposal (81). Monitoring of filters in suspected aircraft should be carried out whenever filter servicing is required and protective safeguards are employed against employee contamination.

Polar detonation of nuclear devices could cause local atmospheric concentration of radioisotopes in the transpolar and North Atlantic air-traffic routes. Similarly, continental detonations could contaminate domestic routes to well above average concentrations for an indeterminate period.

It would appear that monitoring of civil and military aircraft should continue at least until a more definitive picture is obtained in order to detect levels of aircraft contamination greater than those predicted by present experience. Present studies would indicate that even potential hazards are minimal and that these are restricted to flight-line and overhaul personnel. They can be avoided by reasonable monitoring of aircraft and personnel and the maintenance of reasonable standards of personal hygiene among employees.

**Fallout.** In the event of nuclear warfare, gross surface contamination of runways, flight aprons, and parked aircraft will be of great concern. Aircraft taking off and landing on contaminated surfaces predictably will have radioactive dusts thrown into wheel wells or sucked into engines and air ducts. Very high levels of radiation exposure to aircrews and maintenance personnel could ensue even in areas remote from a nuclear detonation.

Similarly, aircraft engaged in testing of nuclear explosions may be contaminated by flying through heavily seeded areas or in operations to and from contaminated air fields.

**Direct Exposure of Aircrews to Radiation in Combat Flight.** Combat aircrews potentially are exposed to ionizing radiation from their own nuclear-weapon bursts and from those used defensively against them. Protection is largely a matter of tactical and strategic deployment because of weight limitations to shielding against neutrons and gamma rays.

**Nuclear-propelled Aircraft.** Specific considerations of radiation hazard in nuclear-propelled aircraft are heavily shielded by security classification. Equally heavy physical shielding of the nuclear reactors involved would alleviate any concern for health hazards.

There are three major factors peculiarly related to nuclear flight, each dealing with radiation hazards: (1) protection of aircrew, (2) protection of construction and maintenance personnel, and (3) protection of the public in the event of accident.

From the standpoint of protection of aircrews, the significant difference between ground and airborne reactors lies in the marked limitation on weight in the latter. Since the effectiveness of shielding is closely related to the mass of the shielding material, the types and energies of the radiations from nuclear reactors require large masses for their diminution to allowable limits of exposure. The problem is alleviated only in part by the lower weight in fuel requirements in nuclear as compared with chemically fueled aircraft.

If shielding limitations are insurmountable, the permissible maximum exposures of military aircrews for training, peacetime operation, and combat missions become highly important as separate considerations.

Protection of maintenance and servicing personnel provides problems essentially different only in detail from those met in stationary or naval shipboard reactors. The same statement applies to accidents involving the reactor.

Public protection is largely a matter of operational decisions. There is already a formidable literature on each of these subjects.

## Microwave Radiation

One could dismiss microwave radiation as unimportant in the operation of jet aircraft at the present time, because significant exposure of an aircrew does not occur. Some discussion of the subject seems necessary, however, because of the real hysteria that has been caused by unguarded speeches, misquotations in the press, immoderate safety regulations, and publication of unverified "accidents."

Microwave radiation, the name given to the electromagnetic frequencies used in radar equipment, is of concern in the field of aviation medicine. This form of radiation is also used in medicine to achieve heating of bodily tissues.

The entire microwave region is said to cover the frequency range from 300 megacycles to about 150,000 or 200,000 megacycles (99). Megacycle refers to 1,000,000 cycles per second (91). Frequencies can be converted to wave lengths by the equation $FL = C$, where $F$ is the frequency, $L$ is the wave length, and $C$ is the velocity of light. This velocity is expressed conveniently, though not exactly, by $3 \times 10^{10}$ cm/sec. The frequency is expressed in megacycles and wave length in centimeters.

From this equation it is seen that a frequency of 10,000 megacycles is equivalent to a wave length of 3 cm. It happens that this particular frequency and wave length is that which has been used for some time and continues to be used to a major extent in airborne radar equipment. The 3-cm to 10,000-megacycle region has been termed the "X-band." Other radar equipment uses the C-band (5 cm, 5,000 megacycles) and the S-band (10 cm, 3,000 megacycles). Medical microwave diathermy uses a 12.2-cm wave length (2,450 megacycles) as specified by the Federal Communications Commission.

Not only is frequency important to technical and biological systems, but the power, or the amount of energy contained in the radiation, is of importance. Many of the radar systems now in use are limited to 250,000 watts (w), but ground installations and some airborne radar exceed that by a factor of 10 or 20, and research is directed at power sources in excess of 100,000,000 watts.

In common with other electromagnetic radiation, microwaves can be reflected or refracted in the course of their contact with matter.

On being absorbed by matter, microwave radiation loses its energy by excitation, that is, by adding energy to orbital electrons in the absorbing atoms which then may return to their prior state by giving off radiation. The energies represented are, however, far below those necessary for ionization (110).

That non-thermal effects in tissue can be produced by microwaves is indicated by intracellular changes affecting chromosomal and other cellular particles in the absence of demonstrable heating. The changes are said to resemble those produced by mitotic poisons or ionizing radiation (93). Specific effects seem to be frequency-dependent.

In a literature which is already becoming formidable in amount, it has been pointed out that there are rather complex relationships between frequencies of microwave radiation and the percentage of its absorption by matter but that, in connection with bodily tissues, certain general statements can be made with respect to absorption. These generalizations have been summarized by Schwan and Li (106) as follows:

1. The percentage of absorbed energy is near 40 per cent at frequencies much smaller than 1,000 and higher than 3,000 megacycles. In the range from about 1,000 to 3,000 megacycles, the coefficient of absorption may vary from 20 to 100 per cent.
2. Radiation of a frequency below 1,000 megacycles will cause deep heating, not well indicated by the sensory elements in the skin and, therefore, considered especially dangerous. Radiation whose frequency exceeds 3,000 megacycles will be absorbed in the skin. Radiation of a frequency between 1,000 and 3,000 megacycles will be absorbed both in body surface and in the deeper tissues, the ratio being dependent on parameters involved.

From these conclusions it can be seen that much of the present radar equipment is operating at frequencies largely reflected or absorbed in the very first few millimeters of bodily tissue. The conversion of this energy to heat within the skin layer activates the heat-sensitive thermal organs and therefore provides some notification of the presence of the radiation.

There are certain consequences of this ability of microwave radiation (90) to heat bodily tissues which are, as usual in exposures of any sort, concerned with the degree and length of the exposure (83, 87, 100, 105, 107). Because of the possible physiological responses by the body, however, the effect varies with the tissue. Vascularized tissues (those provided with a blood supply) are capable of absorbing much greater quantities of the radiation than are non-vascularized tissues such as the lens of the eye. In the former, as heat is added, there is a reflexive increase in the amount of blood flow through the area. More and more reserve blood vessels are opened up, and those that are already active become more widely dilated; the increased blood flow carries away the added heat.

The lens and the intraocular fluid have no such blood supply, nor does urine held in the bladder, intestinal contents, surgically implanted metal plates, cartilage, or certain kinds of bone. These can gain heat rapidly and, if heated excessively, can be damaged or cause damage to surrounding tissues. Poorly vascularized or heat-sensitive tissue, such as the testes, are similarly susceptible to damage. It can be appreciated that the thermal stress imposed on a local tissue, if that tissue has a good blood supply, can within limits be readily dissipated by the spreading of the heat through the blood and ultimately by surface loss all over the body.

Where the entire body is exposed to radiation, however, each portion has a thermal burden that it cannot readily share with another (104). If the total heat dissipation possible through use of the body temperature-regulating systems is less than the heat gained because of radiation, then the body temperatures will continue to rise as long as the radiation is present. With tremendous energies and direct exposure it is conceivable that an intolerable rise in body temperature could occur without early warning. The atmospheric environment can become important to the whole-body effects of microwave radiation. Any combination of atmospheric conditions that would tend to prevent heat loss from the body would increase the effect of microwave heating, especially in the event of whole-body exposure.

Certain other factors concerned with the operation and maintenance of radar equipment affect microwave-radiation dosage. A radar beam emanates from an antenna which concentrates the energy much as a concave mirror concentrates a headlight beam. As a consequence the power radiated does not fall off in the usual inverse-square relationship with distance from the radiating source but remains rather high for a distance spoken of as the *near field* of an instrument.

Two other aspects of radar operation are of importance to human exposure. These are the interruption or pulsing of the beam and the angular sweep through which the antenna is operated. Because of the interruption of the beam, the average power is below that of the peak power of the instrument. Any heating effects of microwave radiation are dependent on the average power available. In addition, if a microwave-radiation device is scanning, the period within which an object in the field is exposed will be followed by a period of no heat gain during which heat loss is possible.

Before proceeding to an examination of the possible interactions between microwave radiation and human tissues, it might be profitable to explore the physical implications of this type of energy. Heat, in the physical sense, is an expression of the amount of energy contained in a system. It is a measure of the work that could be accomplished were this heat converted into work. Thus, it may be possible to transfer the total amount of energy in the form of heat from one system to another without regard for the time during which this transfer takes place. The nature of the problem of the transfer of microwave energy to the human body requires that a time factor be introduced, for it is conceivable that a total amount of heat transferred during one period of time will have an effect different from that which is transferred during a much shorter period of time. This relationship can be expressed by the adoption of the proper units.

Radiation in its passage through space is often thought of in terms of flow or flux, and, to reduce the flow to terms of measurement, one can choose the unit of energy passing through a unit area for a unit period of time. The first two units can be combined by selecting a unit of flux or flow that expresses the amount of energy transferred in a period of time. Such a unit, a unit of power, is the watt (w), which is defined as $10^7$ ergs per second. The unit of area chosen is the square centimeter ($cm^2$). It is not proper to speak of the energy of such a flux in terms of heat for the reason that heat is produced only as a result of interaction between the radiation and the matter with which it comes in contact, and many variables enter

into the percentage of this energy that is so transferred. If it is possible to determine the actual percentage of energy transferred to
heat, then it is possible to express the amount of heat transferred to
an exposed body in terms of large calories, the unit commonly used
in relation to body heat.

Since the body produces heat by its own processes and is limited
by the mechanisms by which it loses heat, these factors present a
possible means of calculating tolerances to whole-body microwave
radiation. If one assigns a total body surface of 2 $cm^2$ to the so-
called average man as a convenient approximation, making no allow-
ances for the effects of body contours, and likewise assumes that the
person is exposed with the radiation beam normal to the front of
the body, a total absorptive area of 1 $cm^2$ is obtained. (DuBois
(88) assigns to the average man a surface area of 1.74 $cm^2$.) Assuming 100 per cent absorption of the incident radiation, it would
be necessary only to measure the energy flux at the site of an exposed
body to determine the total heat transfer. Measurements in the
Boeing Airplane Company of the energy flux produced by radar
equipment in common use on the company planes indicate that the
flux rises to 0.01 w/$cm^2$ within the beam about 37 ft. from the antenna as the antenna is approached.

The consequences of such a whole-body exposure may be represented in the following manner: The energy flux of 0.01 w/$cm^2 =$
0.1 kw/$m^2$, the area of the exposed surface. This is equivalent to
0.143 Cal/min, *large calories per minute* being the expression ordinarily used in reference to body metabolism. This figure of 0.143
Cal/min is equal to about 1/10 the metabolic heat produced by the
average body in a quiet, standing position. The heat added by the
microwave radiation would be equivalent to the metabolic heat
burden that would be added by the initiation of light handwork by
the person standing. It would be necessary to increase the radiant
flux 10 times in order to double the total heat gain of the body due
to metabolism alone, which would amount to producing a condition equivalent to the total metabolic demand of driving a car.
It would require 50 times as much radiation, or 0.5 w/$m^2$, to create
a total body heat from basal metabolism, plus the heat from the
radiation, to equal that produced by metabolism alone in the effort
of felling trees or climbing steps (92).

Thus, it would appear at first glance that the figure chosen would
give an extremely large safety factor in ordinary environmental cir-

cumstances. The relationship of this arbitrary level of safety requires further exploration in terms of actual experimentation on human subjects, particularly in view of the generally unreliable extrapolation of data obtained from the use of small animals. Experiments on dogs are particularly subject to critical evaluation because of the marked limitation of evaporative heat loss in this animal.

Ely and Goldman (89) have exposed two persons to whole-body radiation at a flux of 0.1 w/cm² at the center of the beam, the peripheral exposures falling off rapidly because of the geometry of the set. They calculated the power at approximately 250 w in the entire profile (exposed) area. The ambient temperature was found to be 24° C. The rectal temperature actually dropped 0.4° C during an exposure of 48 minutes. A second exposure of 0.22 w/cm² in the center of the beam and about 400 w over the exposed profile in an ambient temperature of 25° C for a period of 48 minutes, produced a rectal temperature drop of 0.15° C. Using a profile of 1 m² and assuming 100 per cent absorption, this 400 w would amount to 0.4 kw/m² or 0.57 Cal/min. This is equivalent to the metabolic burden of heat that would be added by going from a reclining position to a sitting position involving light handwork. The exposure in this experiment was to S-band radiation of 2,880 meg/sec or 10.4-cm wave length.

Schwan and Li (106) have stated that a flux figure of about 0.3 w/cm² must result in intolerable temperature rise when the irradiated area is larger than 100 cm². These authors assume that 0.03 w/cm² is dangerous if at least half the body is exposed. The experiments just quoted, however, indicate that on the average the whole-body profile received 0.04 w/cm² without any rise in deep-body temperature. Had the experiments been conducted under conditions of high air temperature and high relative humidity, significant rise in body temperatures might have occurred. Apparently, the microwave-radiation flux level, which is defined by the Air Force as the maximal allowable exposure, contains a very large safety factor under ordinary circumstances (109). The implications of this factor for local-tissue exposures should be examined. Most of the research performed on local tissues has been directed at the lens of the eye and the testes (85, 94, 96, 98, 101, 103).

It has been said that microwave radiation affects the body through the production of heat. One important biological effect involves a phenomenon called "denaturation of protein." This amounts to a disorganization of the chemical structure of the protein molecule to a degree that it cannot be reconstituted. This phenomenon is demonstrated every time an egg is boiled. The clear portion of the egg (its protein material) becomes the white of the egg on heating, and, comparably, the clear lens of the eye becomes the cloudy cataract with the denaturation of its protein.

A temperature of 45° C has been suggested as the upper limit of the temperature to be permitted within the human eye if damage is to be avoided (108). This is more than 2° C below temperatures at which lenticular opacities have been produced in the eyes of experimental animals and thus would appear to provide a safe margin to this degree. Williams (110) carried out a series of rabbit-eye exposures in which he found a threshold for cataract formation which ranged from 5 minutes of exposure at 0.59 w/cm² to 90 minutes exposure at 0.29 w/cm². No cataract formation followed 0.5 hour of exposure at 0.12 w/cm², but severe ocular damage was caused by 0.22 w/cm² for the same length of exposure. Threshold exposures were accompanied by vitreous temperatures between 49° and 53° C. Richardson (102) found that opacities of the lens were induced by ocular temperatures at the posterior surface of the lens of 54.8° C and above. All the experiments just referred to were carried out in the microwave diathermy frequency used in medicine.

Much of the concern shown by male radar technicians with regard to the consequences of microwave-radiation exposure has been directed at the testes. Imig, Thomson, and Hines (97) exposed rat testes to temperatures varying between 30° and 47° C, using medical diathermy of 12-cm wave length, and found that all animals showed degenerative changes when the testicular temperature was raised to 35° C or higher. Fifty per cent of the testes showed changes in the range of 31° to 35° C. Ely and Goldman (89) found that the threshold temperature of 37° C was the lowest damaging temperature found in their studies on dogs. The radiation flux required to maintain this temperature was 0.005 w/cm² in the most sensitive animals. At this threshold temperature tubular degeneration of the testes was observed in a 1-hour exposure.

These authors point out the difficulty in evaluating these findings insofar as any permanent effects on the testes are concerned. They and others (97) have pointed out the probable high temperatures sustained by the testes in prolonged hot bathing such as engaged in by the Japanese. The hardiness and the procreational ability of this nationality do not seem to have been affected (nor do those qualities of other groups addicted to parboiling, such as the Finns).

It should be stated that no single case of fully verified injury to radar personnel has been discovered as a result of their work to date as far as this writer is aware. Barron (82) examined a total of 335 employees with a history of potential exposure to radar over a period up to 14 years. He was unable to associate this exposure with any pathological effect in comparison with 100 control subjects. This study also compared the proportion of offspring produced by the two groups without discovering any significant variation.

The opening statement of this section, about dismissing microwave radiation as unimportant in connection with jet aircraft today, is justified in the light of the above discussion when it is realized that the aircrews of present jet aircraft are not in any way exposed to the direct radiation of their own radar equipment. The potential hazard to microwave technicians is real but remote except in special circumstances (84, 86, 95). Very simple precautions have been taken empirically by industrial physicians for many years. Safety regulations direct that technicians stay away from the field in front of a radiating antenna and prohibit direct viewing of an operating source.

Another potential hazard associated with the power sources is that of possible x-ray exposure. The electrons that produce the microwave radiations are capable of producing x-rays in their interaction with materials in the generating devices used, provided their energies are high enough. As voltages rise, shielding becomes more difficult because of the more intense x-radiation produced. Uncontrolled, this form of exposure is possibly a greater potential hazard than the microwave radiation itself.

## Acceleration

In the old days of running boards, one could (and did) "bail out" of a moving automobile without danger, provided the speed was low. With increasing speed the hazard increased, beginning with skinned hands and knees and ending with skull fractures and worse. These were injuries produced by contact with a solid, the ground.

It is now possible to bail out of a jet aircraft at high speeds and to suffer severe injury by contact with the air, that soft nothingness of everyday experience.

In these cases two essential forces are at work. One is that of the direct mechanical action of one substance on another, resulting in the excessive stretching, shearing, or compression of tissue and producing the familiar cuts, bruises, fractures, and avulsions. The second is less easily comprehended but can result in the same types of injuries. It is the force due to relative acceleration or deceleration of the bodily tissues (118; 122, pp. 18-34; 123; 130).

In the 1930's Hugh De Haven (114) began collecting a remarkable series of cases involving falls from heights ordinarily considered lethal. Some of the people involved were unharmed or suffered only minor injuries. It was plain that these persons had undergone an enormous decelerative force; yet the time over which the force acted and the circumstances surrounding the application of the force were in some way protective.

De Haven's investigations revealed factors common to each of the falls. In one instance the person spread-eagled from a height of about 55 ft. into a freshly spaded flower bed, landing in a near-supine position and creating a depression about 4 in. deep. In another similar case the fall was 93 ft. and the depression in the soft earth was 6 in. In the first case De Haven calculated a velocity at contact of 54 ft/sec (37 mph) and an average decelerative force of 140 g. In the second the velocity at contact was 73 ft/sec (50 mph) and the minimum decelerative force 166 g. Traveling at an initial velocity of 54 ft/sec, the body would come to a halt in about 1/80 sec. in 4 in. and at 73 ft/sec initially in about 1/75 sec.

In each case the surface gave way before the falling body, spreading the area of contact and bringing the body to a halt gradually, in a manner of speaking. This gradual halt at the speeds involved permitted the tissues to retain their relative positions, that is, not pull away from each other as the result of unequal decelerations. In addition, the spreading area of contact distributed the mechanical compressive forces over a large area, so that a small area of skull or body did not have to take the full force of the blow. A most important circumstance was that the surface on which each body struck was inelastic. Had it been elastic, the body would have been accelerated in the opposite direction. Since a body does not respond as a unit to such an elastic rebound and since parts of it would be reversing direction as compared with other parts, disruptive forces would develop.

In this regard one can imagine a water-filled balloon dropped from a height onto a hard surface. It is obvious that the water molecules at the bottom of the balloon will tend to come to a sudden halt. As elastic particles they will also tend to rebound in the opposite direction. The molecules higher up will act to prevent this, but will also be acted on both from below and above. The resultant molecular movement will be in the direction of the least pressure. Initially, this is toward the sides of the balloon which will bulge transversely to the axis of fall as the water molecules are displaced laterally. If the force exerted by the water molecules exceeds the cohesive forces holding together the rubber molecules, the balloon will rupture. If not, one could say that no damage has resulted.

The balloon model, however, is not a true analog of the body. Except for its "skin" the balloon is entirely without structure. The human body differs in that its tissues and its individual cells have structural integrity necessary for normal function.

In the body the comparatively rigid structure of the skeleton rapidly transmits decelerative forces so that its parts distant from the point of impact tend to be halted more rapidly than the soft tissues supported by them. When the difference in the deceleration between the bony structure and the soft-tissue masses creates forces that exceed the elastic limits of the soft tissues, tearing of the latter structures occurs (118).

The mass of soft tissue and the decelerative difference together can create stresses capable of fracturing the bony supports. For example, in the upright seated position, a pilot who crash-lands will have decelerative forces rapidly transmitted upward along the long axis of his spine. The upper part of the spine therefore tends to stop much more quickly than the non-rigid masses of the mediastinum and abdomen. The continuing downward momentum of these masses and of the other tissues anterior to the spine acts through the supporting tissues to create bending moments on the spine, which flexes anteriorly unless adequately restrained. If sufficiently large, the resultant forces can cause rupture of the posterior spinal ligaments, compression fractures of the vertebrae, and tearing of organs such as the liver, heart, and lungs. Although it matters little how the molecules of water in the balloon end up in relation to one another (since they have no functional relations), the blood in the body fails its purpose outside the blood vessels, and the liver functions poorly in the pelvis.

Other phenomena may be associated with sudden deceleration. Shock waves can be set up in the body and disrupt tissues. If a tissue mass is set in periodic motion at the resonant rate of the mass, internal or supportive structures can be ruptured at less than non-resonant energies (126).

**Crash Landings and Ditchings.** The decelerations involved in landing accidents or in crash landings of present commercial jet aircraft, and therefore the problems involved in passenger and crew protection, are essentially the same as those in conventional civil aircraft. In combat jet aircraft landing speeds may be significantly greater. It becomes increasingly important to provide combat aircrews with seats and harness that will give protection to the limit of tolerance for decelerative stresses (119, 132). In ejection at high-subsonic and at supersonic speeds, it is necessary to know accelerative tolerances in order to prevent injury as a result of ejection forces as well as of the ram air pressures met outside the aircraft.

There is no single parameter by which these tolerances can be expressed. They vary according to the axis of the body through which a force is acting and also according to anatomical and physiological variables. The time over which the forces act and the speed with which they develop are especially important (115, 120, 127, 134, 136).

As it became apparent that the human body could withstand rather large accelerative forces, interest arose in the provision of maximum protection for passengers and crews in the event of crash landings and ditchings. The maximum force that the body could withstand, however, exceeded that which engineers felt could reasonably be designed against in the aircraft structure. For example, if the body adequately restrained could withstand 30 g in a fore or aft direction, the total force on the seat would be very large. The seat's attachment to the aircraft would thus have to be designed to withstand the total of the forces created by the combined weight of the seat and the body multiplied by 30. (This approach does not consider peak accelerations or forces created by the geometry of the attachments of the seat and restraining harness.) A 200-lb. passenger would himself act as a 6,000-lb. weight under an average deceleration of 30 g.

With a number of simplifications, some idea may be obtained of the rather drastic circumstances that would have to exist in order to create a linear deceleration of only 20 g. The term "linear" refers to a situation in which the force is applied in one direction only, in this case from front to back, so that there is no change in course of the impelled body.

Linear acceleration (deceleration is negative acceleration) can be expressed as follows: $a = \dfrac{v^2 - v_o{}^2}{2s}$, where $a$ is the acceleration (rate of change of velocity), $v_o$ is the velocity at the beginning of acceleration, $v$ is the velocity at the end of acceleration, and $s$ is the distance over which the acceleration takes place. If $v_o$ and $v$ are expressed in feet per second, then $a$ is expressed in feet per second per second.

If an airplane traveling at 150 knots (250 ft/sec) in a landing approach strikes nose down in the bay at the end of the runway, at which distance and in what time does it come to a halt if the average deceleration is 20 g, assuming the unlikely circumstance of a strictly linear deceleration? $v_o$ becomes 250 ft/sec, $v = 0$ ft/sec; $a$ is 20 g or $20 \times 32.2$ ft/sec$^2$, and $s$ is unknown. In this case, g is decelerative and therefore negative.

$$-20 \times 32.2 \text{ ft/sec}^2 = \frac{0 - (250 \text{ ft/sec})^2}{2s \text{ ft.}}$$

$$s \text{ ft.} = \frac{-(250 \text{ ft/sec})^2}{-2 \times 644 \text{ ft/sec}^2}; \; s = 48.5 \text{ ft.}$$

Since the average velocity over the distance $s$ is $\dfrac{250 - 0}{2}$ or 125 ft/sec, the time of deceleration is 48.5 ft. divided by 125 ft/sec or about 0.4 sec.

A total of 4,000 tons of force would be exerted on a 200-ton aircraft subjected to 20 g. Even disregarding how this force would be distributed, an airplane cannot reasonably be designed to stay together under these circumstances in the present state of the art if it is to retain other safe-flying characteristics. Consequently, it would be meaningless to protect passengers against 20 g of linear deceleration when the aircraft would disintegrate under the same stress.

An airplane at the same speed, maintaining a straight and level course in a crash landing, would have to stop within 100 ft. to be subjected to a force of 10 g. Stopping within 2 seconds in 500 ft. would subject the passengers to only 2 g. Structural strength of present commercial jets permits stressing of passenger seats against linear deceleration to about 10 g.

In striking the ground or water, an airplane obviously would have some velocity in a downward as well as in a horizontal direction. In the equation $a = \dfrac{v^2 - v_o^2}{2s}$, $s$ would represent the distance in which the airplane would be stopped in its vertical motion. As $s$ becomes smaller, the deceleration $a$ becomes larger for a given value of $v_o$ ($v = o$). On a hard surface, such as a concrete runway, $s$ could be very small and the deceleration quite large. In a controlled crash landing the pilot can flare out the landing so that the downward velocity can be rather small and in this manner counteract the effect of the small decelerative distance.

If not well controlled, the decelerative force due to the vertical velocity on landing would be large if the aircraft structure were not to give way. (In a normal landing the shock-absorbing "oleos" of the wheels give way to diminish the peak deceleration.) For example, with a downward velocity of 10 ft/sec and a decelerative distance of 0.1 ft. on concrete (a completely arbitrary choice), the equation above becomes $a = \dfrac{10^2}{2 \times 0.1} = 500$ ft/sec$^2$, if there is no elastic rebound.

If the underportion of the fuselage gives way in such a manner as to increase $s$ to 3 ft., the change in $a$ is marked:

$$a = \frac{10^2}{2 \times 3^2} = 5.5 \text{ ft/sec}^2$$

Thus, by proper design the fuselage can provide protection by permitting a degree of controlled collapse, so that the total stress from vertical deceleration on the passengers and crew is minimized.

Purely linear decelerations are seldom met in aircraft accidents. Depending on how the accident progresses, extremely complex forces can be generated about seat attachments should twisting or bending of structural elements or rotation of the aircraft occur. A designer is obliged, however, to see that seat integrity is maintained up to the limit of the structural integrity of the aircraft if he is to act in the best interests of passenger safety. However, concern with seats should not obscure the fact that aircraft structure is a primary contributing factor in safety. This is illustrated by the case of one World War II single-place aircraft that was so designed that the pilot's seat attachment was stronger than the structure surrounding the cockpit. In crash landings the cockpit would tend to collapse, either dashing the pilot's head into the gunmount or, by completely shearing in two, leaving the pilot exposed, securely strapped to the seat, to whatever lay in the path. The plane was designed to stay together in flight and on normal landings, but not to give adequate protection in crash landings.

Crashes have occurred in which major structural integrity was maintained, but injuries and deaths occurred because seats and seat attachments were unable to withstand equal stress. In the design of jet aircraft, the lessons learned from such accidents have been used to advantage. The flight stresses on jet aircraft are such that the structure must be stronger than that of slower propeller-driven planes. The powerful jet engine is capable of compensating for the increased weight involved in the added structural strength. Given the stronger framework, the designer is able to provide significant increases in the protection given passengers and crew. The occupants are encased in a stronger container and are secured more strongly within the container.

At faster landing speeds, the advantages thus gained are overcome by the greater forces that can develop in crash landings and ditchings. In commercial jet aircraft the landing speeds are kept close to those of modern propeller-driven planes. In very high-performance military jets, landing speeds may be considerably greater, so that attention must be given to "beefing up" the crew's seats well beyond the limits possible in commercial jets. Here again the structural strength demanded for performance makes possible greater stressing of the pilot's equipment.

**Accelerative Forces Associated with Maneuvers, Catapult, and RATO Launchings.** The high maneuverability required of some combat aircraft imposes accelerative stress. In a high-speed turn the decelerative force on an aircrewman is directed toward his head (positive g stress). In a dive and pull-up or inside loop, the direction of deceleration is the same. In an outside loop or inverted spin there is accelerative force in the direction of the feet (negative g stress) (123).

In the first instance the body is moving in the direction of the seat while the seat is moving toward the body. Three decelerative effects are possible. Significant injury to tissue is improbable in that stress sufficient to cause such injury is well beyond the capacity of the pilot either to remain conscious or to maintain muscular control during the extended time associated with the type of maneuver under consideration.

Since the blood is free to exert pressure along the longitudinal axis of the long vessels of the body and since there is no force of significant degree acting to return blood to the heart from a position below the heart, blood will "pool" in the elastic vessels of the lower part of the body. In addition, the same decelerative force will hinder blood flow to the brain through the hydrostatic pressure it induces within the heart, a pressure that can exceed the heart's muscular capacity to impel the blood.

The net result of the hydrostatic-pressure effect in positive g stress is to prevent blood from reaching the brain so that cerebral hypoxia and blackout or unconsciousness ensue.

When the force is in the opposite direction, as in an outside loop, the hydrostatic effect is toward the head. The static blood pressure in the head is increased in proportion to the amount of deceleration. The thin-walled vessels of the head and neck and the rigid skull are important factors in the low tolerance to negative g (135).

Decelerative stress increases the weight of the extremities and may exceed their muscular capacity to maintain control of the aircraft (112). Jet aircraft of the fighter type are strongly stressed for performance and are capable of very high speed, but propeller-driven fighters also are capable of exceeding human g tolerance in maneuvers. The forces involved and their magnitude have been widely discussed.

In catapult launchings and RATO (rocket-assisted take-off), linear accelerative forces are exerted on the crew. These forces in themselves are well below tolerance for injury but may interfere with muscular control and hence control of the aircraft. Indirectly, they have been responsible for injury by causing poorly mounted auxiliary equipment to fly free from its mountings.

The launching force is in a direction which approaches the optimum for tolerance in the forward-facing pilot. For other crew positions, possibly not so advantageously placed, adequate restraints are required for protection, a fact overlooked in some World War II aircraft.

**Ejection.** Combat aircraft require special attention to matters of survival. Their rigorous use in training and the hazards of battle damage make it essential that the crew be able to escape. As their speeds increased, it became more and more difficult for unassisted crewmen to abandon combat airplanes. At about 250 mph the pressure of the air and the inability to clear structures such as the vertical and horizontal stabilizers made successful escape improbable (126). An ejection mechanism became mandatory (124, 125, 128, 129, 131).

At still greater speeds ejection had to be accomplished with increasing force. Now the ejection force itself posed a hazard (125).

The human spine with its curved architecture and spongy pads between the vertebrae is hardly an ideal structure to absorb thrusts along its long axis without suffering insult in the bargain. Its tolerance to accelerative stress in this axis is appreciably less than that of the body in general across its transverse axis.

In ejection the speed with which the accelerative force develops is highly important in causing spinal injuries. This rate of change of acceleration varies with the method of providing the impulse. An explosive force tends to produce a very high rate of change at the initiation of the explosion. A rocketlike mechanism, as is apparent to those who have watched missile launchings, has a slow accelerative force initially with a more rapid increase later in the launching. In explosive ejection, however, the acceleration lasts for only a short time and so does not expose the body to stress over a long period. With slower onset the exposure necessarily is spread over a longer period if adequate clearance of aircraft structures is to be successful. The parameters of tolerance of the spine both as to the rate of onset of acceleration and as to the time of exposure, therefore, are needed to design efficient ejection mechanisms (126).

Still other factors have been found that can aggravate or alleviate the stress imposed by ejection. As noted above, an elastic surface, although it may give initially before a body that strikes against it and may therefore reduce the rate of deceleration at this point, "pushes back" at the end of its compressions. This rebound is added to the force of deceleration already existing and can develop at a high rate. In an otherwise tolerable ejection, the added stress due to rebound of an elastic cushion beneath the pilot can cause spinal injuries.

On the other hand, a compressible, inelastic surface that gives gradually but does not spring back will lower the rate of change of the deceleration and tend to protect the spine (126). Additional protection may be afforded by restraining the body in such a way that spinal flexion is minimized.

An ejective force necessary to clear a 40- to 50-ft. vertical fin of a large bomber could be avoided if ejection were to be made downward. Unfortunately, many emergencies develop too near the ground to permit downward ejection, separation of man and seat, deployment of the parachute, and significant reduction of the man's downward and horizontal velocity before his contact with the ground (125). On the other hand, ejection from an inverted aircraft near the ground poses a similar problem if ejection normally is upward.

Ejection is also associated with accelerative forces due to contact of a body with the air and through the tendency of an ejected body to rotate (117, 135, 136). The physical factors acting on an ejected body vary complexly with its velocity, weight, cross-sectional area and configuration, and with the density of the air (122, pp. 18–34).

As the weight increases, so does the kinetic energy at a given initial velocity. An opposing force, represented by air resistance, would thus have to act over a longer period of time to cause equivalent slowing of the heavier of two bodies, assuming equivalent cross-sectional areas. This means that the duration of the decelerative stress on the heavier body would be greater, an important point in regard to human limits of tolerance. The total weight of the man, his equipment, and the escape device are therefore of consequence in this respect alone.

If air density decreases, as with increasing altitude, the opposing force caused by the air is decreased. If weight and area are unchanged, it would be necessary to increase the velocity of an object as altitude increases in order to keep the force the same. It is possible, therefore, for ejections to be made at increasing speeds as altitude increases without increasing the decelerative stress, but the time over which the stress acts will be greater (113, 120, 121).

High rotational rates of an ejected body can develop immediately on ejection. It is possible for the rotation to cause rapid and marked g stresses in those parts well away from the center of rotation of the mass, so that in rotations about the transverse diameters of the body (tumbling), a man's head and viscera suffer severe fluctuations in g forces (130). Depending on the geometry of the rotation in relation to the direction of the ram air pressure, the angular accelerative forces variably add to and subtract from the decelerative force due to the ram air pressure.

As a result vibratory fluctuations of soft-tissue masses of the body are set up. In unstabilized configurations of ejection equipment and occupant, the forces developed may vary from plus 30 or 35 g to low positive or even negative g values several times a second for a bodily region well away from the center of rotation, such as the head. Such forces are intolerable even for a very short period. At high altitude the poor damping effect of thin air prolongs the period. At low speeds the use of aerodynamic stabilizers, such as fins, becomes ineffective.

Further g forces face the ejected pilot. Contrary to "common sense" evaluation, a parachute opening at high altitude provides a more severe deceleration than at low altitudes in spite of the less dense air (122, p. 30; 133). In addition, the greater the horizontal component of the pilot's air speed, the greater the force developed on the opening.

No precise g-tolerance limit is possible for activation of the parachute, because prevention of injury is in part dependent on body attitude at the time of its opening.

As ejection speeds approach the speed of sound, survival by means of a man-seat configuration is problematical or, perhaps one should say, providential. One cannot assume that circumstances will permit slowing of the aircraft prior to ejection. Experience would indicate the contrary (125).

It should be noted that the use of an ejection capsule does not necessarily protect against the accelerative forces noted above, although it provides protection against windblast. Just as with the ejection seat, it must decelerate within tolerance limits of force and duration and must be stabilized against rotation.

Since the critical region of escape with or without capsulation is at low altitude, rapid slowing of the escape-package is essential. This means that advantage must be taken of the upper limits of man's decelerative tolerance if lives are to be saved at low altitude (130).

Published limits for linear deceleration above 25 g front to back are (134):

    (a) Threshold for impact shock related to rate of change of deceleration: 1,000 g per second at 30 g for 0.16 second or less of duration.

(b) Limit of tolerance for rate of change of deceleration: 1,500 g per second at 40 g for 0.16 second duration or less.
(c) Tolerance limit for magnitude of force: 50 g attained at 500 g per second rate of onset and duration of 0.2 second or less.
(d) Duration limit: one second for forces averaging 25 g or more, at 500 g per second rate of onset.

Studies of prolonged acceleration indicate that 15 g can be safely withstood for 5 seconds (116). For optimum body position, 12 g for 5 seconds' exposure down to 4 g for 12 minutes' exposure using restraint suits were found in one series of experiments (113). For longer exposure the transverse g tolerance falls below this level (122, p. 37). Irreversible accelerative shock was produced in chimpanzees at values of 40 g maintained for 15 seconds in a foot-to-head (positive) direction (111). Extrapolations from this and other maximum g-stress studies were applied to humans.

For acceleration along the long axis of the spine, the suggested limit of tolerance is 300 g/sec rate of change of acceleration with a maximum peak acceleration of 25 g (126).

For simple angular rotations around a transverse axis, 3 to 10 seconds at 160 rpm with the heart as center of rotation were found to produce complete unconsciousness. With the center of rotation at the *iliac crest, petechiae* were produced at 90 rpm for 3 seconds and at 50 rpm for 2 minutes. The rate of rotation was limited to 125 rpm because of the onset of pain (135).

Hydraulic effects due to accelerative force apparently do not become effective below about 0.2 second's duration of the force.

That these limits cannot be applied in aircraft design without regard for the effect of one upon the other has been indicated. Their adequate evaluation and application, however, can be negated by human factors attendant on operational circumstances, such as inadequate indoctrination of aircrewmen and careless maintenance and overloading of escape facilities.

## Noise

**Characteristics of Noise.** Noise (138–140) is a form of energy convertible to mechanical force. In the production of the sensation of sound, this energy, through its action on the ear drumhead, sets in motion the mechanical transducers of the middle ear, the ossicles. These in turn transmit their vibration to a fluid within which lies the cochlea or hearing organ. Within the cochlea are specialized cells which react to vibration by setting up neural discharges. These discharges on transmission to the brain are interpreted as sound.

Sound waves impinge on the drumhead of the ear and on the body as a whole. If the energy of the sound is great enough, it can cause stimulation of the hearing organ without acting by way of the ear drumhead. The energy is transmitted by other bodily tissues. Thus, intense sound can bypass the normal hearing channel, but in so doing its energy is cut down by the "damping" action of the tissue. Because of this added route of transmission, however, the amount of protection that can be afforded the cochlea by protective equipment, short of enclosing the entire body, is limited.

The normal mechanism of transmission is much more sensitive. The pressure of sound waves on the tympanic membrane (the ear drumhead) can create the sensation of sound at extremely low energies. The so-called normal ear can be stimulated by pressures of less than 0.0002 dynes per square centimeter (equivalent to a weight of less than 2/1,000,000 gm or less than 1/10,000,000 oz.).

The important differences between pressures compared at the lower end of the decibel scale and those compared at the higher end were clarified by the work of Tonndorf (145). These throw light on the implications of increasing noise at the higher noise levels for producing injury to the ear. To examine these differences, it is necessary to state the equation for the sound pressure level (SPL), which is the measure commonly used in comparing different noise levels as they affect the ear:

$$\text{SPL (in decibels)} = 20 \times \log_{10} \frac{\text{existing sound pressure } p}{\text{reference sound pressure } p_o}$$

All decibel (db) notations are in reference to 0.0002 dynes per square centimeter.

If one chooses the SPL of a quiet office, say, 60 db, and that of a quiet residential area, say, 40 db, it appears that there is a difference of 20 db. The actual difference in pressure can be calculated as follows:

$$(1)\ \ 40 = 20 \log_{10} \frac{p_{40} \text{ db}}{0.0002 \text{ dynes/cm}^2}$$

$$2 = \log_{10} \frac{p_{40} \text{ db}}{0.0002 \text{ dynes/cm}^2}; \text{ or } 10^2 = \frac{p_{40} \text{ db}}{0.0002 \text{ dynes/cm}^2}$$

$$p_{40} \text{ db} = 10^2 \times 2 \times 10^{-4} \text{ dynes/cm}^2 \text{ or } 0.02 \text{ dynes/cm}^2$$

$$(2) \quad 60 = 20 \log_{10} \frac{p_{60} \text{ db}}{0.0002 \text{ dynes/cm}^2}$$

Similarly,

$$p_{60} \text{ db} = 10^3 \times 2 \times 10^{-4} \text{ dynes/cm}^2 \text{ or } 0.2 \text{ dynes/cm}^2$$

Note that the ratio of $\dfrac{p_{60} \text{ db}}{p_{40} \text{ db}} = \dfrac{0.2}{0.02}$ or 10:1; but that the actual pressure difference is 0.18 dynes/cm². 

At about 60 ft. in front of a 10,000- to 12,000-lb. thrust engine operating at full power (dry), the broad-spectrum (over-all) exposure is about 120 db. Moving from this position to that of a trim mechanic standing directly beneath the engine increases the over-all exposure to about 140 db. It is possible to calculate the pressure ratios and differences of these different engine SPL's in the same manner as above:

$$(3) \quad 120 = 20 \log_{10} \frac{p_{120} \text{ db}}{0.0002 \text{ dynes/cm}^2}; \ p_{120} \text{ db} = 200 \text{ dynes/cm}^2$$

$$(4) \quad 140 = 20 \log_{10} \frac{p_{140} \text{ db}}{0.0002 \text{ dynes/cm}^2}; \ p_{140} \text{ db} = 2,000 \text{ dynes/cm}^2$$

Note that here the *ratio* of the pressures is still 10:1, but that now the pressure *difference* is 1,800 dynes/cm² instead of only 0.18 dynes/cm². Thus, in going from 120 db to 140 db, the compressive and decompressive force to which the ear is exposed is more than 1,800 times greater than experienced in going from 40 to 60 db. Carrying the illustration further, to go from 140 db to 160 db entails a pressure increase of 18,000 dynes/cm².

This pressure increase of 18,000 dynes/cm² has immediate and serious consequences, since it is in this range that rupture of the tympanic membrane can occur. Even short exposures at this SPL range can result in some permanent hearing loss.

Jet-engine sound pressure levels currently are great enough to create disruptive forces in the ear. These forces can result in rupture of the tympanic membrane without other trauma to the hearing apparatus, in dislocation of the ossicles, in partial or complete destruction of the hearing organ, or in a combination of these. In contrast to these acute effects of a single exposure, the prolonged action of lower levels of sound energy can, without injury to other structures of the ear, cause increasing degeneration of the special cochlear cells concerned with sound detection and so lead to gradual hearing loss.

**Sources of Noise Associated with Jet Aircraft.** Noise levels of considerable magnitude attend the manufacture, testing, maintenance, and operational flight of jet aircraft. Because of the number of people involved and their more or less continuous noise exposure, the industrial physician is more concerned with the manufacturing phases than with those of the test, maintenance, and flight. Conversely, in most instances the manufacturing phase is of lesser consequence to the medical personnel of the airlines and the Armed Services. Their concern is with maintenance and operational noise. On the ground the important sources of noise in jet aircraft are from the jet engine and accessories such as ground-power and starting carts. In the air both aerodynamic and engine noises may be of consequence.

Accessory power plants on the ground are tending more and more to use the gas-turbine engine as the power source. Unshielded, these sources can produce noise exposures hazardous to the human ear. The noise produced lies in a relatively narrow band of frequencies and is high-pitched. The same comment applies to noise produced during ground testing of power packs permanently mounted in jet aircraft.

From the standpoint of maintenance, there are two types of noise produced by jet engines. One is a high-pitched, almost pure-tone whine developed by the compressors at idle power. This noise is projected chiefly ahead of the engine. At this power the jet gases issuing from the afterend of the engine cause relatively little noise. At full power the turbine whine increases in pitch and tends to be drowned out (masked) by the high-frequency noise of the total noise spectrum developed by the jet itself. The noise issuing from the jet stream is produced by turbulence at the boundary between the jet gases and the surrounding air (142). The frequencies produced vary from subsonic to ultrasonic. The maximum noise is produced along an angle of about 45 degrees away from the jet-exhaust axis to either side of the engine. At equal distances from the engine, it is found that noise intensities drop as one proceeds forward from this position. Small increases in noise levels attend the use of water injection, and large increases accompany the use of afterburners in the operation of jet engines.

In flight very little engine noise is transmitted to the cabin, except to the rear of the aircraft, in those with wing-mounted jet engines. In flight at cruising speed, suppressors reduce engine noise to levels below those of the aerodynamic noise of jet airliners, so that at such speeds cabin-sound levels are those produced only by the turbulence of the air next to the "skin" of the aircraft. In multiengine aircraft without noise suppressors, noise in the aftercabin can be high enough to warrant the wearing of ear protectors in the event of flights of several hours' duration. In certain multijet craft rearward mounting of the engines prevents engine-noise transmission to the cabin in flight.

**Protective Measures: General.** The method of noise attenuation most appealing to the industrial physician is that of reducing the noise level at its source. Carried far enough, this method avoids the many difficulties attendant on other measures. Unfortunately, it is not often possible because of expense or other obstacles. This approach includes both treatment and isolation of the source. An example of the former is the use of noise suppressors on an engine; the latter principle is used in housings developed for testing engines apart from the aircraft or during test or maintenance operations on small, easily handled jet aircraft. The solution is not practical for large, multijet planes.

Noise transmission to the broader environment can be combated in part by acoustic treatment of the surroundings. Such a method is not protective of persons immediately exposed to the source but does reduce the exposure of persons in the area. For example, a riveter would not be shielded from the noise of his own rivet gun but would be subjected to a lessened amplitude of noise developed by guns in the general area. Out-of-doors use of blast fences for jet engines, plantings of trees and shrubs, and placement of buildings may be helpful in reducing the directional high frequencies but accomplish little reduction of low-frequency noise energy. Cost and obstacles to utilization limit these approaches on land, and such methods are out of the question at sea.

Protective measures directed at the individual are his isolation by complete enclosure, removal from the source, limitation of exposure time, and use of personal protective devices. Each of these may have significant obstacles to its use.

**Reduction of Noise at the Source.** The source largely determines the means by which noise reduction is possible. When riveting cannot be replaced by welding, damping of the riveted material or the rivet gun may appear attractive; but too often it interferes with access to the work, increases work time, or offers too small attenuations. Riveting at ultrasonic speeds appears advantageous and reduces riveting noise to little more than a moderate hissing sound but so far is limited to soft rivets. Present transducers are incapable of transmitting sufficient energy for deforming the hard rivets used in aircraft manufacture.

In source reduction of noise on aircraft engines, the total energy available for engine thrust must not be decreased significantly or there will be penalties on range, fuel cost, and safety if the suppressive device is to be operative in flight. This consideration places a significant limit to the amount of attenuation to be achieved by such devices.

Experimentally, attenuations of more than 25 db in parts of the jet-noise spectrum have been developed by detachable suppressors for use during ground engine runs. Practical limitations are those of cost, size, time consumed in attachment and detachment, and the like.

**Isolation of the Individual.** It has been possible to construct portable observation booths useful in gun-turret test firing and capable of more than 35-db attenuation at the peak impact over-all sound pressure levels produced by the guns. Combined with the use of ear inserts and muffs, these booths have provided adequate protection for observers in impulse sound pressure levels produced by gunfire of about 170 db.

Such test firing is ordinarily restricted to short bursts and the total firing is limited, but this method of combined protection would seem applicable against sound pressure levels produced by future jet engines were it not for the lack of mobility imposed on the protected person. Nevertheless, some such approach has seemed attractive in relation both to the difficulties in communication between exposed persons and to the hazard to hearing. Acoustic "armor" has been tested as a substitute for an isolation booth and deserves further study in prospect of increasing engine noise, especially for flight operations aboard ship.

**Removal of Personnel from the Source.** One would not ordinarily consider removing a Marine from his rifle as a means of hearing conservation. Certain operations do permit remote control by an operator, however, and jet-engine testing is one of these, if the necessary provisions are made.

Exposure of personnel wearing hearing protection against jet-engine noise below the levels involving risk of hearing loss may occur and may be accompanied by irritability and fatigue. For this reason and because engines of increasing power were to be expected, the writer several years ago advised the development of a device for the remote control of engine trimming. The device, called a "remote-trim actuator," permitted engines to be trimmed from the cockpit or from special housing and effectively removed the mechanic from direct exposure to the engines. Mechanics noted a definite lessening of fatigue.

Each new engine model, however, resulted in relocation of trim screws, and previously developed actuators were of no use in these models. It became difficult and then impractical to build continuously new models of the actuator, and it was necessary to return to manual trimming at the engine.

Exposure to present J-57 engines, even with their increase in thrust from 10,000 to 13,500 lbs., does not appear to offer a significant increase in risk of hearing loss with available safety practices. However, with engines now available or under development in the 25,000- to 30,000-lb. thrust class, it would appear that engine manufacturers must assume the responsibility of providing remote-control trimming. The danger to personnel at these higher energies will become acute; yet, unless anticipatory action is taken to remove men from the engine, some will surely be forced to expose themselves.

Too many responsible persons in the aviation industry have taken the attitude that research on prevention of hazardous noise exposure is not their concern. However, the responsibility for such research must be assumed if only because the aviation industry creates technical conditions which outstrip present knowledge of biological parameters or known preventives and is the first to expose humans to these hazards.

**Limitation of Exposure.** Limitation of exposure may be accomplished by controlling the time during which a noisy operation is carried out or by arbitrarily reducing the individual's time in the noise field.

Before jumping to conclusions in regard to either possibility, a thorough study of the operation producing the noise is advisable. In view of the fact that recovery time is necessary to the ear exposed to noise, it is particularly important to determine whether or not it is possible to perform the noisy part of an operation in less time. For example, a hard-faced rivet gun may be found to require only half the number of blows, as compared with a soft-faced gun, to deform a rivet head. Riveting exposure with such a gun could be reduced and recovery time increased if the operation is not one of continuous riveting.

In one situation thorough study of jet-engine test runs revealed that the time of runs could be reduced by 50 per cent, permitting a significant reduction in personnel exposure and in cost as well.

Reduction of time in a high-noise-level field may be impossible without duplication of personnel or rotation of persons skilled in a non-noisy task as well as in the noisy operation. In practice the reverse situation may be the case, and overexposure of a crew may result because of lack of personnel skilled in the noisy operation.

Proper discipline is necessary to limit the exposure of persons not truly necessary to the operation.

**Hearing-Protection Devices.** Even when reducing the noise at its source or removing the individual from the source may not be possible, personal hearing-protection devices such as earplugs and muffs can permit varying degrees of attenuation. The limitation of this attenuation by bodily tissue transmission of noise in very high-noise levels was mentioned above, but this is minor in comparison with other factors that limit the theoretically attainable attenuation in the practical use of earplugs and muffs. In the first place, employees customarily adjust the devices for comfort, not protection. They may even cut off the inner ends of the inserts so as to fool a superior or drill holes through them in order to hear conversation better in between bursts of noise. They trade plugs until they find some more comfortable than those so carefully fitted in the dispensary. If they detect any leniency of superiors toward wearing hearing protection, they often keep the plugs in their pockets.

The industrial physician and the safety engineer will recognize immediately that the issues involved in providing a workable hearing-conservation program are exactly those of protecting workers against any hazardous environment. An effective program requires continual educational efforts as well as the imposition of unequivocal regulations and discipline in their enforcement. The institution of a poorly conceived, vacillating, and unenforced program is worse than none at all, for it encourages inattention to, and violation of, all safety programs in an industry.

Muffs may provide problems similar to those of ear inserts because of head shape and comfort factors. Sweating occurs readily under the devices that give the best seal to the head; spring pressure may cause discomfort, or there may be imperfect sealing of the cup to the head.

In short, the manner in which the devices customarily are worn may give less than one-quarter of the best attenuation, as measured in the laboratory for the frequencies below 2,000 cycles per second (cps). Mutilation of the devices may result in no attenuation. It is for these reasons that other measures of protection must be given serious consideration.

Helmets developed for hearing conservation that have been examined in the laboratory show no more noise attenuation than the average muff, but mechanics who prefer the helmets refer to a lessening of fatigue when they are worn during jet-engine exposure. It is possible that enclosure of the head may reduce the total energy absorption by the head or prevent resonant frequencies from reaching the head and so be associated with the experience noted. Certain unsympathetic persons have dismissed this argument in favor of one which states that with a helmet the mechanic thinks he looks like a jet jockey.

High-pitched noises are absorbed or damped much more readily than low-pitched noises. Almost any hearing-protection device available will exhibit two to three times as much noise-attenuating capability for frequencies above 2,000 cps as for sounds below that level. The employee who wears earplugs may be well protected against the higher frequencies of the broad jet-engine noise spectrum but poorly shielded against the low frequencies. Thus, the present method of engine-noise suppression may benefit the mechanic through the attenuation accompanied by a shift in the noise spectrum toward the higher frequencies as well as by total reduction of the noise level.

**Criteria for Limitation of Exposure.** Exposure has been mentioned without specific reference to time or severity. Methods of relating these factors have been attempted (137, 143, 146). The first of these references seeks to establish "damage risk criteria" for the unprotected ear for continuous exposure during the eight-hour-day, five-day-week working lifetime. In essence it states that, for exposure to wide-band noise in the energy levels above the 75- to 150-cps octave, the SPL of each octave band should not exceed about 95 db. Somewhat higher SPL's would be permitted at the lower frequencies. For narrow-band or pure-tone noise such as is encountered in planers and other high-speed rotating gear, levels of about 85 db would be the limit beyond which a lifetime of exposure of 40 hours per week could possibly cause some hearing loss.

These criteria, as misinterpreted by some workmen's compensation board personnel and otologists, have been thought to refer to *over-all* noise levels. As a result it has been argued that exposure to an over-all SPL of wide-band noise at 95 db is sufficient to cause hearing loss. The criteria have also been misapplied to short-range exposures in contradiction to their intent. The criteria are helpful to those concerned with determining the existence of a possible hazard to hearing but are not applicable to the medicolegal situations arising from industrial noise exposures except in the relatively uncommon circumstance of continuous exposure.

Eldred, Cannon, and Von Gierke (137) recommended criteria for short exposures to jet-engine noise with and without protective devices in use. Using the damage-risk criteria referred to above for eight hours of daily exposure, they stated that for shorter exposure times the permissible SPL exposure can increase 3 db for each halving of the exposure time for the unprotected ear.

Such criteria are not known to be applicable to impulse noise such as produced by riveting, drop-hammer operation, and gunfire. In other words, it may be that impulse peak levels cannot safely be integrated with the associated lower levels as a means of assessing the hazard to the hearing organ but must be considered by themselves. Further investigation is needed before exposure criteria for impulse noise can be formulated.

In practice, when dealing with exposures about 130 db (over-all), regardless of what personal hearing-protection devices are worn, it is advisable to conduct time-of-exposure studies. These should be correlated with audiometric tests performed before and after exposure of the subject employees, so as to detect possible temporary threshold shift (decrease in hearing acuity), its degree, and the period required for recovery. Usually, a temporary threshold shift exhibits a two-thirds recovery within 30 minutes and almost complete recovery within the first 16 to 24 hours following exposure.

Marked shift or prolonged recovery time may reveal inadequate protection or unusual susceptibility to hearing loss. Fortunately, the "tin ear" is not common. The noise-susceptible individual who suffers rapid and permanent hearing loss within a noise environment hazardous to his fellow workers only after years of exposure exists possibly in the ratio of no more than 1:10,000.

At any rate, no criteria can presently be recommended as substitutes for audiometric monitoring of exposed personnel.

**The Future.** Engines are now available or under development that can produce thrusts of from 25,000 to 30,000 lbs. Along with this power there will be produced increased noise levels. It can be calculated that, depending on certain factors, exposures considerably in excess of 160 db are possible in those positions near the engine that are now occupied by trim mechanics, fire-bottle operators, and other personnel. Such sound pressure levels exceed human tolerance, no matter what protective equipment is worn. Remote control of fire hazard and engine trimming will be required for unsuppressed and possibly even for suppressed engine operation on the ground.

Suppressors for in-flight use on these advanced engines will probably not achieve attenuations important to maintenance personnel exposed on the ground. Voice communication for such personnel, at borderline intelligibility with some present engines, may become impossible. Non-auditory effects become increasingly of concern above 150 db.

The turbofan engine may help to relieve the problem of increasing noise with increasing engine power. Such an engine moves a greater mass of gas at less velocity, achieving greater thrust with less noise because of the fact that noise in the jet is a function of its velocity, varying approximately as the eighth power.

It is possible, then, to expect noise reduction in such engines, but it is unlikely that considerable net reduction will be accomplished. The air-transportation industry would be interested in the use of the full power of the turbofan engine unhampered by noise suppressors. Its greater power should permit more rapid climb-out, thus reducing the time of noise exposure to communities.

A further matter, primarily one of public relations but one that could seriously affect airline operational practices, is that of sonic boom (141, 144, 147). This phenomenon is a percussive effect of shock waves propagated from various surfaces of aircraft traveling at speeds above that of sound. At ground level the pressures exerted by these waves are a complex function of aircraft speed, size, shape, distance from the ground, air pressure at flight altitude and at ground level, and meteorological and other factors.

There is no simple relationship between distance and attenuation of the shock wave. It is known that aircraft flying supersonically at altitudes of from 60,000 to 80,000 ft. can produce a significant change of pressure on the ground, significant in that it could rattle windows and startle the unwary or uninformed.

National Aeronautics and Space Agency observers have indicated that pressures above 1 lb/sq ft can be objectionable. Just what criterion was used for the objection was not stated. Presumably, as has been noted following the introduction of jet operations, the initial reaction of the population subsides quickly as experience with the related noise increases. Youngsters and an increasing number of adults quickly learn to identify and discount sonic booms in areas of present high-altitude supersonic military operations.

Low-altitude supersonic flight can produce shock waves capable of breaking windows and causing structural damage to light frame construction. Flight patterns may have to be arranged so as to avoid low-altitude supersonic effects, but restricting low-altitude operations could be very costly of fuel.

At present there seems to be no design solution to the sonic boom. Community reaction to engines of increasing power will be interesting to watch. Without preplanning, the noise barrier may be more important to the aviation industry than the heat barrier.

## Human Factors in the Control of Aircraft

Sometime ago an aeronautical engineer watched his nine-year-old son folding paper airplanes and casting them into erratic and disastrous flight. With that "papa knows best" approach, he folded a plane, stuck pins about for weight balance, tore and folded here and there, and came up with a product which flew straight and level. Turned over to the young pilot, the expertly designed craft soon met the same fate as the others. It had experienced the introduction of the human equation at the operational level.

No one would think of turning over a jet aircraft to a youngster of nine, but it would be nice to know what are the characteristics of the person to be placed in control.

.

**The Basic Material.** Each individual inherits not only characteristics obviously different morphologically but a functionally unique organism in which is hidden myriad systems of enzymes and hormones, blood and cellular constituents, and neural and other components of variable make-up and efficiency (161). In addition, there are the effects of intrauterine influences which are only now beginning to be appreciated.

Molding this constitutional framework from the moment of birth are the physical and social environments which add immeasurably to the singular nature of the individual. Finally, the organism is subjected to the residual effects of disease and the changes of aging.

The human substrate places a limit on the maximum developmental possibilities of the organism, but throughout the life of the organism, an interchange between the substrate and the environment is necessary for developing and maintaining the integrity of the organism.

**The Nervous System—Some Considerations.** The neural substrate carries with it a certain structured reactivity common to living material in general and to higher forms more specifically, but the dynamics of the human substrate are such that an enormous matrix of unstructured "form" resides within the nervous system.

Incoming stimuli are transmitted to the central nervous system. These stimuli evoke ancient structured responses such as reflex withdrawal from a painful contact. At the same time, however, the brain receives an impression that goes far beyond the simple perception of pain. Stimuli proceeding from the environment through the other sensory systems are associated with the pain, and the entire series of events occurring in the nervous system within a certain temporal span surrounding the painful stimulus is impressed to greater or lesser degree on the hitherto unstructured matrix in the young organism.

It is the peculiar essence of the nervous system that it reacts to a repeated stimulus or sequence of stimuli in a manner such that the associated series of events in the system assumes a structure or pattern. This pattern contains both stimuli and response and, through later events having superficially only a remote association with the original sequence, can be triggered to produce the entire original response and its associated physical and emotional reactions. In other words, some of the neural elements in the brain that are part of one structured response may be a part of another, so that either or both of the reactions of the overlapping matrices may be brought into play by a stimulus common to both.

The temporal span referred to above is in itself extremely complex in extent. For example, the burned child perceives not only the hot object responsible for his pain but also the sympathy or lack of it expressed by the parent, the trip to the doctor's office and its ramifications, the limitation on his play, the taunts of his playmates, and so on.

The nervous system thus has the capacity to take in a very large number of sequential data which become structured according to the importance to the organism of the data. This importance in turn is determined by the innate structure and the imposed structure.

It would seem logical to assume that confusion or, in terms of neural activity, blocking of an established pattern could arise out of disordered or conflicting stimuli originating either within or without the nervous system. The organism, impelled to respond in opposing directions, is immobilized, vacillates, or is driven in one direction by the more firmly established reaction pattern. In some manner the neurochemical and hormonal mechanisms may likewise be disturbed in such instances as well as in strong or repeated traumatic experiences of other types. In these situations the response may have no direction in the ordinary sense but consists of a state commonly referred to as anxiety.

As the basic neural matrix resolves itself into a vast complex of submatrices, interlocking, overlapping, opposing, complementary, and supplementary, a supermatrix evolves out of which arises a reaction of the entire organism to the whole environment. It is this intrinsic state that determines how the world is perceived, that determines "why one individual sees the doughnut and another the hole," as the saying goes.

Anxiety in its chronic form is thus a dramatic aspect of this total state, or set, as it has become known, but it is also associated with a tendency of the "anxious" nervous system to overreact to all stimuli.

Over all this function the human *cortex* imposes a capacity to anticipate events far beyond the anticipations imposed by the set of the organism. Insofar as the activity of the cortex is dissociated from neural patterns having an emotional tone, it may be purposeful and productive. But if cortical function activates neurons that lie within such patterns, the new activity may elicit or come to have emotional coloring. Conversely, the highest cortical function can act to reduce emotional context.

The anatomical and physiological foundations for these functional structures are being elucidated at an increasingly rapid rate (149). We are told that the *midbrain* of man is essentially the most advanced part phylogenetically and that it is also the most advanced part of lower forms now living. It becomes increasingly overshadowed in higher forms by the development of the cortex.

The midbrain and other structures within its immediate vicinity are important to the neural reactions that, by projection to the highest levels of the cortex, are experienced as emotion. These structures form a functional system that has been called the *mesodiencephalic activating system* (MAS) and that gives emotional tone to certain kinds of stimuli arising both outside and inside the body (153, 160). The cortex modifies the general tone of the emotion by its memory of past events (160).

Each of the primary sensory systems (pain, touch, etc.) responds to only one type of stimulus and when stimulated conducts its messages rapidly and directly to a specific receptor region in the cortex. In contrast, the MAS responds to all the sensory systems (150). It also receives inputs from the cortex. It is capable of increasing or decreasing the strength of the signals received before passing them on as well as modifying the signals by imposition of other intrinsic signals.

It would appear that the midbrain acts as a superswitchboard operator who ordinarily determines what shall get through to "Mr. Big" (the cortex) but who can be cut in on by Mr. B who also has private lines to the sensory organs. It is as if, in most circumstances, the midbrain takes a quick look at many of the incoming signals and modifies them or cuts them off if they are not important. Otherwise, the cortex would be overwhelmed by all the messages that impinge on man's senses.

The midbrain is not the sole determinant in distinguishing the importance of stimuli to a particular individual. Neurosurgery and psychopharmacology are beginning to push aside some of the mystery associated with the sensation of pain as apart from the emotional context of pain. It is possible for drugs to suppress the latter (for example, depression and dread), while not interrupting the pathways by which the brain experiences the pain itself. On the other hand, surgery of the brain can actually stop pain but fails to remove the emotional impact of the condition having caused the pain, for example, the knowledge that the victim has cancer.

Electrical stimuli from electrodes placed in the brains of humans have substituted for sensory or intrinsic neural activity in producing inhibition or intensification of reaction. The MAS is known to modify incoming signals in either direction, depending on the strength of the new neuronal activity aroused by associated inputs. This selective capability must be considered a function of the entire central nervous system, however, not of one portion alone.

From these and other considerations one investigator postulated that the cortex can, through recollection of past painful stimuli, further activate the lower brain structures which in turn "feed back" intense signals of high emotional context and so interfere with the higher faculties of the cortex, such as judgment (160, p. 2).

In addition, the ability of the cortex to anticipate the future can similarly act upon the lower brain. For example, the naval aviator who, only a few minutes before, was blasting the smokestacks of an enemy vessel with carefree abandon may become a serious, calculating, and troubled airman on learning of the arrival of his first-born. An inhibiting factor—a new responsibility—becomes stamped within his brain to throw out neural signals interfering with the finely co-ordinated patterns of reaction already developed. Here nothing was changed in the external environment.

Similarly, intrinsic initiation of neural signals can occur by other means. A recurring dream related by a patient may be illustrative:

> The dream began with his lying on a thick rug by the fireside of his childhood home. He would then hear the purring of his old gray cat and see it stretched in front of the fire. As he reached out his hand to stroke the cat, the animal was no longer a cat—it was a lion. At this point the patient would awaken in the midst of a violent reaction. He would be bolt upright in bed with a constriction in his throat, a dry mouth, profuse perspiration, the hair on his neck prickling, a cry strangled in his throat, and his arms sharply withdrawn against his chest.

The recollection of the soft purr, the visualization of his pet, and the neural associations or memories aroused by these stimuli were sufficient to facilitate neural reaction patterns resulting in the outstretched hand and the relaxing emotional response associated with home, Tabby, and fireside. On the other hand, the visual impact of the lion, whether originating in the retina or in the visual memory, and the neuronal activity arising out of the brain's interpretation of "lion" combined to pour a flood of impulses into the response-control systems of the brain, inhibiting the initial reaction and inducing withdrawal and fear reactions.

The figure of a lion is perhaps unfortunate as an example in that it is universally associated with danger. How does one account for variations among humans in response to a task such as flying? On the one hand, there is the farm boy who reacts to a dangerous combat flying assignment as if it were just one more of the chores. On the other hand, there is the superb athlete of near-genius who vomits before even routine flights, in the absence of prior flying emergencies or other direct threats associated with flying.

It is clear that in the latter case the developing neural patterns have associated flying and danger to a degree that aroused abnormally intense emotional reaction. In other words, the past experience of the nervous system had led to a certain "set" or a state of expectation which gave its own unique interpretation of the stimulus provided by the flying task (151, p. 1273).

Far more numerous are the subtler reactions controlled by less dramatic events in the nervous system. These can be more difficult to evaluate or predict, because they are more readily influenced by other phenomena and hence can be ambiguous as to direction.

**Development of the Material.** Reposing in the basic material is only a *promise* for the individual's ultimate capacity to respond to the environment. The experiences of the individual as he probes the environment or as the environment forces itself upon him create the perceptual state referred to above. The picture thus obtained may constitute a challenge or a threat and lead to participation or to withdrawal.

A positive response, however, may be concentrated or diffuse. A crude illustration of this might be the response leading on the one hand to the development of an instrumental virtuoso and on the other to the conductor of a symphony. In the latter instance there is the achievement of an encompassing intellectual integration, in the former one of predominantly neuromuscular integration. Such responses may represent the organism's and possibly the species' near-limit of development in one direction.

A positive response does not indicate the degree of achievement. For example, different types of diffuse response can lead to the development of either a symphony conductor, a Jack-of-all-trades, or a dilettante.

The environment, physical or social, can restrict and extend limits to response on the part of the individual: it may contain little to elicit response, it may categorically prohibit response, or it can exceed the individual's capacity to respond. Conversely, it can extend the number and scope of situations within which the individual can probe and either develop effective responses or withdraw.

**Perception, Motivation, and Response: Some Physiological and Psychological Aspects.** A challenge or task imposed by the environment is modified perceptually by the individual. It is analyzed in respect to the value it has to the person in satisfying a need. It is not necessary that this need be recognized by anyone as being real. It may be as pragmatic as climbing a hill to obtain the other side or as immaterial as climbing a mountain because it is there.

Perception, then, is seen to be important to motivation. Motivation may be equally immaterial and yet result in an achievement which, expressed in terms of human capacities, sets a very high standard of accomplishment.

Any task, pragmatic or otherwise, that becomes defined in terms approaching the species limitations restricts the fraternity to which the task is accessible, no matter what the motivation. This fact may have little consequence in flagpole sitting or pie-eating contests, but it assumes wide importance if it deals with the abilities of a nation's scientists or its pilots. It has certain implications to be discussed.

A little circumspection will reveal that tasks must be defined in terms of the persons capable of accomplishing them as well as of the underlying attributes which provide the ability. With very few exceptions formal definitions have not even been attempted and then only in a very general way. The reasons are manifold. The number and complexity of the basic variables involved in the accomplishment of a task already have been indicated.

It would appear that definition is possible only by retrospect, that is, by noting the characteristics of the persons capable of doing a job and finding out how they got that way. It is not enough to know that four-minute milers have a certain minute respiratory volume and cardiac output and can stand so much oxygen debt. It is just as necessary to know that for years they have run twenty-five miles a day, run up sand dunes fifty times a day, don't smoke, and maybe put pepper on their ice cream. (All this still tells us nothing about why they want to run a mile even in ten minutes.) Short of motivation, however, defining the requirements for running the four-minute mile is simple compared to defining the task of flying (and immediately one wants to know, flying what?).

Over the years large numbers of persons have gravitated to aviation, having convinced themselves they wanted to fly. Since flight training costs money, the pull was toward the Armed Services. The Services spent millions of dollars examining student and combat pilots in order to discover what it took to fly. As a result it was reported that the basic ability to fly can be predicted by test with over 80 per cent reliability. Basic ability to fly may mean flying a "Yellow Peril" and landing it at 35 knots. This is not quite the same thing as playing tag with the enemy at 60,000 ft. and coming in at 135 knots nor coming in on an instrument-landing approach with 150 passengers aboard.

As the task complexity increases, new standards of accomplishment are imposed. Again, evaluation of the individual's ability to meet these standards must be retrospective in the same sense as before. Unfortunately, the behavioral sciences do not seem to offer much hope of avoiding this approach. They can assist in two directions, namely, by saying something about empirical requirements and by helping simplify a task, but other factors beyond their scope (in the narrow sense) also impose significant limitations on the individual's capacity to develop and respond.

The nervous system's reactions are governed not alone by the system's own structural make-up. They are also under the influence of other body mechanisms, functional and pathological. These are on the whole of undramatic nature in the ordinary course of events and readily overshadowed, but they are nonetheless important and perhaps decisive at critical points in the total response of the organism.

Response is affected by the metabolic state and hence by all the factors entering into metabolism, including the so-called physiological rhythms and cycles (155-159), diet, activity, and humoral mechanisms. It is further modified by disease and abnormal functional states, including those occasioned by aging.

Behavioral studies, unsophisticated as they are at the present state of development, tend to ignore such factors almost of necessity (154, p. 62). They are concerned with developing empirical means of measuring responses and cannot yet be expected to be constructed on the basis of controlling factors such as the above. In fact, it may be difficult or even impossible to isolate these latter influences. By considering their number, direction, interrelationship, and the effect of attempts at control, they may provide a problem equivalent to that arising from the uncertainty principle of Heisenberg. Consequently, the outlook is largely for the continuing development of statistical generalizations not too reliable for application to the individual human being.

Response studies demonstrate that the nervous system can fail to respond because of an overload of stimuli or through the failure to observe infrequent stimuli.

The capacity of the human nervous system to distinguish disparate stimuli is excellent. In this, however, it depends on a certain complexity and order or sequence in the incoming signals. The ability to recognize a single voice among hundreds of others is illustrative. The highly complex and ordered series of events that make up the quality of the particular voice have been associated with the mental picture of the owner. The entire complex is stored in the brain in such a way as to permit its differentiation from other voice-owner complexes.

On the other hand, one telephone bell may sound like any other. Three telephones each with the same type of bell placed side by side could hardly be distinguished as to an incoming call. Separating the bells would provide two extra dimensions for differentiation, namely, directional and amplitudinal components of the sound, but background noise or position of the listener in the room could cause failure to identify the source. By changing one bell to a buzzer and a second to a gong, the three signals could much more easily be distinguished even if kept together spatially. More than two added dimensions are available here. The entire complex of each sound, in particular the timbre as well as amplitude and pitch, provides a readily differentiated pattern.

**Monitoring.** The foregoing fact may be lost sight of in the design of systems that are supposed to alert a monitor to infrequent signals. Without regard for other psychophysiological aspects of "vigilance" or "alertness," it becomes apparent that in a complex field the fewer the distinctive components of an incoming signal, the more liable the monitor is to fail to identify it or place it in its proper context. And, since the human being is a multisensory organism and depends on multiple inputs for orientation and recognition, the complexity and order of any stimulus are important to its recognition. Unistimulatory devices used as warning signals may make recognition difficult, and confusion results. If bells or horns of a single tone and amplitude or lights of single shape and color serve to warn of different kinds of trouble, the neural responses of the monitor are burdened by the additional task of determining the source. In an urgent situation the delay of recognition sets up psychic and hormonal stresses that disrupt neuromuscular response mechanisms.

Applied to monitoring, this approach would require that attention be given to the make-up of the monitored signal so that it can be made sufficiently complex and ordered to permit identification with minimal training and reinforcement.

The use of frequent artificial signals as a means of maintaining vigilance for infrequent real signals has been proposed (154). Such a suggestion could apply only to simple individual tasks and not to one that is merely a part of a much broader complex of tasks such as flying. The use of artificial signals in this manner would seem to pose the secondary problem of "Wolf! Wolf!" and to add a multiplicity of sensory inputs that could overwhelm the monitor. Monitoring of infrequent events in flying would appear to be more susceptible of treatment by making the infrequent signal more reliably recognized and identified.

The discrimination of individual signals is only one aspect of the stimulus-response mechanism. The integration of the signals leading to a response is the more demanding one, especially in the temporal sense, and can be disturbed readily. Various mechanisms can serve to disrupt even a well-established stimulus-response pattern. An illustration from the juggler's art is perhaps helpful in indicating how neural overload may be brought about.

Assume that a juggler has learned to handle up to six balls with high reliability. If a seventh ball were suddenly introduced, one could predict a serious impairment or loss of control, although through practice the juggler might learn to have the seventh ball introduced with greater and greater reliability of response.

A loud noise or other unexpected extraneous sensory stimulus also could disturb control of the six-ball cycle.

If the juggler were required only to respond to an unexpected introduction of a third ball into a two-ball cycle, his reliability of response should be greater, because his nervous system is monitoring and controlling fewer items and has greater leeway in time. However, if the third item is introduced in association with an added sensory stimulus, the reliability of response to the dual-load factor may be no better than that of the addition of the seventh ball to the more complex six-ball cycle, a single-load factor.

In these illustrations two types of interfering stimuli have been considered. One is that of a familiar object out of sequence in an established pattern. The other is a stimulus foreign to the pattern and capable of calling forth a natural reflex occurring involuntarily. In an airplane an electrical-system malfunction could activate a warning device during operation of a complex stimulus-response pattern and cause the response to fail.

Another type of interfering stimulus might be examined. Let us say that our juggler now performs reliably with six red balls and with the introduction into the pattern of a seventh red ball. Without his knowledge let us introduce a peeled tomato in place of the seventh red ball. In the brief scanning period available to the juggler, the tomato is a familiar object—another red ball. His first appreciation of its foreign nature is when the wet, flabby object strikes his hand.

Such a stimulus in sequence may have as great a disruptive influence on response as the introduction of a familiar item out of sequence. The first recognition of the foreign nature of the seventh object comes too late for adequate response and sets up interfering or inhibiting neural stimuli.

In part the tomato is seen as a red ball, because the juggler expects to see a ball. Had he been forewarned, he would have augmented his differentiating capacity by requiring more visual dimensions to be satisfied before accepting any of the objects as a red ball. He would more critically examine for shape, sheen, surface markings, and the like, and his cortical centers with the new "set" and early recognition would act to override the tactile sensory stimuli from the hand which, differing widely between tomato and ball, would otherwise set up interfering signals within the central nervous system.

One could further complicate the task by introducing a red ball made of lead. The juggler would lose the advantage of early visual discrimination, and, forewarned or not, his first recognition would occur as the very heavy object struck his hand. Since his neuro-muscular expectation was not prepared, he would probably drop the lead ball.

Aviators can "drop the ball" under similar circumstances. How critical the circumstance must be depends on the temporal and spatial arrangements as well as the complexity of the entire stimulus-response field. Should the booster mechanism for control systems in aircraft be so designed that booster failure suddenly could cause unexpected demands to be made counter to the pilot's reflex patterns at a critical moment, another accident might mistakenly be ascribed to pilot error.

One cannot demand hypercritical monitoring for a number of reasons. First, the nervous system is so constituted that close attention to a given task will largely exclude attention to others. (See Chap. 4.) In this respect all persons have one-track minds. As demands are made to increase the scope of monitoring, less and less attention can be given to any part of the field, and fewer and fewer dimensions of each part can be examined critically. If each of the parts has high significance, real or emotional, to the observer, a state of anxiety will be set up for the reason that the need to encompass all parts is accomplished with the threatening realization that the examination of each part is inadequate.

The need for training in complex tasks recognizes this fact. As monitoring of, and response to, simple systems are relegated to reflex patterns, the trainee is capable of handling a wider and wider field of tasks, provided nothing acts to disrupt seriously any one of the patterns. The moment that such disruption occurs there is danger that scanning of the rest of the field will be impaired or blotted out with disastrous consequences. Thus, to ask that a pilot give hypercritical attention to one aspect of landing, as might be demanded for exact touch-down on a short field, is to invite neglect of other aspects of landing.

**Physiological Rhythms and Cycles.** Studies of rhythmic variables in animal and human physiology have revealed factors that may affect flight safety. The diurnal nature of the usual human mode of existence carries with it a waxing and waning of metabolic function (155, 157, 158). The associated patterns of rise and fall in temperature, neural excitability, and "efficiency" tend to persist for a time when the day-night cycle is altered artificially or by rapid change of longitude. Individual metabolic differences are apparent both in adjustment to a changing timescale and in the time of day when peak efficiency is reached.

For example, some people are slow starters. Mental and physical activity continues at low ebb for an extended period after waking. Their alertness picks up as the day goes on and may reach a peak in the afternoon or evening. Others develop an early peak and then seem to run down as the day progresses.

Prolonged loss of sleep results in disturbances of behavior, hallucinations, and changes in attitude and personality (148, p. 272). How shorter periods of sleep deprivation might act to further compound illusory sensations such as can be met in flight is not adequately known. Disturbances in the diurnal cycle leading to loss of sleep could possibly act to reinforce illusory sensations.

A non-rhythmic or, in Kleitman's terms, a cyclic variable also is found in the metabolic state during muscular activity and in sedentary situations. Some people show a rather marked drop of metabolism during inactivity, although their metabolic rate during activity is commensurate with that of others. It is as if metabolic fires were banked and required physical activity to stoke them. This would seem to have implications for the degree of alertness or ability to respond to extrinsic stimuli or integrative mental work.

Such variables as the diurnal and active-inactive metabolic states are thus important to airline operations (152). What, for example, are the consequences of placing a man in control of an airplane within a short period following waking or during his lowest diurnal metabolic level regardless of his waking time? What errors in judgment may arise when fatigue factors of prolonged flight coincide with this metabolic nadir? Are these factors sufficiently important to require the determination of individual pilots' metabolic patterns? These are not entirely idle questions in view of the jet airplane's ability to reverse completely the day-night cyle in a single flight.

The development of sophisticated flight simulators gives airlines the capability to study some of these questions in the safety and comparative economy of a ground operation. While it is possible that such factors may be so influenced by still other factors that detailed concern is of little importance, the possibility requires validation.

The effects of cyclic variables in pilot physiology are not the only items needing exploration. Pilot habit patterns, including consumption of coffee, alcohol, drugs, and food, become increasingly important as demands on pilots are complicated by speed, heavier air traffic, and greater passenger loads. In addition, greater information on and attention to food and rest problems at foreign destinations are required.

**External Factors in the Control of Aircraft.** Thus far the discussion has dealt with intrinsic factors in the control of aircraft. The extrinsic factors in the aircraft system and the general environment provide the field of external stimuli to which the individual must respond. The complexity of this field, the method, sequence, and speed of its presentation will determine in large degree the effectiveness of the human response.

It has been said that man is a good differentiator but not a good integrator. Even at his most alert and efficient state of response, he is markedly limited in the amount of information he can receive and integrate within a given period of time (151, p. 186). As the time period decreases, which it does with the increasing speeds of aircraft, he approaches the limit of his integrating and reacting capacity. One means of overcoming in part the human limitation is to substitute mechanical or electronic extensions of human senses and muscles. Another is to decrease the complexity of the job.

A fortuitous advantage of the jet aircraft arises out of the jet engine. Its simplicity of operation has permitted elimination of a number of monitoring and control devices necessary to the piston engine. Since the field stimulus complexity is at a maximum in landing and take-off, elimination of a number of devices that must be monitored or controlled at this time favors an increase in the reliability of the pilot's responses.

The fortuitous nature of this simplification is emphasized for the reason that some would believe that aircraft are designed primarily around the human being. Actually, aircraft are designed around performance capabilities and requirements. The pilot might like to land at 35 knots—it's safer—but he'll take 135 and like it if his Mach 2 fighter won't stay in the air under that speed. If the designer, on the other hand, doesn't realize that this landing speed means trouble in the presence of other complicating factors, he will not act to simplify the pilot's over-all task.

Unfortunately, there is a tendency of some designers to select maximum human-performance data for applying human parameters and to design against these without realizing that the human organism is not capable of maximum function in all its systems simultaneously. At the opposite extreme is the apparent desire of some pilots to operate in a zero-stress environment. Neither extreme is conducive to human reliability.

There is the combined requirement, therefore, for an operator, civil or military, to match aircrews and operating conditions against an aircraft system and for an aircraft manufacturer to match aircraft performance and control to a reasonable level of human capability and operational circumstances. Governmental agencies, aircraft operators, and manufacturers are chiefly responsible for protecting the flying public. Once selected, however, the airmen themselves carry a significant burden of this responsibility.

It is obvious that the man-machine concept is a bit too simple to encompass the *human factors* involved in aviation. Reliability must include the extended field of regulatory, operational, and political factors involved in flight. Thus, to limit attention to the man or to the machine as providing the only human factors deserving consideration is to make an absurd simplification.

The design engineer cannot give primary attention to regulatory and operational human factors outside his control. His primary concern is to design for machine reliability, and his secondary goal is to provide monitoring and control devices that singly or in concert do not overburden the aircrew in circumstances reasonable within the basic performance concept. As long as he can adopt controls proved adequate for previous aircraft designs and adapt these with minimum changes to the new design, he is on rather safe ground; the human factors have been worked out through trial and error. When he must provide new control systems, however, he is faced with all the uncertainties of human reaction to strange situations plus whatever new factors have been introduced by the performance capabilities of the aircraft itself. And, insofar as he has not forewarned his colleagues in the biological sciences as to what to expect machine-wise, they may well be at least as much in the dark as he is about what these reactions will be.

The operator, that is, the command or airline that operates aircraft, has the responsibility for choosing competent aircrewmen.

Tests of intelligence, neuromuscular co-ordination, mechanical aptitude, and physical fitness are available and have been shown to be adequate predictors of control of aircraft in the past. Insofar as aircraft systems change, the prediction-test batteries must be re-examined and possibly revised.

In some respects aircrew and, particularly, pilot selection is a negative process to the extent it is based on arbitrary standards whose real importance to the ability to fly have not been demonstrated. As training and experience progress following initial selection, a weeding-out process follows the trainee, and later the pilot, by trial and error. This same trial and error attests to the reliability of the tests.

Unfortunately, the absence of pathology does not guarantee continued good health, nor do the red-lens and depth-perception tests really tell if a man will be able to make a night carrier landing with reasonable consistency. Athletic ability and "physical fitness" do not *assure* an ability to perform the requirements of flying.

Aptitude tests are at best only indirect measures of motivation. And motivation measurement is baffling; an individual's score at any one time may have little relation to the apparent level or direction of motivation on other occasions.

Many psychological tests are used uncritically by persons who should know better, and their results are presently worthless for practical personnel administration. Psychological testing of personality and motivation, in particular, is in its infancy, and applications should be monitored by rigorous experimental studies in the hands of qualified investigators. The reliance of some large companies on unvalidated tests for selection and advancement of personnel is merely an indication of gross ignorance of these facts. In some cases the results are completely dependent on the scorer, whose accuracy of prediction of an acceptable criterion may never have been tested. A number of "objective" tests, scored automatically, have not been shown to have any connection with the demonstrated behavior of the individuals tested.

The Federal government has accepted the responsibility of determining physical standards for civil aircrewmen. The seriousness of this undertaking has unfortunately not been paralleled in the nature and extent of the supporting research necessary to the creation of such standards nor by the separation of the designated professional agency from political pressures. It remains to be seen what the creation of the new Federal Aviation Agency will accomplish in this area.

Finally, the pilots themselves carry a responsibility not always made clear by the actions of their spokesmen in the Airline Pilots Association. Maintenance of efficiency and postponement of aging and its concomitants are the responsibilities of the individual pilot, but the development and dissemination of the knowledge by which he may accomplish this is not.* His union can be effective toward making this possible by statesmanlike action. As the pilots bargain themselves into a position of an economic elite, they can also examine their claims of greater responsibility in the light of what this responsibility means personally. At the least it means maintaining the status of a physiological and psychological elite as well.

These considerations demonstrate the need for a greater coordination of effort in dealing with human factors as the jet age advances, proceeding from aircrew selection through aircraft and component-system design and operation and governmental regulation. While some accomplishment has been made, one is reminded of the story in which the agricultural expert was sent out to teach modern farming techniques. As he explained his program to one marginal operator, the farmer commented, " 'Twon't do no good, mister. I don't farm as good as I know how now!" One suspects that, in the interests of flight safety, we're not operating as well as we know how now.

---

* The great majority of airline pilots are highly responsible men who recognize their need in this regard and seek instruction on how best to accomplish it. An effective program could be contained in a manual on physical and mental fitness. Consultation as necessary should be available to assist the pilot. Inculcation of high self-maintenance standards should begin with the new pilot and be reinforced throughout his career.

# References

## Air Conditioning

1. BEDFORD, T. 1946. *Environmental Warmth and Its Measurement.* (War Memo. No. 17.) Med. Research Council (U.K.), H.M. Stationery Office, London.
2. BEDFORD, T. 1954. Heating and ventilation, requirements and methods. In MEREWETHER, E. R. A. (ed.). *Industrial Hygiene and Medicine.* Butterworth & Co., Ltd., London. Pp. 272–307.
3. BEST, C. H., and TAYLOR, N. B. 1955. *Physiological Basis of Medical Practice.* 6th ed. Williams & Wilkins Co., Baltimore. Pp. 620 ff.
4. BLOCKLEY, W. V., McCUTCHAN, J. W., and TAYLOR, C. L. 1954. *Prediction of Human Tolerance for Heat in Aircraft: A Design Guide.* (WADC Technical Report 53–346.) USAF, Wright-Patterson Air Force Base, Ohio.

5. BROUHA, L. A. 1955. *Protecting the Worker in Hot Environments.* Trans. Ind. Hyg. Foundation, 20th Annual Meeting, Nov. 16–17, 1955. Mellon Institute, Pittsburgh.

6. BUETTNER, K. 1950. Effects of extreme heat on man. *J. Am. Med Assoc. 144:* 732–738.

7. BUETTNER, K. Effects of extreme heat and cold on human skin: I. Analysis of temperature changes caused by different kinds of heat application. *J. Appl. Physiol. 3:* 691–702, 1951; II. Surface temperature, pain and heat conductivity in experiments with radiant heat. *J. Appl. Physiol. 3:* 703–713, 1951; III. Numerical analysis and pilot experiments on penetrating flash radiation effects. *J. Appl. Physiol. 5:* 207–220, 1952.

8. BUETTNER, K. 1953. Thermal stresses in modern aircraft. *Symposium on Frontiers of Man-Controlled Flight.* Inst. Transportation and Traffic Engr., University of California at Los Angeles. Pp. 7–12.

9. CHRENKO, F. A. 1957. The effects of the temperatures of the floor surface and of the air on thermal sensations and the skin temperature of the feet. *Brit. J. Indust. Med. 14:* 13–21.

10. DuBois, E. F. 1951. Physiological aspects of heating and ventilating. *Heating, Piping and Air Conditioning 23:* 134–136.

11. HABER, F. 1952. Adiobatic compression and friction. In WHITE, C. S., and BENSON, O. O., JR. (eds.). *Physics and Medicine of the Upper Atmosphere.* University of New Mexico Press, Albuquerque. Pp. 75–87.

12. HABER, H. 1954. *The Physical Environment of the Flyer.* USAF, Air University, School of Aviation Medicine, Randolph Air Force Base, Tex. Pp. 46, 110, 129–134.

13. HERRINGTON, L. P. 1958. The biotechnical problem of the human body as a heat exchanger. *Trans. Am. Soc. Mech. Engrs. 80:* 343–346.

14. HOUGHTEN, F. C., and YAGOGLOU, C. P. 1923. Determining lines of equal comfort. *Trans. Am. Soc. Heat. Engrs. 29:* 116–163.

15. HUMPHREYS, C. M., IMATIS, O., and GUTBERLET, C. 1946. Physiological responses of subjects exposed to high effective temperatures and elevated mean radiant temperatures. *Heating, Piping and Air Conditioning 18:* 101–106.

16. KELLEY, J. B. 1956. Heat, cold and clothing. *Sci. American 194:* 109–116.

17. LINDES, DEA. 1951. Requirements for protection against thermal hazards of high speed flight. *J. Aviation Med. 22:* 358–364.

18. LLOYD-SMITH, D. L., and MENDELSSOHN, K. 1948. Tolerance limits of radiant heat. *Brit. Med. J. 1:* 975–978.

19. McCUTCHAN, J. W., and TAYLOR, C. L. 1951. Respiratory heat exchange with varying temperature and humidity of inspired air. *J. Appl. Physiol. 4:* 121–135.

20. McCUTCHAN, J. W., and TAYLOR, C. L. 1954. *The Effect of Reduced Pressure upon Evaporation and Perspiration in Nude, Resting Man.* (WADC Technical Report 54–72.) USAF, Wright-Patterson Air Force Base, Ohio.

21. MAYO, A. M. 1952. Basic environmental problems relating man and the aeropause. In WHITE, C. S., and BENSON, O. O., JR. (eds.). *Physics and Medicine of the Upper Atmosphere.* University of New Mexico Press, Albuquerque.

22. MUNRO, A. F., and CHRENKO, F. A. 1948. The effects of air temperature and velocity and of various flooring materials on the thermal sensations and skin temperature of the feet. *J. Hyg.* (Cambridge) *46:* 451–465.

23. MURPHY, A. J., PAUL, W. D., and HINES, H. M. 1950. A comparative study of the temperature changes produced by various thermogenic agents. *Arch. Phys. Med. 31:* 151–156.

24. NEWBURGH, L. H. (ed.). 1949. *Physiology of Heat Regulation and the Science of Clothing.* (Prepared at the request of the Division of Medical Sciences, National Research Council.) W. B. Saunders Co., Philadelphia. P. 457.

25. PASSMORE, R., and DURNIN, J. 1955. Human energy expenditure. *Physiol. Revs. 35:* 801–840.
26. POLLACK, H., CONSOLAZIO, C., and ISAAC, G. J. 1958. Metabolic demands as a factor in weight control. *J. Am. Med. Assoc. 167:* 216–219.
27. QUIMBY, F. H., PHILLIPS, N. E., CAREY, B. B., and MORGAN, R. 1950. Effect of humidity on the change in body temperature during exposures to low atmospheric pressure. *Am. J. Physiol. 161:* 312–315.
28. SEELEY, L. E. 1940. Study of changes in the temperature and water vapor content of respired air in the nasal cavity. *Heating, Piping and Air Conditioning, 12:* 377–388.
29. STILL, E. W. 1957. Air conditioning in aircraft. *J. Roy. Aeronaut. Soc. 61:* 727–755.
30. STILL, E. W. 1957. *Into Thin Air.* Sydenham & Co., Bournemouth, England.
31. TAYLOR, C. L., and BUETTNER, K. 1955. Influence of evaporative forces upon skin temperature dependency of human perspiration. *J. Appl. Physiol. 6:* 113–123.
32. TILLER, P. R., GREIDER, H. R., and GRABIAK, E. 1957. Effects of pilots' tasks on metabolic rates. *J. Aviation Med. 28:* 27–33.
33. VEGHTE, J. H., and WEBB, P. 1957. *Clothing and Tolerance to Heat.* (WADC Technical Report 57–759.) (ASTIA Doc. #AD142248.) USAF, Aero-Medical Laboratory, Wright-Patterson Air Force Base, Ohio.

## Toxicology

34. *Aviation Toxicology.* Committee on Aviation Toxicology, Aero Medical Assoc. The Blakiston Co., New York. 1953.
35. *Liquid Propellant Safety Manual.* Liquid Propellant Information Agency, Silver Spring, Md. 1958. (Prepared under the auspices of Dept. of Defense.)
36. ROBBINS, C. 1958. Some Health Hazards Associated with the Manufacture of Commercial Jet Aircraft. Paper presented before 3rd Annual Meeting of the Pacific Northwest Section, Am. Ind. Hyg. Assoc., Seattle, Sept. 13, 1958.
37. ROUSH, G., JR. 1959. The toxicology of the boranes. *J. Occup. Med. 1:* 46–52.
38. STILL, E. W., 1957. Air conditioning in aircraft. *J. Roy. Aeronaut. Soc. 61:* 727–754.
39. WILKINS, E. W. C. 1958. *Ozone as a Hazard in High Altitude Flying.* (AGARD Report 203.) (Available through the Natl. Adv. Comm. for Aeronautics, 1512 H St., N.W., Washington, D.C.)

## Decompression

40. EKBERG, D. R. 1958. Rapid decompression in aircraft during high speed flight. *J. Aviation Med. 29:* 609–610.
41. FULTON, J. F. 1951. *Decompression Sickness.* W. B. Saunders Co., Philadelphia.
42. GORDON, B. (ed.). 1957. *Clinical Cardiopulmonary Physiology.* Grune & Stratton, Inc., New York.
43. HABER, F. 1950. *On the Physical Process of Explosive Decompression.* Special Report. USAF, Air University, School of Aviation Medicine, Randolph Air Force Base, Tex.
44. HABER, F., and CLAMANN, H. G. 1953. *Physics and Engineering of Rapid Decompression.* (Project No. 21–1201–0008, No. 3.) USAF, Air University, School of Aviation Medicine, Randolph Air Force Base, Tex.
45. KARSTENS, A. I. 1957. Trauma of rapid decompression. *Am. J. Surgery 93:* 741.
46. PASSMORE, R., and DURNIN, J. 1955. Human energy expenditure. *Physiol. Revs. 35:* 801–840.

47. SIMONS, D. G., and ARCHIBALD, E. R. 1958. Selection of sealed cabin atmosphere. *J. Aviation Med.* 29: 350–357.
48. STILL, E. W. 1957. *Into Thin Air.* Sydenham & Co., Bournemouth, England.
49. *Submarine Medicine Practice.* Bureau of Medicine and Surgery, U.S. Navy. Government Printing Office, Washington, D.C. 1956.
50. TILLER, P. R., GREIDER, H. R., and GRABIAK, EDNA. 1957. Effects of pilots' tasks on metabolic rate. *J. Aviation Med.* 28: 27–33.

## Ionizing Radiation

51. BRADT, H. L., and PETERS, B. 1950. The heavy nuclei of the primary cosmic radiation. *Phys. Rev.* 77: 54–70.
52. CHASE, H. B., and POST, J. S. 1955. Damage and repair in mammalian tissues exposed to cosmic ray nuclei. *J. Aviation Med.* 27: 533–540.
53. FREIER, P. S., ANDERSON, G. W., NAUGLE, J. E., and NEY, E. P. 1951. The heavy nuclei of the primary cosmic radiation. *Phys. Rev. 84:* 322–331.
54. GLASSTONE, SAMUEL. 1958. *Sourcebook on Atomic Energy.* 2nd ed. D. Van Nostrand Co., Inc., Princeton, N.J.
55. GRAY, L. H. 1947. The distribution of the ions resulting from the irradiation of living cells. *Brit. J. Radiol., Suppl. I*, pp. 7–15.
56. HABER, H. 1954. *The Physical Environment of the Flyer.* USAF, Air University, School of Aviation Medicine, Randolph Air Force Base, Tex. Pp. 114–153.
57. INGLIS, D. R. 1958. *Future radiation dosage from weapon tests. Science 127:* 1222–1227.
58. KINSMAN, S. 1958. Background radiation exposures of the general population. *Am. Ind. Hyg. Assoc. J.* 19: 8–14.
59. KORFF, S. A. 1957. The origin and implications of the cosmic radiation. *Am. Scientist 45:* 281–300.
60. KREBS, A. T. 1952. The biological effects of laboratory radiation. In WHITE, C. S., and BENSON, O. O., JR. (eds.). *Physics and Medicine of the Upper Atmosphere.* University of New Mexico Press, Albuquerque. Pp. 267–289.
61. LAUGHLIN, J. S., and PULLMAN, J. 1957. *Gonadal Dose from the Medical Use of X-rays.* Natl. Acad. Sci.-Natl. Research Council, Washington, D.C.
62. LIBBY, W. F. 1955. Dosages from natural radioactivity and cosmic rays. *Science 122:* 57–58.
63. LOCKHART, L. B., JR. 1958. Concentrations of radioactive materials in the air during 1957. *Science 128:* 1139.
64. Radioactivity of watches with luminous dials. *Med. Sci. 3:* 713, 1958.
65. MORGAN, W. E. 1959. Personal communication (Radiological Safety Officer, Boeing Airplane Co., Seattle).
66. MULLER, H. J. 1955. How radiation changes the genetic constitution. *Bull. Atomic Scientists 11:* 329–337.
67. NEHER, H. V. 1957. Cosmic rays near the north geomagnetic pole in the summer of 1955 and 1956. *Physiol. Revs. 107:* 588–592.
68. RUSSELL, W. L., RUSSELL, L. B., and KELLY, E. M. 1958. Radiation dose rate and mutation frequency. *Science 128:* 1546–1550.
69. SCHAEFER, H. J. 1951. The diurnal intensity variation of the heavy primaries of cosmic radiation and its consequences for the hazard to health in flight at extreme altitudes. *J. Aviation Med.* 22: 351–357.
70. SCHAEFER, H. J. 1952. The biologic effects of cosmic radiation. In WHITE, C. S., and BENSON, O. O., JR. (eds.). *Physics and Medicine of the Upper Atmosphere.* University of New Mexico Press, Albuquerque. Pp. 290–315.
71. SCHAEFER, H. J. 1954. Theory of protection of man in the region of the primary cosmic radiation. *J. Aviation Med.* 25: 338–350.
72. SCHAEFER, H. J. 1955. Biological significance of the natural background of ionizing radiation observed at sea level and extreme altitudes. *J. Aviation Med.* 26: 453–462.

73. SCHAEFER, H. J. 1956. *Exposure Hazards from Cosmic Radiation in Flight in Extra-atmospheric Regions.* Trans. Inst. Radio Engrs. on Med. Electronics.
74. SCHAEFER, H. J. 1956. Optimum altitudes for biological experimentation with the primary cosmic radiation. *J. Aviation Med. 27:* 513–521.
75. SPECIAL SUB-COMMITTEE ON RADIATION OF THE JOINT COMMITTEE ON ATOMIC ENERGY. 1957. *The Nature of Radioactive Fallout and Its Effect on Man.* U.S. Government Printing Office, Washington, D.C. (May 27, 28, 29; June 3, 1957.) Part I.
76. SPECIAL SUB-COMMITTEE ON RADIATION OF THE JOINT COMMITTEE ON ATOMIC ENERGY. 1957. *The Nature of Radioactive Fallout and Its Effect on Man.* U.S. Government Printing Office, Washington, D.C. (June 4, 5, 6, 7; 1957.) Part II.
77. SPIERS, F. W. 1956. Radioactivity in man and his environment. *Brit. J. Radiol. 29:* 409–417.
78. UNITED KINGDOM MEDICAL RESEARCH COUNCIL. 1956. *Hazards to Man of Nuclear and Allied Radiation.* H.M. Stationery Office, London.
79. UNITED NATIONS SCIENTIFIC COMMITTEE ON THE EFFECTS OF ATOMIC RADIATION. 1958. Excerpts from summary and conclusions of report. *Science 128:* 402–406. (See also comment entitled Pathologic Effects of Radiation. *Science 129:* 377–378, 1959.)
80. VAN ALLEN, J. A. 1952. The nature and intensity of the cosmic radiation. In WHITE, C. S., and BENSON, O. O., JR. (eds.). *Physics and Medicine of the Upper Atmosphere.* University of New Mexico Press, Albuquerque. Pp. 239–266.
81. Waste disposal: Congressional atomic energy group studies waste disposal problem. From News of Science, *Science 129:* 375–376, 1959.

## Microwave Radiation

82. BARRON, C. I., LOV, A., and BARAFF, A. 1955. Physical evaluation of personnel exposed to microwave emanations. *J. Aviation Med. 26:* 442–452.
83. BOYSEN, J. 1953. Hyperthermic and pathologic effects of electromagnetic radiation (350 mc). *A.M.A. Arch. Ind. Hyg. Occup. Med. 7:* 516–525.
84. CLARK, J. W. 1950. Effects of intense microwave radiation on living organisms. *Proc. Inst. Radio Engrs. 38:* 1028–1032.
85. COGAN, D. 1950. Lesions of the eye from radiant energy. *J. Am. Med. Assoc. 142:* 145–151.
86. DAILY, L. E. 1943. A clinical study of the results of exposure of laboratory personnel to radar and high-frequency radio. *U.S. Naval Med. Bull. 41:* 1052–1065.
87. DAVIS, T. R. A., and MOYER, J. 1954. Use of high frequency electromagnetic waves in the study of thermogenesis. *Am. J. Physiol. 178:* 283–287.
88. DUBOIS, E. F. 1951. Physiological aspects of heating and ventilating. *Heating, Piping and Air Conditioning 23:* 134–136.
89. ELY, T. S., and GOLDMAN, D. E. 1957. *Heating Characteristics of Laboratory Animals Exposed to Ten-Centimeter Microwaves.* (Research Report, Project NM 001.056.13.02.) Naval Med. Research Inst., Natl. Naval Med. Center, Bethesda, Md.
90. FREDERICK, J. N., and OSBORNE, S. 1948. Heating of human and animal tissues by means of high frequency current with wave-length of 12 cm. *J. Am. Med. Assoc. 137:* 1036–1040.
91. GINZTON, E. L. 1958. Microwaves. *Science 127:* 841–851.
92. GORDON, E. E. 1957. Energy costs in the prescription of activity. *Modern Med. (Minneapolis) 25:* 83–91.
93. HELLER, J. H., and TEIXEIRA-PINTO, A. A. 1958. Further investigation into radiofrequency effects which appear to be active on the RES in whole-body irradiation. *RES Bulletin 4:* 10–11.

94. HERRICK, J. F., and KRUSEN, F. H. 1953. Certain physiologic and pathologic effects of microwaves. *Elec. Eng. 72:* 239–244.
95. HINES, H. M., and RANDALL, J. E. 1952. Possible hazards in the use of microwave radiation. *Elec. Eng. 71:* 879–881.
96. HIRSCH, F. G., and PARKER, J. T. 1952. Bilateral lenticular opacities occurring in a technician operating a microwave generator. *Arch. Ind. Hyg. Occupational Med. 6:* 512–517.
97. IMIG, C. J., THOMSON, J. D., and HINES, H. M. 1948. Testicular degeneration as a result of microwave irradiation. *Proc. Soc. Exp. Biol. Med. 69:* 382–386.
98. INSTITUTE OF RADIO ENGINEERS. 1956. Symposium on Physiologic and Pathologic Effects of Microwaves. *IRE Trans. on Med. Electronics,* PGME-4 (entire issue).
99. MONTGOMERY, C. G. 1947. *Technique of Microwave Measurements.* McGraw-Hill Book Company, Inc., New York.
100. MURPHY, A. J., PAUL, W. D., and HINES, H. M. 1950. A comparative study of the temperature changes produced by various thermogenic agents. *Arch. Phys. Med. 31:* 151–156.
101. PATTISHALL, E. G. (ed.). 1957. *Proceedings of Tri-Service Conference on Biological Hazards of Microwave Radiation* (July 15–16, 1957). (Air Force Contract 18 (600)–1180, Project #57–13.) George Washington University, Washington, D.C.
102. RICHARDSON, A. W., DUANE, T. D., and HINES, H. M. 1949. Experimental lenticular opacities produced by microwave irradiations. *Arch. Phys. Med. 29:* 765–769.
103. SALISBURY, W. W., CLARK, J. W., and HINES, H. M. 1949. Exposure to microwaves. *Electronics 22:* 66–67.
104. SCHWAN, H. P. 1956. The biophysical basis of physical medicine. *J. Am. Med. Assoc. 160:* 191–197.
105. SCHWAN, H. P., and LI, K. 1953. Capacity and conductivity of body tissues at ultrahigh frequencies. *Proc. Inst. Radio Engrs. 41:* 1735–1740.
106. SCHWAN, H. P., and LI, K. 1956. Hazards due to total body irradiation by radar. *Proc. Inst. Radio Engrs. 44:* 1572–1581.
107. SCHWAN, H. P., and LI, K. 1956. The mechanism of absorption of ultrahigh frequency electromagnetic energy in tissues as related to the problem of tissue dosage. *IRE Trans. on Med. Electronics,* PGME-4, pp. 45–49.
108. SCHWAN, H. P., and PIERSOL, G. M. 1954. The absorption of electromagnetic energy in body tissues. *Am. J. Phys. Med. 33:* 371–404.
109. UNITED STATES AIR FORCE. 1958. *Radio Frequency Radiation Hazards.* (USAF Technical Order 31-1-80, 15 April 1958, revised 15 May 1958.) U.S. Dept. Air Force, Washington, D.C.
110. WILLIAMS, D. B., MONOHAN, J. P., and NICHOLSON, W. J. 1955. *Biologic Effects Studies on Microwave Radiation: Time and Power Thresholds for the Production of Lens Opacities by 12.3 cm. Microwaves.* (Report No. 55–94.) USAF, Air University, School of Aviation Medicine, Randolph Air Force Base, Tex.

## Acceleration

111. BECKMAN, E. L., ZIEGLER, J. E., DUANE, T. D., and HUNTER, H. N. 1953. Some observations on human tolerance to accelerative stress: II. Preliminary studies on primates subjected to maximum simple accelerative loads. *J. Aviation Med. 24:* 377–392.
112. BROWN, J. L., and LECHNER, M. 1956. Acceleration and human performance. *J. Aviation Med. 27:* 32–49. (Review article with 98 references.)
113. CLARKE, N. P., BONDURANT, S., and LEVERETT, S. 1959. Human tolerance to prolonged forward and backward acceleration. *J. Aviation Med. 30:* 1–20.

114. DE HAVEN, H. 1942. Mechanical analysis of survival in falls from heights of fifty to one hundred and fifty feet. *War Med.* 2: 586–596.
115. DIXON, F., and PATTERSON, J. 1953. *Determination of Accelerative Forces Acting on Man in Flight and in the Human Centrifuge.* (Project No. NM 001 059.04.01.) U.S. Naval School of Aviation Medicine, Naval Air Station, Pensacola, Fla.
116. DUANE, T. D., BECKMAN, E. L., ZIEGLER, J. E., and HUNTER, H. N. 1955. Some observations on human tolerance to accelerative stress: III. Human studies of fifteen transverse G. *J. Aviation Med.* 26: 298–303.
117. EDELBERG, R. 1953. *Problems of Emergency Escape in High Speed Flight: Tumbling.* (WADC Document #53WC–1470.)
118. FASOLA, A. F., BAKER, R. C., and HITCHCOCK, F. 1955. *Anatomical and Physiological Effects of Rapid Deceleration.* (WADC Technical Report 54–218.) (WADC Aug. 1955.) USAF, Wright-Patterson Air Force Base, Ohio.
119. GAUER, OTTO. 1950. The physiological effects of prolonged acceleration. In *German Aviation Medicine World War II.* Government Printing Office, Washington, D.C. Vol. I, pp. 554–583.
120. HABER, F. 1952. Bailout at very high altitudes. *J. Aviation Med.* 23: 322–329.
121. HABER, F. 1952. *Escape and Survival in Space Travel.* (Am. Rocket Soc. Paper No. 68–52.) New York.
122. HABER, H., and HULBERT, S. (eds.). 1955. *Escape From High Performance Aircraft: A Symposium.* (Los Angeles, Calif., Oct. 7, 1955.) Inst. of Transportation, University of California at Los Angeles.
123. HENRY, J. P. 1950. *Studies of the Physiology of Negative Acceleration.* (AF Technical Report No. 5953, Oct. 1950, and attached bibliography.) USAF, Air Materiel Command, Wright-Patterson Air Force Base, Ohio.
124. HEYMANS, R. J. 1956. Crew Survival in the Jet Age. Paper presented at the SAE National Aeronautic Meeting, April 9–12, 1956, New York. (Published by the Society of Automotive Engineers, Inc., 29 W. 39th St., New York.)
125. KILGARIFF, T. G.. 1957. Escape from high-performance aircraft. *Aeronaut. Eng. Rev.* 16: 59–64.
126. LATHAM, F. 1957. A study in body ballistics: Seat ejection. *Proc. Roy. Soc.* (*London*) 147B: 121–139.
127. LATHAM, F. 1957. *Linear Deceleration Studies in Human Tolerance.* (FPRC 1012). Institute of Aviation Medicine, Royal Air Force, Farnborough, England.
128. MOSELY, H. G., and SHANNON, R. H. 1958. *USAF Ejection Escape Experience.* (Publication No. M–12–58, 10 November 1958.) USAF, Directorate of Flight Safety Research, OTIG, Norton Air Force Base, Calif.
129. RICKARDS, M. A. 1957. *A Study of the Unstabilized Aft-facing Ejection Seat.* (DR 5609.) Weber Aircraft Corporation, Burbank, Calif.
130. ROMAN, J. A., COERMANN, R., and ZIEGENRUECKER, G. 1957. Vibration, buffeting and impact research. *J. Aviation Med.* 30: 118–125.
131. ROOT, D. M. 1958. Some Fundamental Considerations in the Selection and Design of Escape Capsules. Paper presented at the SAE National Aeronautical Meeting, Los Angeles, Calif., Sept. 29–Oct. 4, 1958. (Society of Automotive Engineers, Inc., New York.)
132. RUFF, S. 1950. Brief acceleration: Less than one second. In *German Aviation Medicine World War II.* Government Printing Office, Washington, D.C. Vol. I, pp. 584–597.
133. SCHEUBEL, F. N. 1950. Parachute opening shock. In *German Aviation Medicine World War II.* Government Printing Office, Washington, D.C. Vol. I, pp. 599–611.
134. STAPP, J. P. 1955. Effects of mechanical force on living tissues. *J. Aviation Med.* 26: 268–288.
135. WEISS, H. S., EDELBERG, R., CHARLAND, P. V., and ROSENBAUM, J. I. 1954. Animal and human reactions to rapid tumbling. *J. Aviation Med.* 25: 5–22.

136. WIANT, H. W. 1956. *The Effects of Simultaneous Deceleration, Tumbling and Windblast Encountered in Escape from Supersonic Aircraft.* (WADC Technical Note 54–18.)

## Noise

137. ELDRED, K., CANNON, W., and VON GIERKE, H. 1955. *Criteria for Short Time Exposure to High Intensity Jet Aircraft Noise.* (WADC Technical Note 55–355.) USAF, Wright Air Development Center, Wright-Patterson Air Force Base, Ohio.
138. GLORIG, A., JR. 1958. *Noise and Your Ear.* Grune & Stratton, Inc., New York.
139. HARRIS, C. M. (ed.). 1957. *Handbook of Noise Control.* McGraw-Hill Book Co., Inc., New York.
140. *Industrial Noise Manual.* The American Industrial Hygiene Assoc., Braun-Brumfield, Inc., Ann Arbor, Mich. 1958.
141. MAGLIERI, D. J., and CARLSON, H. W. 1959. *The Shock-Wave Noise Problem of Supersonic Aircraft in Steady Flight.* (NASA Memorandum, 3–4–59L.) National Aeronautics and Space Agency, Washington, D.C.
142. RICHARDS, E. J. 1953. *Thoughts on Future Noise Suppression Research.* (Proc. 3rd AGARD Gen. Assembly, Sept. 7–10, 1953, London.) (Available through the Natl. Advis. Comm. for Aeronautics, 1513 H St. N.W., Washington, D.C.)
143. ROSENBLITH, W., and STEVENS, K. 1953. *Handbook of Acoustic Noise Control.* (WADC Technical Report 52–204.) Wright Air Development Center, Wright-Patterson Air Force Base, Ohio. Vol. II, p. 219.
144. TALBOT, J. M. 1955. Breaking the sound barrier and its effect on the public. *J. Am. Med. Assoc.* 158: 1508–1512.
145. TONNDORF, J. 1953. *Some Implications of the Decibel Scale.* USAF, Air University, School of Aviation Medicine, Randolph Air Force Base, Tex.
146. UNITED STATES AIR FORCE. 1956. *Air Force Regulation 160–3.* Hazardous Noise Exposure. Washington, D.C.
147. WITZE, CLAUDE. 1959. Learning to live with the sonic boom. *Air Force*, January, 1959. Pp. 35–38.

## Human Factors in the Control of Aircraft

148. BARTLEY, S. H., and CHUTE, E. 1947. *Fatigue and Impairment in Man.* McGraw-Hill Book Company, Inc., New York.
149. FLOYD, W. F., and WELFORD, A. T. (eds.). 1953. *Symposium on Fatigue.* H. K. Lewis & Co., Ltd., London.
150. FRENCH, J. D. 1958. The reticular formation. *J. Neurosurg.* 15: 97–115.
151. GEORGE, F. H. 1958. Machines and the brain. *Science 127:* 1269–1274.
152. HANNISDAHL, B. 1949. Maximum flying time for aircrews. *J. Aviation Med.* 20: 257–259.
153. HIMWICH, H. E. 1958. Psychopharmacologic drugs. *Science 127:* 59–71.
154. HOLLAND, J. G. 1958. Human vigilance. *Science 128:* 61–67.
155. KLEITMAN, N. 1939. *Sleep and Wakefulness.* University of Chicago Press, Chicago.
156. KLEITMAN, N. 1949. Biological rhythms and cycles. *Physiol. Revs.* 29: 1–30.
157. KLEITMAN, N. 1949. The sleep-wakefulness cycle of submarine personnel. In *Human Factors in Undersea Warfare.* National Research Council, Washington, D.C. Pp. 329–341.
158. KLEITMAN, N. 1952. Sleep. *Sci. American 187:* 34–38.
159. STRUGHOLD, H. 1952. Physiological day-night cycle in global flights. *J. Aviation Med.* 23: 464–473.
160. UPJOHN COMPANY. 1955. Physiology and pharmacology of emotion. *Scope 4:* 1–8.
161. WILLIAMS, ROGER. 1953. *Free and Unequal.* University of Texas Press, Austin.

# 12

# The Engineered Environment
# of the Space Vehicle

HANS G. CLAMANN, M.D.*

## The Problem

A decade ago a "space vehicle" would have meant to most people a vehicle capable of carrying man to a far-distant interplanetary destination. At that time the term "space" was almost exclusively used by astronomers with reference to distances of interplanetary magnitude.

In the meantime manned aircraft have attained higher and higher altitudes. With each increase in altitude of about 53,000 ft., the atmospheric pressure decreases to a tenth of its previous value. The density of the atmosphere decreases at the same rate. This decrease in density means fewer molecules of air per unit of volume and consequently less oxygen, despite the fact that the proportion of oxygen remains constant at 21 per cent of the volume of air.

Both the power plant of an aircraft and its passengers need oxygen to function. If the air becomes too thin to provide enough oxygen, either air compression to higher density without added oxygen or addition of oxygen to the non-compressed air may correct the deficiency. The enormous quantities of air at sufficient pressure needed to supply oxygen for the "thousands of horses" of an airplane engine dictate the use of powerful high-speed compressors. Man, less powerful with barely one-tenth of a horsepower for continuous physical work, is relatively modest in oxygen consumption.

* Professor of Biophysics, School of Aviation Medicine, USAF, Brooks Air Force Base, Texas. This chapter was originally prepared for an Air Force symposium on "The Human Factor in Space Travel" and appeared in slightly modified form in the *Air University Quarterly Review*, Summer, 1958.

But he lacks the structural strength of an engine; his weak chest muscles will not allow pressurization of the lungs by much more than 5 per cent of atmospheric pressure. Therefore, pressurization has to be extended to the whole cabin, which is then referred to as a "pressurized cabin." In contrast to an engine, for which pressurization serves only the purpose of oxygen supply, a pressurized cabin has to be ventilated for removal of carbon dioxide, water vapor, odors, and possible traces of noxious gases (for instance, carbon monoxide). The two latter factors increase ventilation requirements almost tenfold.

The other possibility, of breathing oxygen-enriched air, to maintain man at altitudes above 10,000 ft. may just be mentioned. Its main advantage lies in the protection it affords against bends at altitudes above 25,000 ft. Also, in combination with partially pressurized cabins, this procedure protects the airman against failure of pressurization and rapid decompression and keeps him prepared for emergency bail-out.

Above 80,000 ft., where the atmospheric pressure is reduced to 3.5 per cent of that at sea level, present air compressors become increasingly bulky, heavy, power consuming, and inefficient to provide both a high pressure ratio and a large mass flow. In addition, there is a problem of high temperatures caused by the high pressure ratio.

Therefore, both the power plants and the passengers of aircraft flying above such altitudes must rely completely on an oxygen supply rather than on pressurization. The reciprocating engine and the jet must be replaced by the rocket, carrying its own fuel and oxidizer. Instead of the pressurized cabin a completely sealed cabin must separate the passengers from the outside rarefied atmosphere or vacuum. An oxygen supply and the means for removal of carbon dioxide, water vapor, etc., have to be carried along.

Since the sealed cabin constitutes the only means to keep man alive from 80,000 ft. and outward to any realm of space, it is well justified to say that for man "space" begins at 80,000 ft. and to call any craft cruising at such altitudes a spacecraft. With reference to oxygen supply alone, even lower altitudes may be called "space equivalent."

Actually, man has other needs for protection in addition to oxygen. Even on earth, without protective clothing, housing, and heating and cooling systems, he would be restricted to a rather small geographical area. For full physical performance and even more for full mental performance, he has always needed an "engineered environment." In modern aircraft, especially military aircraft under operational conditions, and likewise in future space vehicles, fast sensory reactions, alertness, and good judgment are paramount.

Thus, the so-called comfort conditions with respect to all environmental factors are no longer a luxury but a necessity. As an example, studies of radio operators showed that errors in receiving radio code increased 80 per cent above normal after the first hour when the operator was exposed to a room temperature of 98° F as compared to a normal of 78° F. Even excessively loud noises have been shown to decrease mental performance.

## The Sealed Cabin

The predominant factor in the sealed cabin seems to be the confined environment. Studies of confined environments are generally regarded as an outcome of the space age. Actually, however, such studies on man and animals had been carried out long before the idea of a sealed cabin came close to practical applicability. For instance, as early as 1870 Paul Bert, the French physiologist who is recognized as the father of aviation medicine, put sparrows in sealed glass jars of various sizes filled with normal air and with various air-oxygen mixtures to study the effects on their survival.

It has been known for a long time that the ratio of the volume of exhaled carbon dioxide to the volume of consumed oxygen is, on the average, close to 0.85. This important ratio is known as the respiratory quotient (RQ). In other words, with reference to volume, about 15 per cent more oxygen is absorbed from a surrounding atmosphere than is replaced by exhaled carbon dioxide. Thus, a pressure drop is produced in a confined space, provided there is no interference by changes in temperature and humidity. If temperature and humidity are kept constant and carbon dioxide is completely absorbed, the pressure drop in this case provides a simple means of monitoring the proper oxygen supply in a sealed cabin.

In a sealed cabin of 50 cu. ft. occupied by one man at rest with no oxygen supply or absorption of carbon dioxide or water vapor, the oxygen percentage will drop after four hours to about 14 per cent, corresponding to 10,000 ft. equivalent altitude, while the carbon dioxide concentration will rise to 6 per cent. Complete water-vapor saturation, or 100 per cent humidity, will be obtained within the first quarter hour. This example demonstrates that the rise in carbon dioxide concentration is the decisive factor for survival under such conditions.

While there is little doubt as to the lowest permissible concentration of oxygen, approximately 12 per cent for the unacclimatized man, there is less agreement on the highest permissible concentration of carbon dioxide. The main reason is probably the neglect of the time factor. Two human subjects spent three days in a sealed cabin in an atmosphere of 3 per cent carbon dioxide with apparent signs of acclimatization. Animals were kept for two weeks in a sealed cabin while the carbon dioxide rose to 11 per cent. They lost their appetite but recovered rapidly when they were brought back to normal conditions.

These examples show the influence of long exposure time on acclimatization to carbon dioxide concentrations. Eleven per cent carbon dioxide would be intolerable during acute exposure. For the human carbon dioxide concentrations up to 1 per cent may still be regarded as maximum. Theoretically, acclimatization to low oxygen and acclimatization to high carbon dioxide concentration may not be compatible with each other. While acclimatization to either low oxygen or high carbon dioxide partial pressure would aid in tolerating emergency situations in a sealed cabin, such acclimatization would not help to decrease either oxygen consumption or production of carbon dioxide. Such decrease alone would be decisive in reducing weight of oxygen and of carbon dioxide absorbents.

Physiologically, normal atmospheric pressure and composition of gases would be most desirable. From the viewpoint of the design engineer, a lower than normal pressure may be preferable for two reasons. First, a pressure differential of less than 14.7 pounds per square inch (psi), such as would exist between the external vacuum of space and the interior of the cabin, may be required for structural reasons. Second, if uncontrollable leakage of cabin air should occur, the best situation to minimize such leakage would be a pressure differential as small as possible.

In conclusion, the discussion of these general problems of the sealed cabin indicates the predominant influence of the time factor or, in other words, the influence of the duration of an excursion into space upon the construction and equipment of a space cabin. For short flights (in magnitude of hours or several days), many problems are not very different from those of ordinary high-altitude flights in space-equivalent conditions.

**Man as an Energy Converter.** Before considering in detail the supply problems of sealed cabins, it is necessary to take a closer look at the primary energy converter: man. In principle, man like other living beings obtains the various forms of energy necessary to sustain life—for instance, all muscular work—by converting chemical substances of high energy into those of lower energy. As an example, carbohydrates and fats are converted to water and carbon dioxide. Such conversions are called "metabolic conversions" and the total process "metabolism." A kind of standard man has been created, and his metabolic conversions are quantitatively shown for the state of rest with occasional light muscular activity, as in the case of a pilot in flight.

It is well known that in man the daily metabolic turnover undergoes considerable fluctuation. The oxygen consumption in particular may vary anywhere from 360 l per day at complete body rest (sleep) to more than five times as much at heavy muscular work. Next to muscular work eating and the subsequent processes of digestion constitute a powerful stimulus to metabolism. Metabolic processes are speeded up by environmental temperature.

For a pilot of an airplane, a consumption of 535 l of oxygen per day has been reported. While it is impossible to arrive at a single figure for oxygen consumption without showing correspondingly accurate figures on all the factors mentioned above, an oxygen consumption of 603 l per day has been tentatively set for our standard man, assuming that the activity of a "space pilot" may resemble closely that of his counterpart in the troposphere. In reality the pilot of a large spacecraft with more room and greater occasion for muscular exercise may consume considerably more oxygen than the pilot of a conventional aircraft. In any case, for determining fairly accurate figures on oxygen consumption, a simulation model, providing complete duplication of all conditions that may occur in the cabin of a spacecraft, needs to be developed and tested. Such duplication simulation could be performed in special sealed cabins, or "space simulators," in a ground laboratory.

One interesting question that is unanswered at the present time is whether or not the state of weightlessness will cause a relative decrease in oxygen consumption, since there are no "weights" to be lifted such as the weight of the body and its parts. Of course there are still "masses" to be accelerated and decelerated.

All the factors of metabolism are closely interlinked. The data shown in Fig. 12–1 are calculated for an assumed average man of about 154 lbs. body weight. Again, while the actual values may fluctuate, they tend to remain constant over a period of time. The mass of all input substances, in particular, must equal exactly the

## DAILY METABOLIC TURNOVER

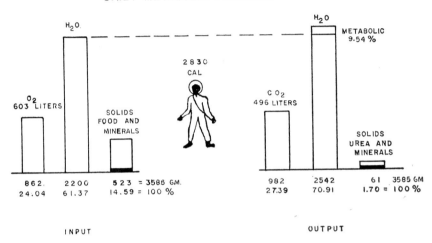

Fig. 12–1. Daily metabolic turnover. This quantitative portrayal of man's metabolic conversions assumes an average man weighing 154 lbs. with a respiratory quotient of 0.82. His assumed diet consists of proteins (80 gm), carbohydrates (270 gm), and fat (150 gm).

output mass, since the body mass of a healthy adult remains practically constant and no substance can vanish. The only "loss" consists of heat energy (2,830 Cal. per day).

Consequently, all the water consumed on the intake side has to reappear quantitatively in the output, whether as part of the urine, feces, perspiration, or exhaled water vapor. But added to this output is the water produced metabolically by the oxidation of food. With the diet chosen for the "standard man," the metabolic water surplus will amount to about 10 per cent of the total water turnover. The percentage of metabolic water depends on the type of food. Fat, for instance, would produce more metabolic water than carbohydrates or proteins.

This example of a single metabolic factor (water balance) demonstrates how closely biological problems and problems of the engineered environment are interlinked. To keep the weight and space requirements of equipment to a minimum, it is necessary to consider carefully all the factors involved in maintaining a proper balance. An increase of fat in the diet with its high caloric value would save weight on the food supply, but it would also increase the amount of oxygen and water absorbents needed. In any case the amount of water in a space cabin will constantly increase with time.

Basically, for a self-sustaining ecological system as constituted by the sealed cabin, everything needed to support life has to be stored before departure of a spacecraft. With increasing duration of a flight into space, the necessary storage will increase correspondingly. To minimize the mass of storage, it is desirable to develop as absorbers for carbon dioxide and water, materials that can be used again. Such "regeneration" can be carried out for some absorbers by heating. The ideal process would be the complete "recycling" of the metabolic waste products back to food, of carbon dioxide and water back to sugar and starch, of nitrogen compounds (for instance urea in the urine) back to proteins.

An ideal prototype in this respect is the earth. Because of its gravity, the earth can afford to have its atmosphere on the outside, thus killing four "problem birds" with one stone: leakage, solar radiation, cosmic radiation, and meteorites. There is also a perfect recycling process between oxygen and carbon dioxide, which is based on photosynthesis, as well as one for nitrogen and water.

While such ideal conditions appear to be beyond the possibility of even the largest spacecraft, regenerating and recycling processes have been taken into consideration.

**Oxygen.** The three main sources of oxygen available at present are: (1) compressed gaseous oxygen, (2) liquid oxygen, and (3) chemical compounds that liberate oxygen. Gaseous oxygen has the advantage of the best and most complete flow control. Contained in metal cylinders, it has the disadvantage of a high dead weight of between 80 and 90 per cent. Considerably smaller dead weight may possibly be achieved by the development of containers based upon synthetic resin material.

Liquid-oxygen converters have a much better dead-weight ratio compared to cylinders filled with compressed gaseous oxygen. As shown in Fig. 12–2, only from 50 to 60 per cent of their poundage is lost to dead weight. The main problem with them is to avoid evaporation. Normally, only good thermal insulation can prevent excessive losses. In a spacecraft with controlled position toward the sun, the cold "shadow side" may support thermal insulation by minimizing the temperature gradient. If the rate of evaporative losses is smaller than the rate of requirement for gaseous oxygen, this would

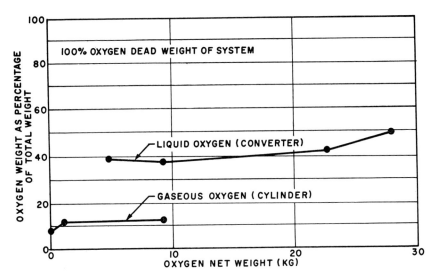

Fig. 12–2. Comparative weight of oxygen in two systems.

not be harmful for a sealed cabin in contrast to a normal airplane where free gaseous oxygen is not retained. Special precaution would have to be taken to prevent liquid oxygen from entering the evaporator during the state of weightlessness.

Oxygen supply from chemical sources, such as hydrogen peroxide ($H_2O_2$), sodium chlorate ($NaClO_3$), sodium superoxide ($Na_2O_2$), and other superoxides, has two disadvantages: (1) oxygen release cannot be controlled and (2) there is explosive hazard in the possibility of contact with organic material. In the state of weightlessness, a drifting of organic particles is likely to occur at any time. As to the dead-weight factor, chlorate candles, for instance, must be listed between gaseous- and liquid-oxygen systems.

To represent the multipurpose processes, potassium superoxide ($KO_2$) may serve as an example of an oxygen producer that at the same time acts as a carbon dioxide absorber. According to the equations

and
$$4KO_2 + 2H_2O = 4KOH + 3O_2$$
$$4KOH + 2CO_2 = 2K_2CO_3 + 2H_2O$$

water vapor causes liberation of oxygen and formation of potassium hydroxide, which in turn absorbs carbon dioxide and liberates water. As a net result 3 gram molecules (moles) of oxygen correspond to 2 moles of carbon dioxide, and the RQ of this system is ⅔ or 0.67.

This ratio reveals a problem common to most multipurpose and recycling processes: carbon dioxide and oxygen exchange between man and chemical is not in complete, controllable balance. Here, an excess of oxygen is produced if all the carbon dioxide is absorbed; or if only enough oxygen is released, not all the carbon dioxide will be absorbed. As far as water is concerned, theoretically the same amount is consumed as is produced. Actually some water may be retained as solvent for the potassium carbonate. Such secondary processes are typical for all chemical compounds, whether they are producers or absorbers. Together with physical factors (active area, diffusion processes), they may considerably alter the expected efficiency of a system.

Photosynthesis as a regenerative process, with its unchanging dead weight regardless of the length of time, offers a very attractive possibility of using green plants for production of oxygen by the uptake of carbon dioxide, water, and light energy. With their high amount of chlorophyll, algae seem especially well-suited. In the photosynthetic process, for each mole of carbon dioxide and water, one mole of oxygen is generated. This would result in an $RQ = 1$. But in algae such as *Chlorella*, in which the dry substance consists of 50 per cent protein, it is necessary to assume other synthetic processes indirectly related to photosynthesis. Therefore, theoretically a lower RQ should be expected. Indeed RQ's of from 0.9 to 0.7 have been found, depending on the feeding of the algae with either nitrates or urea. Thus, a certain regulation of the RQ close to man's RQ of 0.82 seems possible, perhaps at the expense of optimum oxygen production.

*Chlorella* algae are most effective in a 1 per cent suspension in water. For the production of 600 l of oxygen per day, 2.3 kg of wet algae in 230 l or 8.1 cu. ft. of water are necessary. Actually this much oxygen is produced only in a rapidly growing algae solution. Growing at a "compound interest" rate, 1 kg of algae would increase to 2.6 kg in one day. In any case a certain amount of algae has to be removed at intervals. How far this "harvest" with its high-protein content can be utilized for inclusion in the nitrogen cycle of man or algae remains to be studied in the future. The nitrogen cycle is the exchange of nitrogen between man and plant: plants convert urea or nitrates into protein, man digests protein and excretes its nitrogen content as urea.

A comparison may be made between the weight of a liquid-oxygen system, sufficient to sustain life for one person for 180 days, and the weight of a tank of algae 8.1 cu. ft. in volume. The former weighs about 800 lbs. and the latter about 500 lbs. In the liquid-oxygen system, the oxygen decreases from 360 lbs. at start to zero, leaving only the dead weight of the converter (440 lbs.) at the end of 180 days. The weight of the algae suspension remains constant, notwithstanding the increase of the weight of the algae proper at simple rate or cumulative rate of growth. The accessories needed for the algae system (tanks, pumps, light systems, etc.) have been omitted, because their weight is very hard to estimate at the present time. But even on this basis of comparison, the weights of the two systems do not approach the same magnitude before 150 days. With accessories added a comparison favoring the algae system may require a considerably extended duration of flight.

As a last possibility to produce oxygen, electrolysis of water may be mentioned. With the use of high-current-density systems, a process of electrolysis using electrodes of relatively small area with electric currents of high amperage, about 40 lbs. of equipment would be required to produce 600 l of oxygen per day. The utilization or removal of hydrogen and the provision of adequate electric power (by solar energy?) are some additional problems of such systems, not to mention the potential explosive hazard of free hydrogen.

**Carbon Dioxide, Water, and Waste.** The conventional absorbers for carbon dioxide belong to the class of the alkaline metal hydroxides. Such absorbers are sodium and potassium hydroxide, Baralyme (a mixture of calcium hydroxide and barium hydroxide), and soda lime (a mixture of calcium hydroxide and caustic soda or sodium hydroxide [NaOH]). About three units of weight are required for the absorption of one unit of weight of carbon dioxide. Lithium hydroxide, on the other hand, requires about one and a half units. Also it retains full reactivity almost down to the freezing point of water. Temperature and humidity exert an influence on most of the absorbents.

Size of the granules, bed height, and velocity of the ventilated air are other parameters that have to be considered for development of an effective absorptive system. It should be emphasized that the exact quantitative behavior of a system cannot be predicted accurately. Experimental testing is necessary to determine performance characteristics.

Other methods of carbon dioxide removal are based upon the high solubility of carbon dioxide in certain liquids. Under high pressure in a special container, correspondingly large amounts of carbon dioxide go into solution. Thereafter, release of pressure liberates the carbon dioxide which is vented to the outside. Such methods, as used in submarines, are not feasible for space vehicles because of weight and bulk. Another method open for future development may be the "freeze out" method. Here, upon the application of temperatures below the freezing point of water, water solidifies (freezes to ice), and at much lower temperatures even carbon dioxide solidifies (dry ice) and can be removed as such.

The alkaline metal hydroxides, such as sodium hydroxide, produce 1 mole of water (18 gm) for each mole of carbon dioxide (44 gm) absorbed. Part of this water is retained by the absorbents, but the rest evaporates and has to be removed by the water absorbents.

Common absorbers for water are the oxides of calcium and barium. They require about ten units of weight for one unit of water. The absorptive quality of silica gel is strongly influenced by the relative humidity: the weight requirement falls from ten to seven units between 10 and 30 per cent relative humidity at 80° F. Silica gel is capable of regeneration by heat. So is Anhydrone (magnesium perchlorate) which, except for lithium chloride, requires the smallest amount in weight (two to three units of weight per unit of water). A disadvantage of Anhydrone is its possible explosive hazard if it comes in contact with high concentrations of organic vapors at high temperature.

The previously mentioned absorbents remove water that is in the form of vapor. But a greater amount of water is produced in urine and in feces. Not much has been accomplished to solve this problem. Urine can be distilled, feces dried. For short flights removal of water does not constitute a serious problem; waste can be stored.

There are a number of issues related to the problem of expulsion of water and solid waste from a spacecraft. Expulsion would mean a certain loss of cabin atmosphere. Any expelled solid material would constitute artificial "meteorites" which might endanger other spacecraft. The loss of mass as such would not alter the course of a spacecraft when it cruises after burn-out of the rocket in a purely inertial orbit. Only the momentum (mass $\times$ velocity) of the ejected material would have an influence on the craft's course in proportion to the momentum of the craft. To prevent this influence, it would be necessary to expel waste material at two opposite points symmetrical to the craft's axis simultaneously in equal quantities.

Based upon the previous discussion, the weight of material necessary to sustain one man for one day in a sealed cabin is presented in Table 12–1.

TABLE 12–1

Weight of Material Necessary to Sustain One Man for One Day in a Sealed Cabin

| Material (Supply) | Weight (gm) | Material (Absorbents) | Weight (gm) |
|---|---|---|---|
| Oxygen | 862 | Lithium hydroxide to absorb 496 l of carbon dioxide | 1,330 |
| Water | 2,200 | Anhydrone to absorb 800 gm of water | 2,400 |
| Food (dry) | 523 | TOTAL ABSORBENTS | 3,730 |
| TOTAL SUPPLY: | 3,585 | | |

TOTAL WEIGHT: $3,585 + 3,730 = 7,315$ gm = 16 lbs.

The total weight indicated in Table 12–1 does not include the weight of containers, blower ducts, etc., which will remain constant for a given period. As a reference figure, a weight of from 15 to 20 lbs. has been calculated by engineers for an absorber blower and circulation blower, including the power supply of half a horsepower per occupant of a space cabin, provided the cabin pressure does not deviate much from the normal value. Special attention has to be directed toward the arrangement of the absorptive material with respect to weightlessness to avoid drifting of material and to secure proper air flow.

No figures can be presented for storage of inert gases in cases in which a constant leakage of a "sealed" cabin would be unavoidable.

**Temperature.** The temperature of an aircraft or of a sealed cabin within such craft is determined by the difference between heat gain and loss. The heat gain is derived from several sources; the heat loss is effected by the usual channels of heat transfer:

*Heat gain:*
>           External sources—Aerodynamic heating, solar radiation
>           Internal sources—Rocket motor (or other propulsion), auxiliary equipment, passengers

*Heat loss:*
>           Conduction (heat transfer through a substance as such), convection (heat transfer by moving substance), radiation, evaporation

For space vehicles that start from the ground, aerodynamic heating by friction during the first phase of their flight seems to be of lesser importance. In passing through the denser layer of the atmosphere shortly after start, the speed of the vehicle is still not high enough to generate much heat by friction. With increasing speed the vehicle soon leaves the atmosphere, thus eliminating friction. During orbital flight the heat balance is completely determined by radiation. With the sun as practically the only outer source of heat energy, it should be possible to maintain a suitable cabin temperature within the area between the orbits of Mars and Venus by varying the area of highly reflective surfaces toward the sun and surfaces of high emissivity (black) in the opposite direction. This requires that the spacecraft maintain a stable position with reference to the sun. For manned satellites orbiting at such distance and speed that time within the earth's shadow does not exceed several hours, protection against heat loss should not be serious.

The most important problem for all space vehicles destined for return to earth is the re-entry into the atmosphere of the earth, reducing a speed of thousands of miles per hour to a tolerable landing speed. At supersonic speed the movement (kinetic energy) of the air molecules is decelerated—mainly on the leading edges—and then converted to heat. If the air molecules come to a complete standstill, the temperature reached by the air is called "stagnation temperature" ($T_s$). The relation between $T_s$ and the Mach number

M (1M equals the speed of sound) has been described by a simplified equation:

$$T_s = 50 \times M^2 \text{ (degrees centigrade)}$$

So at a speed of 3 Mach, $50 \times 9 = 450°$ C would be reached.

But temperature must not be confused with heat, which always can be expressed in units of energy. As an example, a small gas-burner of high temperature may need a considerably longer time to heat a pot of water to the boiling point than a large wood stove of much lower temperature. The stagnation temperature is only one factor. Heat transfer from air to the skin of the vehicle and heat conduction from the skin through the intermediate material to the wall of the cabin constitute another factor. Time is a third factor. Consideration has been given to the question of whether a fast, steep dive or a slow, long-lasting glide would produce the smallest amount of heat. For protection of the cabin, it has been proposed to sacrifice some material to melting and evaporating, while the cabin remains in the "shadow" of a Mach angle cone by means of a suitable shape of the vehicle. Engineers seem recently to have more confidence of achieving tolerable temperature conditions within a cabin during the re-entry phase.

It has been stated that 50 per cent of man's heat exchange is performed by radiation. This is true only if the wall temperature of a room is cooler than the temperature of the skin or clothing. Man's most powerful means of temperature regulation rests with evaporation of water. Each milliliter or gram of water evaporated at a skin temperature of $25°$ C carries away 582 cal. or about 2.25 British thermal units (BTU). This figure demonstrates the importance of keeping the cabin air dry, of making perspiration possible if high temperatures cannot be avoided. The Air Force has had considerable success in developing a heat-reflectant, ventilated suit. As important as studies of heat tolerance under extreme conditions are, it should always be remembered that the maintenance of normal temperature-humidity conditions is necessary for full mental and physical performance.

Heat production of man is about equivalent to that of a 100-w electric-light bulb, 470 BTU per hour. This amount is probably negligible compared to heat production by auxiliary equipment, for which definite values can be given only in concrete cases.

Heat production of the propulsion mechanism is, in the case of the rocket motor, enormous. Since the blast of a chemical rocket carries most of the heat away from the vehicle itself and lasts only a short time, it does not constitute a problem at present.

**Rapid Decompression.** One of the most discussed accident potentials in space travel is the puncture of the hull by a meteorite. Depending on the size of the hole, volume of the cabin, and pressure differential between cabin atmosphere and outside space, the cabin air will leak out more or less rapidly. In contrast to general opinion, the total decompression time increases with decreasing outside pressure and theoretically becomes infinite with an outside vacuum, as exists in space. Also in contrast to the general opinion, in case of a finite counterpressure the speed of the outrushing air reaches its highest value, the speed of sound, at a pressure ratio of about 1.9 and does not increase further. The greatest danger of a rapid decompression to extremely low pressure is the onset of acute hypoxia, with vaporization bubbles in the body fluids above 63,000 ft. In present-day military aircraft the pilot is protected by a pressure suit. For short flights in orbiting vehicles, a pressure suit may also be used. But there is another problem. Cruising in an orbit makes bail-out useless, since after bail-out the pilot himself would remain in the orbit. Therefore, cabins have been designed that can be operated independently of the main vehicle.

In large spacecraft on long flights, the passengers would be unable to wear space suits all the time. Here also the possibility for plugging a leak is much better. But the loss of cabin air may be so severe that the flight cannot be completed. In this case the best solution seems to be to use a "fleet" of spacecraft on such flights instead of just one. This would permit the passengers of a crippled vehicle to board another vehicle of the fleet.

# 13

# Operational Aspects of
# Space Flight

Alfred M. Mayo [*]

Space travel is characterized by close proximity to a completely unfriendly environment of vast distances. Free space environment is totally intolerable to human life, but the problems of providing a satisfactory, even comfortable, microenvironment for a space traveler appear to be mostly solvable (12). New data and much effort, however, will certainly be required. As in the submarine, only the vehicle hull and shielding will separate the crew from quick death. The size of oceans and the fear of being lost have for ages worried sailors and, more recently, fliers. Even so, two-dimensional ocean surfaces are truly minute when compared to distances which exist in three-dimensional space. For example, only about one-sixtieth of a second would be required to travel from New York to Paris at the speed of light. One and one-half seconds would be needed to get to the moon. Five and one-half hours would be required for a trip to the sun's most distant planet, Pluto. Four and one-third years would be consumed in a trip to the nearest star, Alpha Centauri (19). Roughly one billion years would be required to reach the farthest parts of space observed through the 200-in. Palomar telescope.

The atmosphere will be the realm of the initial and terminal phases of many space flights (7, 9, 13) and is of great consequence in most early space exploration. Following successful earth orbital operations, the moon will be an early space goal. Present tech-

[*] Assistant Director for Bioengineering, Office of Life Science Programs, National Aeronautics and Space Administration, Washington, D.C. Formerly, Chief, Equipment and Safety Research Section, Engineering Department, El Segundo Division, Douglas Aircraft Company, Inc., El Segundo, California.

nology does not provide a ready approach to travel beyond the solar system. However, the solar system can provide a challenge adequate to occupy man's effort for some time.

## Trajectories

Space vehicles, like the heavenly bodies, must obey well-known laws of celestial mechanics. One very significant feature of celestial mechanics is the fact that bodies in space are generally not impeded significantly by a physically resisting medium. Velocities once established remain essentially constant except for the attraction of other bodies. The points of departure and destination are themselves moving at such velocities that every voyage becomes an interception in space and time. The flight paths are practically never straight lines between two points.

Once in free orbit and without thrust, a satellite vehicle follows essentially an elliptical path with the earth as one focus. The elliptical orbit is slightly distorted by the attraction of the moon, the sun, and other planets and by the fact that the earth is not precisely a homogeneous sphere. An apparent precession of the orbit results from the rotation of the earth. The orbital time or period of the free satellite depends on its average altitude. It would be about 84 minutes if one could be maintained at sea-level altitude. The average periods of the Sputnik, Explorer, and Vanguard vehicles range from 90 to 150 minutes. At an altitude of 22,000 miles above the equator, the period of a satellite would be about one day, and, if orbiting in the direction of the earth's rotation, it would appear to be stationary above the same spot on the earth's surface. At an altitude of about a quarter of a million miles, equal to the moon's distance from earth, a satellite would have a period of one lunar month.

The conventional procedure for establishing an earth satellite consists of launching the vehicle nearly vertically then gradually steering it into a curved flight path. Several stages of propulsion have generally been employed, and the propulsion stages jettisoned when exhausted. At or near the apex of the ascent, when the vehicle is theoretically horizontal, additional thrust must be applied to convert the vehicle trajectory into an orbit. If the final velocity is horizontal and sufficient speed is attained, the transition point becomes the apogee or perigee of the elliptical orbit, depending on whether the velocity is less than or greater than that required for a circular orbit (16).

If the satellite velocity is increased appreciably above circular velocity, the ellipse becomes greatly elongated; at the escape velocity, which is $\sqrt{2}$ times the satellite velocity, the trajectory becomes parabolic and at higher speed hyperbolic. In the latter case the vehicle, if left to coast, would no longer return to the body of origin. Such a vehicle launched from the earth would not return to the earth but would establish its own elliptical orbit about the sun. To escape from the sun would require a minimum of $\sqrt{2}$ times the minimum orbital velocity about the sun.

A trip to an outer planet, Mars or beyond, would best be initiated by adding thrust in the direction of the earth's orbit around the sun. To visit Venus or Mercury, inside planets, the impulse should be applied in the reverse direction to the earth's orbital velocity.

The prevalent notion that a misdirected space vehicle would fall into the sun is in error. In order for a vehicle to fall into the sun, nearly all its orbital velocity would need to be dissipated. Nearly five times as much energy would be needed to cause the misdirected vehicle to fall into the sun as would be required for it to escape from the solar system.

An infinite variety of trajectories can be established to provide a correct position and time intercept between planets. Such orbits are largely governed by Newtonian forces and are subject to reasonably precise calculations based on well-advanced techniques. Each astronautical objective has a specific orbit of minimum energy, or minimum velocity change, associated with a definite time of travel. For interplanetary travel the minimum energy orbit is the "Hohman transfer" (1, 6). This ellipse has its perihelion and aphelion at the tangent points with the orbits of the planets of departure and destination. In this case departure is so timed that the vehicle will arrive at a point opposite and beyond the sun at precisely the time that the target planet arrives at the same point. For a minimum energy trip departure must be exactly planned to coincide with the synodic interval between the destination and target planet (about 780 days for an earth–Mars Hohman trip). If a greater energy or initial velocity is available, the trip is not only correspondingly shortened, but leeway is also provided in the selection of a suitable departure time.

If it is desired that a space vehicle orbit about its target, additional impulse must be provided at the desired distance to effect the orbit.

If a soft landing is to be effected on the moon or a planet without atmosphere, sufficient additional impulse must be available to kill the orbital velocity in a manner so precise as to arrive at negligible velocity at the instant of contact with the surface. Landings in which atmospheric braking and aerodynamic controls are utilized in the place of added propulsion are possible where a suitable atmosphere exists.

## Propulsion

It has often been said that the prime limitation on space travel is the availability of adequate means of propulsion. A suitable propulsion system must be capable of providing the thrust, in the near vacuum of space, necessary to provide velocities considered fantastic with respect to those achieved near the earth's surface. In addition to extreme environmental requirements, it can readily be envisioned that the space-propulsion system must be capable of reliable operation in some cases after long periods of shut-down and without the benefit of normal ground-crew maintenance.

Space-propulsion systems presently envisioned can be generally divided into categories of "high" and "low" thrust. A high-thrust propulsion system is considered to be one that can develop sufficient thrust to take off from earth. Such systems must generally provide thrust of one to ten times the initial weight of the vehicle.

The low-thrust engines for use in free space may develop thrusts from one-millionth to one-thousandth the weight of the vehicle.

High-thrust engines include the familiar liquid- and solid-propellent chemical rockets and nuclear rockets using the reaction to heat a working fluid (such as hydrogen).

Figure 13–1 illustrates one type of secondary-fluid nuclear engine. Variants of the chemical-rocket motors utilizing free radicals and metastable chemicals utilizing reactions involving inner-ring electrons have been shown to possess considerably higher energy than the chemical systems but have not yet been proved practical.

In the high-thrust class the chemical rockets can produce impulses of from 200 to 450 pound-seconds of thrust per pound of

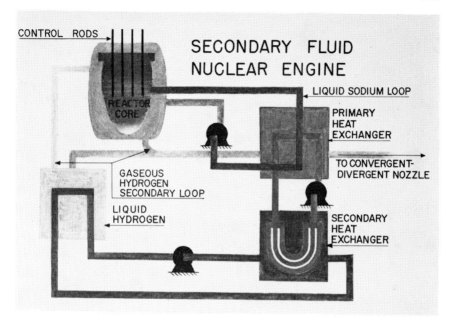

Fig. 13–1. In a secondary-fluid nuclear engine, a fraction of the gaseous hydrogen may be passed through a cooling loop for temperature control of the reactor in addition to the temperature control provided by the liquid-sodium loop. The remaining gaseous hydrogen is heated by the primary heat exchanger which obtains its heat from the liquid sodium. In actual practice many design considerations will influence the final system configuration. Examples of two such considerations are the type of reactor and shielding to be used.

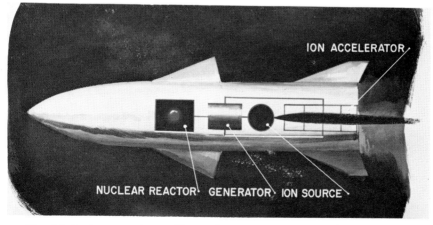

Fig. 13–2. Ion propulsion. The nuclear reactor serves as the primary source of power; the generator converts the primary power to usable electricity which can in turn act to ionize the material and also to operate the ion accelerator.

propellant. The free-radical and metastable chemicals theoretically might double these values. High-thrust nuclear-fission engines may produce impulses in the order of from 800 to 2,000 pound-seconds per pound of fuel.

Present technology places most of the "exotic" engines in the low-thrust category. Prominent among these engines is the ion-pro-

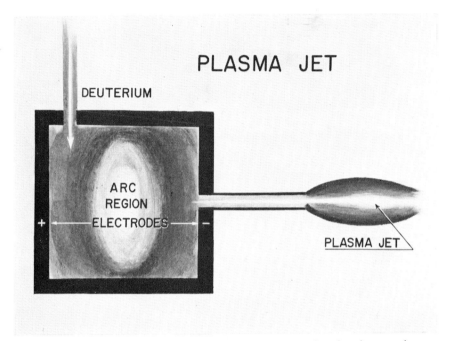

Fig. 13–3. The deuterium or "working gas" enters the chamber as shown. A very high current is discharged across the arc region which ionizes the gas and generates a shock wave. The shock wave is generated due to the fact that the gas nearer the orifice receives less energy than the gas in the arc region. The result is the highly ionized plasma jet. In practice, provisions must be made for cooling and insulation.

pulsion system of Stuhlinger (18) in which a nuclear reactor furnishes electric power to ionize a propellant (usually cesium) and to accelerate the ions and electrons out of a nozzle by means of a linear electronic accelerator. Figure 13–2 diagrams such a system.

The relatively new application of magnetohydrodynamics has produced "plasma jets" (Fig. 13–3) and "plasmoid" (Fig. 13–4) propulsion systems. These systems produce thrust by ejecting material accelerated by electrical currents and magnetic fields, respectively. Based on present technology, these engines also fall in the low-thrust category, but the promise of effecting nuclear fusion by magnetohydrodynamic means and the containment of high-temperature (upward of three hundred million degrees centigrade) reactions in magnetic fields (Fig. 13–5) offers the potential of fantastic

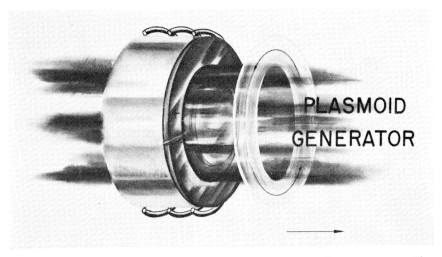

Fig. 13–4. This device generates a plasmoid in the following manner: The plasma attains rotational kinetic energy due to the current. The rotational kinetic energy is transformed into translational kinetic energy due to the gradient in the magnetic field.

levels of available power. It is conceivable that such engines might be capable of eventually producing, for at least short periods of time, high thrust as well as high impulse. Specific impulse values for ionic, plasma-jet, and plasmoid engines fall generally in the range of from 10,000 to 50,000 pound-seconds per pound of fuel.

Another class of low-thrust level engines includes "photonic" (Fig. 13–6) and light-pressure (Fig. 13–7) engines. These devices utilize the thrust from beams of high-intensity light and employ the sun's energy as a "solar sail." Here the specific impulse may range from hundreds of thousands of pound-seconds per pound of fuel to a nearly infinite amount in the case of the sail.

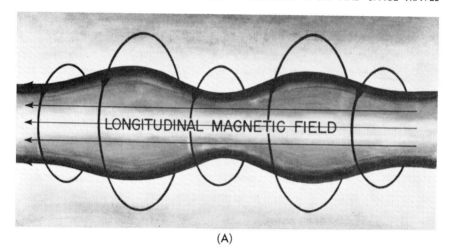

(A)

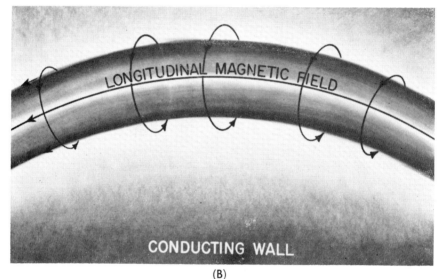

(B)

Fig. 13–5. A very high current is discharged through a contained gas, and the result is a highly ionized conducting gas. Immediately after the discharge, the column of gas contracts (pinches), and certain instabilities follow. These instabilities in the pinched plasma are primarily of two types, the "sausage mode" (A) and the "kink mode" (B).

(A) Once the constriction occurs, the magnetic forces become stronger around the constriction and weaker around the bulge. The normal remedy is to impose a longitudinal magnetic field to stabilize the pinch (long arrows).

(B) Once the kink mode is initiated, the reaction is quickly damped due to collisions with the wall; however, if the wall is made conducting, the circular lines tend to hold the plasma away from the wall.

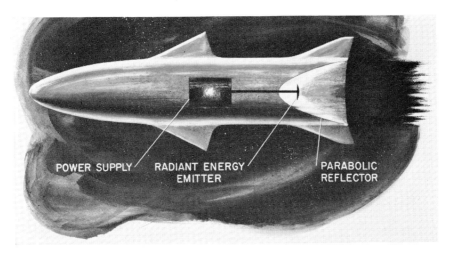

Fig. 13–6. In the photon rocket, thrust may be obtained by the emission of radiant energy from a heated plate. Electrical or nuclear excitation of the plate will heat it, thus generating photons of light required to propel the space vehicle.

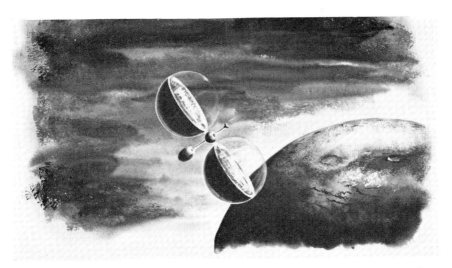

Fig. 13–7. An artist's concept of solar-powered space ship. The solar-powered space ship utilizes energy derived from the electromagnetic radiation emanating from the sun and impinging on the "solar sail."

## Structure

The requirements for structural configuration and material suitable for space operations will vary radically with the time of flight. Another important set of requirements will be governed by the need of some of the vehicles to make a high-speed exit from or re-entry into an atmosphere. In this latter case the structure must be configured to withstand high-acceleration loads and high-friction temperatures associated with aerodynamic heating in addition to those stresses specific to free-space travel. Temperature problems incident to high-speed atmospheric re-entry can be attenuated significantly by proper control of the forward shape of the vehicle (sometimes called "blunting") and by the use of an exterior coating of a material capable of absorbing heat by virtue of its own progressive erosion or destruction. The process of cooling by combined evaporation, erosion, and endothermic chemical decomposition is referred to as "ablation."

Once the spacecraft is established in a free-space orbit, the structural loads associated with gravity and atmospheric loading fall to near zero values. It is because of the elimination of gravitational, aerodynamic, and high-acceleration forces that the space vehicle designed only for flight from one orbit to another can be of a very much lighter structural configuration than the take-off and re-entry vehicle.

Some parts of even the orbit-to-orbit vehicle must nevertheless carry significant mechanical loads. The pressure necessary to provide one earth atmosphere environment for the crew, for example, would equal a load in excess of one ton to each square foot of surface exposed to this pressure. In addition to supporting the pressure loads, the structure of occupied areas must provide a continuous hermetic seal against the loss of vital gases. Figure 13–8 illustrates the possibility of utilizing a self-sealing inner layer to the structure in order that the penetrations of small meteoroids might be self-healing. Additionally, the structure should be configured to resist stresses incident to a substantial temperature gradient in the event one side of the structure was exposed to the sun's radiations for significant periods of time while the shadow side was being cooled by radiant-heat loss.

Meteoroid and space-debris resistance is another desirable quality of a suitable space-vehicle structure (2, 22, 23). For a given expenditure of weight, meteoroid penetration can be improved by increasing the modulus of elasticity, the specific heat, the heat of fusion, the heat of vaporization, the ionization potential, and the binding energy of the structural material while decreasing density. Low-density material allows a longer path of resisting material, to interact with the disintegrating meteoroid particles, for a given weight than do high-density materials (3). In general, the low-

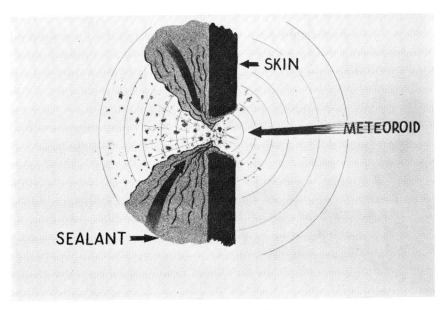

Fig. 13–8. Leak sealing.

density materials can also provide better heat insulation and, if of a low-molecular-weight composition, possibly more effective radiation shielding. While present data on space radiations are clearly inadequate, it has been determined (20) that high-molecular-weight materials cause much greater secondary emission when subjected to high-energy ionizing radiation than do the low-molecular-weight materials (11, 14). Dr. Fred Singer has stated that from this standpoint hydrogen would be an ideal shielding material (15). No practical configuration of a sufficient amount of hydrogen to attenuate certain high-energy particles has yet become common knowledge. Ionization from some of these high-energy particles is still increasing after one foot of lead has been penetrated (21). For these reasons it would appear to be of questionable advisability to utilize materials such as lead for shielding against lower-energy radiation such as x-rays.

On the whole, even though much development and research will be required, the structural problems while clearly formidable do not appear to present insurmountable obstacles.

## Payloads

A wide variety of payloads will be carried by space vehicles. These will range from scientific instruments and human or other

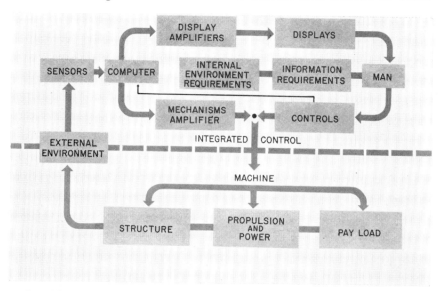

Fig. 13–9. Man-machine system illustrating the over-all relationship of the integrated control system and its human controller.

biological specimens to military weapons and reconnaissance devices. In every case the high energy and effort cost of early space flights will put a great premium on weight savings. Accordingly, each payload item, just as the space vehicle itself, should either be designed specifically for the purpose or, in the case of the crew or biological specimens, should be selected carefully for the required job or function.

## Integrated Control

The integrated control system or "brain" of the space vehicle will provide the link between the system and the brain of its human controller. Proper control and data handling are as important to the success of unmanned space probes as to the manned space vehicle. Figure 13–9 is a block diagram of a man-machine system illustrating this over-all relationship. Figure 13–10 illustrates how a similar system might be utilized for a remotely controlled probe-type vehicle in which telemetering or other electromagnetic communication links are utilized to complete the control loops.

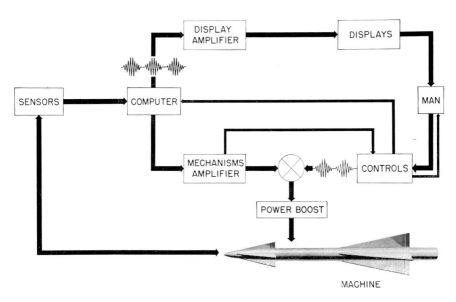

Fig. 13–10. Man-machine system illustrating a system that utilizes communication links to complete the control loops.

Since the space vehicles and missions will be configured from the imagination of human brains and to satisfy human objectives, it appears evident that the value of these systems must be a direct function of the quality of the linkage to the human brains utilizing the vehicles. In many cases advanced mechanical computers can be used to configure data as a function of time into the optimum forms for the operator. On the other hand, it should be remembered that the mechanical computer is inherently stupid in that it can only perform those tasks (however complicated) that it has been precisely programed to perform. New situations and unforeseen obstacles will require intelligent human thought to provide proper reprograming.

The human operator can nevertheless be greatly aided in his tasks if suitable displays are provided to take advantage of his strength and if automatic controls are configured to supplement his limited time-constants and muscular capabilities.

An important relationship between the man and the machine in such a system dictates a proper balance of effort between factors directly affecting the machine and items controlling the efficiency of the human factors (8). Briefly, it may be stated that the over-all effectiveness of any man-machine system is a product function of the effectiveness of the controller times that of the machine. The useful effectiveness can therefore not exceed the value of the least effective part.

On this basis it can be easily visualized that the reliability and efficiency of the machine should be sufficient to provide a high probability of mission achievement. On the other hand, the environment provided, for the human operator to be compatible, must accomplish much more than provide minimum physiological tolerance levels (4, 5, 10, 17). It should also be conducive to logical and rational thinking by the operator in order to provide a compatible brain link with the users of the knowledge gained.

Figure 13–11 is a speculative control station. Orientation, direction, and quantitative data can be presented in an integrated form on a central display on which an imaginary plane surface can serve to aid the earth-trained operator in spatial orientation. A three-dimensional situation display is also provided to give a broad picture encompassing the situation over a longer period of time. Orbital information and alternate computed operation can thus be studied, and decisions as to the necessary reprograming can be made. The controls can serve both as reprograming devices and for emergency remote-control activation.

The control station would be but one important part of the over-all space cabin. Figure 13–12, also speculative, is provided to stimulate thinking and to illustrate some of the combined environmental factors. The control center is designed to permit one man to get the entire picture and to have the necessary controls for both reprograming and emergency over-ride. A computing center, a laboratory, and recreational and living quarters are provided in a manner designed to satisfy both the physiological and psychological requirements for both on-duty and off-duty crew members.

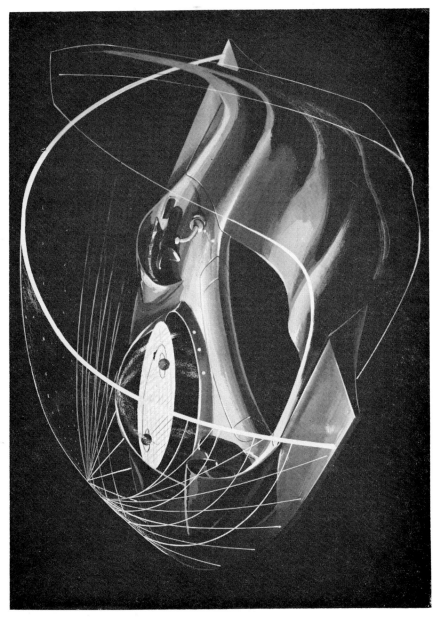

Fig. 13–11. Speculative control station.

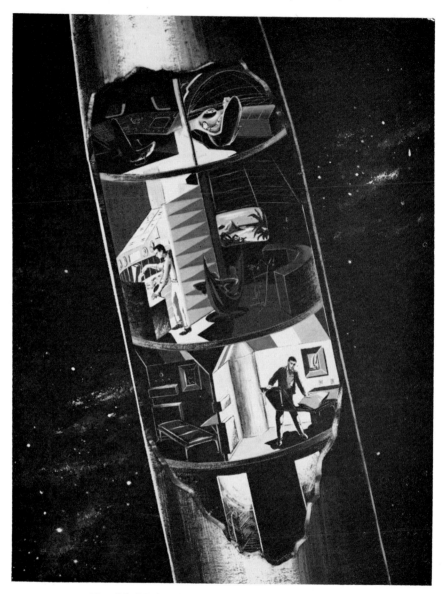

Fig. 13–12. Man's environment in a space cabin.

Duplicate systems and ready access to the equipment are provided to permit the large reliability gains achievable when maintenance and part replacement can be affected during operation.

A constant component of acceleration of sufficient value to be compatible with human-efficiency requirements is provided in a head-to-foot direction.

## Escape

In addition to the normal-function considerations, added hazards, complex systems, and the long flight times of the space operation will increase the likelihood of accidents or failure of the type requiring escape consideration. Even on the launching pad it is possible to imagine explosions, structural failures, or the release of corrosive or toxic materials requiring an escape mechanism. As the spacecraft leaves its launching pad, high speeds, potential control malfunctions, and environmental control failures can add to the list of problems. An escape system for these initial and terminal phases of space flight would, however, have requirements not too different from those of a very high-performance aircraft. This escape device should be configured to allow sufficient separation from a damaged space vehicle to leave behind potential explosions and fires and at the same time to carry with it an adequate short-term environment to insure survival of the crew. To minimize the compromise of the over-all system, it appears that such a device might well be the smallest practical part of the over-all space vehicle capable of protecting the crew during escape and, after landing, until rescue.

A different set of requirements for survival must be met by the craft operating far out in space (8). The great distances are likely to dictate a long waiting time for rescue and the need for maximum provision of long-term environment and ecological needs.

In this case advanced emergency communication systems become essential, and the desirability of staying with the largest safe part of the vehicle then assumes great importance. It seems probable that, for distant space operations, optimum survival probability would be more nearly approached by an escape program in which potentially dangerous components of the over-all system might be selectively severed and ejected from the vicinity of the remainder of the system. An example might be the ejection of a runaway or malfunctioning nuclear reactor or a leaking fuel cell.

Space operations motivated by man's competitive instinct and his desire for knowledge and adventure will be undertaken with full knowledge of the dangers of space environment.

The effectiveness and timing of these operations will be governed by the efficiency with which large numbers and wide varieties of problems can be defined and solved and by the quality of the manner in which human brains can be used in the conception and operation of the devices.

# References

1. EHRICKE, K. A. 1959. Interplanetary operations. In SEIFERT, H. (ed.). *Space Technology.* John Wiley & Sons, Inc., New York. Chap. 8.
2. GRIMMINGER, G. 1948. Probability that a meteorite will hit or penetrate a body situated in the vicinity of the earth. *J. Appl. Phy. 19:* 947–956.
3. HABER, HEINZ. 1957. Personal communication. March, 1957.
4. HENRY, J. P. 1950. *Studies of the Physiology of Negative Acceleration.* (AF Technical Report Nr 5953.)
5. HESS, JOHN, and LOMBARD, C. F. 1957. *The Approximation of the Response of the Human Torso to Large Rapidly Applied Upward Accelerations by That of an Elastic Load and Comparison with Ejection Seat Data.* (DAC Report ES–26472, 1957.)
6. HOHMAN, W. 1925. *Die Erreichbarkeit der Himmelskoerper (Flight to Celestial Bodies).* Oldenburg Publishing Corp., Munich, Germany.
7. HOOVER, G. W. 1958. A Program for Space Flight. Paper presented to American Astronautical Society, Jan., 1958.
8. HOOVER, G. W. 1958. Man's Operational Environment in Space. Paper presented at American Astronautical Society, Aug. 18, 1958.
9. KAPLAN, JOSEPH. 1952. The chemosphere. In WHITE, C. S., and BENSON, O. O., JR. (eds.). *Physics and Medicine of the Upper Atmosphere.* University of New Mexico Press, Albuquerque. Pp. 99–108.
10. LOMBARD, C. F. 1948. *Human Tolerances to Forces Produced by Acceleration.* (Douglas El Segundo Report No. ES–21072.) El Segundo, Calif.
11. MORGAN, K. Z. 1956. Maximum permissible internal dose of radionuclides: Recent changes in values. *Nuclear Sci. and Eng. 1:* 477–500.
12. MYERS, JACK. 1954. Basic remarks on the use of plants as biological gas exchangers in a closed system. *J. Aviation Med. 25:* 407–411.
13. ROBERTS, H. E. 1949. The earth's atmosphere. *Aeronaut. Eng. Rev. 8:* 18–31.
14. SCHAEFER, H. J. 1954. *The Cross Section for Thin-Down Hits from Heavy Nuclei of the Primary Cosmic Radiation in Biological Experimentation.* (Research Report No. NM 001 059.13.07.) U.S. Naval School of Aviation Medicine.
15. SINGER, S. F. 1952. Research in the upper atmosphere with sounding rockets and earth satellite vehicles. *J. Brit. Interplanet. Soc. 19:* 61–73.
16. SIRY, J. W. 1959. The Vanguard IGY earth satellite launching. Trajectories and orbits notes. In SEIFERT, H. (ed.). *Space Technology.* John Wiley & Sons, Inc., New York. Chap. 6.
17. STAPP, J. P. 1955. Effects of mechanical force on living tissues. I. Abrupt deceleration and windblast. *J. Aviation Med. 26:* 268–288.
18. STUHLINGER, E. 1955. Electrical Propulsion System for Space Ships with Nuclear Power Source. Paper presented at the 2nd Annual Meeting, American Astronautical Society, Dec. 1, 1955.

19. *The Space Encyclopedia.* E. P. Dutton & Co., Inc., New York. 1957.
20. TOBIAS, C. A. 1952. Radiation hazards in high altitude aviation. *J. Aviation Med. 23:* 345–371.
21. VAN ALLEN, J. A. 1952. The nature and intensity of the cosmic radiation. In WHITE, C. S., and BENSON, O. O., JR. (eds.). *Physics and Medicine of the Upper Atmosphere.* University of New Mexico Press, Albuquerque. Pp. 239–266.
22. WHIPPLE, F. L. 1952. The contents of interplanetary space-meteoritic phenomena and meteorites. In WHITE, C. S., and BENSON, O. O., JR. (eds.). *Physics and Medicine of the Upper Atmosphere.* University of New Mexico Press, Albuquerque. Pp. 137–170.
23. WHIPPLE, F. L. 1957. The Meteoritic Risk to Space Vehicles. Unpublished report, Harvard College Observatory, 1957.

# 14

## Speculations on Space and Human Destiny

HAMILTON B. WEBB, M.D.*

After a man goes into space, men will go. An objective is to put observatories and laboratories in orbit, to look at the stars, to inquire into the nature of matter and of time and space. After men go into space, mankind will follow. Man, men, mankind—there seems to be no stopping this at all.

Space medicine was first established as a discrete curriculum in 1949, and it consists, in part, of the attempt to simulate on the surface of the earth those conditions that man or mankind will encounter in space. It is possible to simulate almost all these various conditions: the loneliness and the noise, the tremendous accelerative forces, the synthetic atmosphere, and the problems of diet, fluid, gas exchange, and excrement neutralization that the encapsulated man must face. To a certain extent even that neutralization of gravity which occurs during free fall in orbit can be achieved. A fast airplane flying a carefully calculated parabola can leave a man unstressed by gravity for as much as a minute.

Gravity is man's oldest enemy. The infant, from the time he first tries to toddle across the floor, is in a lifelong struggle against gravity and one from which he can win only a temporary victory. A few seconds or even a few minutes of freedom from its pull does not really simulate the gravity-free environment. Much has been learned from this brief experiment; but the long-time neutralization of gravity is one thing that cannot be simulated biologically or in any

* Colonel, USAF, MC, Director of Base Medical Services, Otis Air Force Base, Massachusetts.

engineering way on the surface of the earth. Increased gravity is simulated in a centrifuge, but there is no "negative centrifuge" that can diminish the pull of gravity and its action on the human body.

One can only speculate on what will happen as a result of the neutralization of gravity, but these speculations are very interesting. It is known, for example, that if a developing human being is not subjected to the stresses of gravity, his bones will not form in the way characteristic of an adult. The most typical example of this, perhaps, occurs in the femur. If a femur were never the weight-bearing axis of the body, then that peculiarly Gothic type of lamellar architecture in the neck and trochanter would not develop. It will develop, however, after the individual begins to put stress, that is, begins to bear weight, on that bone.

From this observation the awesome hypothesis is suggested that if man should multiply in space, as will happen in the foreseeable future, he will not, in the absence of gravity, develop the anthropological characteristics that are familiar on earth. His bones and muscles will grow a little bit differently, deprived of the formative stresses that weight provides. Observation of creatures on earth which live in neutralized gravity makes it possible to speculate on what will happen to mankind by analogy. The whale, for example, was a primordial pig. He grew to an indefinite age and to an enormous size. Fish, in whose lives gravity is neutralized by buoyancy, grow through indefinitely long lives to relatively enormous sizes. Some fish that develop from an egg the size of a pinhead exceed a thousand pounds when full adult size is reached.

It may be that mankind put into an environment from which gravity's influence has been removed may find himself undergoing changes of the same degree of magnitude, changes in his physical appearance and capabilities. At the same time there is a penalty involved in this. The beached whale dies because, unbuoyed by water, he no longer can breathe; he no longer retains the strength to expand and contract his chest when his enormous weight is held imprisoned by gravity. Perhaps man will have to face this fate, too, at some indefinite point in the future. If he, too, thoroughly adapts to an environment in which gravity is minimum, he may never be able to return to the surface of a 1-g planet.

It is also known that the continual fight against gravity takes an enormous amount of energy. The g force must be opposed with an equal and opposite muscular force, and it has been estimated that of man's total energy production one-third is utilized for this. Before he can begin to accomplish any useful work, he must spend one-third of his energy unproductively in the mere opposition of gravity. What is mankind to do with those surplus energies when he is relieved of this burden, when he no longer needs to expend energy combating gravity? Perhaps the diminished stress will confer a longer survival. Perhaps the surplus energies will become available for the mental activities of a less fatigued mind, for sustained concentration or meditation, or for feats of endurance and pertinacity impossible to one chained by gravity.

These concepts require us to change our thinking about ourselves. We have been accustomed to thinking of mankind as a terrestrial creature. Once man thought of himself as having been created a few centuries ago, of earth, fire, and water. More recently the concept has been held of man as the final product of an inversely manlike series of primates and rodents, formed in the ebb and flow of glaciers and deserts. The creative process has been dated earlier, in the shallow seas of the earth half a billion years ago. Man has thought of himself as created in Mesopotamia or formed in Europe as a member of a nation or of a race. Recently man has come to the conclusion that he is a creature of the whole planet earth and that man has finally reached his maturity in encompassing and adapting for his use the whole planet on which he was created.

But when it is realized that man's future, his greatest fulfillment, may lie in the cosmos and not on the surface of the earth at all, then it is strongly suggested that mankind has not reached maturity but only completed gestation. Man is a creature not merely of the earth. Man's creation began as a turbulence in a cloud of gas in infinite space and proceeded by condensation into a galaxy, stars, planets, and finally the seas and continents of the earth.

These speculations lead inescapably to the concept that man is the creature of the cosmos, not of the earth; that the earth is only his womb, his chrysalis perhaps. It follows that man is now not about to mature but to be born; that man's first 100,000 years or 500,000,000 years are just the beginning of the life of a race which is preparing itself to inherit the realm of the cosmos. This is perhaps an exceedingly long extrapolation, but there is little doubt that space medicine and the other space-orientated sciences have indicated the direction of progress. Mankind is going out into space. It appears certain that the experience is going to change him. No one knows what mankind is going to be like when he becomes an inhabitant of the cosmos. But we look forward to this as a greater, perhaps the ultimate, fulfillment of man's destiny.

# Name Index

# Subject Index

Acceleration, 284; *see also* Gravity
  in crash landings, 287
  in ditchings, 287
  in ejection, 292
  in inverted spin, 290
  in jet aircraft, 284–95
  linear, 288, 289
  loss and mass increase, 16
  negative; *see* Deceleration
  in outside loop, 290
  positive, 105, 290
  prolonged, 295
  seat integrity and, 289, 290
  in space travel, 168
  tolerance of, 36, 38, 287
Accidents
  aircraft, 117, 214
  behavioral factors in, 230
  causes of, 217
  cockpit arrangement and, 227
  compromises affecting, 225
  and disorientation, 221
  dysbarism and, 220
  environmental adversities in, 229
  errors of judgment in, 222
  fatigue as a factor in, 221
  hypoxia in, 220
  incapacitation in, sudden, 220
  instrument interpretation in, 227
  instrument malfunction in, 227
  investigation of, aeromedical, 228
  linear deceleration in, 288, 289
  loss of life due to, 214
  and opportunity, 224
  physiological compromise in, 220
  pilot in, 218, 219
  pilot's attitude and, 223
  pilot's capacity and, 222
  pilot's emotional stability and, 222
  pilot's experience and, 222
  pilot's performance and, 223
  potential, in sealed cabins, 344
  prevention of, 230, 233, 235
    cockpit improvement in, 234
    physiological compromise in, 232

    screening of aircrew applicants in, 231
  seat integrity in, 289, 290
  types of, 216, 217
Advisory Group for Aeronautical Research and Development, 13, 22
Aerophagia, 198
Age limit for pilots, 146, 188
Air
  irritants in, 247
  moisture in, 241
  still, comfort chart for, 108
  temperature of, and altitude, 244
Air ambulances, 156
Air conditioning, 209
  factorial interactions in, 243
  ground-level comfort and, 248
  humidity control in, 247
  in jet aircraft, 238
  physical factors in, 239
  physiological factors in, 242
  psychological factors in, 243
Air evacuation, 156
*Air Force Pamphlet 160-5-15*, 160, 164
*Air Force Regulation 50-27*, 142, 148, 153
*Air Force Regulation 160-52*, 157
Air-insulation, principle of, in clothing, 239
*Air Service Medical Manual*, 136, 163
Air transport
  of aged, 163
  of infants, 163
  of patients, 156–63; *see also* Transportation of patients
Air Transport Association Medical Committee, 159
Aircraft
  accidents, 214; *see also* Accidents
  catapult launchings of, 291
  comfort at ground level, 248
  control of
    external factors in, 319
    human factors in, 306, 320
    monitoring in, 314